Craniosacral Therapy

Craniosacral Therapy

JOHN E. UPLEDGER, D.O., F.A.A.O. AND JON D. VREDEVOOGD, M.F.A.

Eastland Press
SEATTLE

To Our Families

Dianne, Leslie, John Matthew, Mark, Mike and Rob

and

Kim and Jon

Table of Contents

Foreword

Craniosacral therapy, as explained and taught in this volume, throws light on the interface, or area of blending, that lies between intervention medicine and self regulation medicine, between traditional allopathic-osteopathic medicine and psychophysiologic self regulation. In other words, this book throws light on mechanisms that lie "between body and mind," if such an inappropriate expression can be used when the differentiation between mind and body is rapidly disappearing in physics, biology, psychology and medicine.

In the Preface to this book, John Upledger states that "people . . . continue to suffer even though they have passed through the portals of some of the finest health care facilities in the world. Why? This is so because orthodox medicine has yet to recognize the existence of the craniosacral system and its pathophysiologic significance."

This forceful statement about the craniosacral system, and its implications for craniosacral therapy, are subscribed to by this writer (having seen many remarkable—some would say inexplicable—results of the discipline in the last three years). But those words do not summarize Upledger's whole story, and since he has allowed me room for comment, I will focus on what I think is an especially important feature of this book, the "V-spread" technique. The practical and theoretical significance of this therapeutic technique might not be noticed by the rapid reader, but in my estimation this, or similar techniques, will be studied in many research projects during the next ten years, and by the turn of the century will be implemented in most hospitals and medical schools.

From the practice of palpation in craniosacral therapy there is emerging an "energy therapy," for want of a better name, the rationale for which cannot be developed or elucidated by reference to anatomic and neurophysiologic texts. In studying the references in this book to the "V-spread" technique, I am especially struck by the many parallels between the sensings and manipulations in Upledger's "direction of energy" and the sensings and manipulations of "body electricity" in yogic theory and practice, both in yogic intervention and in yogic self regulation. It is not surprising, therefore, that this "direction of energy" technique and some of the visualization methods for self regulation should find common ground. At present, these therapeutic modalities have a number of physiologic correlates that remain without satisfactory explanation if we do not hypothesize the existence of a kind of "body electricity" that can be "transferred" from therapist to patient (in the "V-spread" technique) or can be self manipulated by a patient trained in visualization therapy, one of the self-regulation methods of psychophysiologic therapy.

Since self-regulation phenomena perfuse almost all of intervention medicine (witness the placebo effect in drug studies, for instance), a crucial question is raised immediately after the reality of the "V-spread" data is accepted: Are the phenomena merely the result of psychophysiologic self-regulation, conscious or unconscious, by the patient?

It is a well known fact that the placebo effect, a real biochemical and electro-physiologic change in a patient's body, is a subdivision of the general visualization effect (even though the patient is completely unconscious of having generated it). Much is known about how a patient consciously or unconsciously uses imagination (visualization) to induce biochemical and electrophysiologic change in the body. And admittedly, much is not known. But one thing is certain: *without mental imagery, conscious or unconscious, nothing can be self-initiated or self-controlled.* It is also known that placebos and self-regulation methods do not work with babies and dogs. Those creatures do not know what we are talking about. In them, inside-the-skin mechanisms can not be self-directed through visualization.

But the "V-spread" technique *does* work with babies and dogs. It is clearly inter-vention. Self-regulation may handle the same energy in a different way, but in both cases we find it useful to hypothesize the existence of a non-neurological and non-classical "body electricity" to account for results.

Returning to consideration of the placebo effect: Often when the "direction of energy" technique is used the patient does not know what is happening, and has no idea of what is "supposed to happen." The changes described by Upledger (and which are observed by workshop students, including myself) take place *without* the patient's own visualization. And since visualization is the *sine qua non* of self-regulation in both its aspects, conscious or unconscious, self-regulation can be ruled out as a satisfactory explanation of "V-spread" phenomena.

In Chapter 8, Upledger says, *"This technique works.* Although it may sound a bit strange as described, you should try it before rejecting it out of hand." To me, however, one who has long been interested in this area, it rings a familiar note. It brings to mind the explanations of yogis whom we (The Voluntary Controls Re-search team of The Menninger Foundation) studied in India in 1974 with a portable psychophysiology lab. Those self regulation adepts who were willing (and able) to explain, maintained that everything they did "inside and outside the skin," however strange to Western psychology and medicine, was accomplished through the manipulation of a non-neurologic electricity of the body, which they called "prana."

According to classic yogic theory, the body's neurological network is a correlate, or reflection, of a more primary network of "nadis," which are filaments of superphysical, but real, substance not yet detected by instruments. These filaments are constructed, it is said, of "dense prana," and they conduct a more subtle form of "prana" throughout the physical structure. Acupuncture channels (meridians) are said to be significant parts of this non-neurologic structure. In any event, according to yogic adepts, *psychophysiologic phenomena* are inside-the-skin examples of *psycho-kinetic phenomena* which, mediated by "prana" and directed by "mind" (conscious or unconscious) are found both inside and outside the skin. Thus, the former are special cases of the latter.

The theory that best accounts for Upledger's facts is, in my estimation, this theory from classic yoga. It is consistent with the data of modern visualization therapy and self-regulation, hypnosis, healing by therapeutic touch (the laying on of hands), t'ai chi (the "energy" dance of China), the martial arts (kung fu, karate, judo, akido), acupuncture and traditional Chinese medicine, Philippine psychic surgery (in certain cases), traditional East Indian medicine (Ayurvedic medicine) and traditional American Indian medicine. In addition, the theoretical "body electricity" has characteristics similar to those of the "vital physical body" of Aurobindo (which the "dense physical body" is said to servily obey), and is similar to the "auric body" of psychics, reported much these days in "out of body" and "near death" experiences.

It is interesting to note that in the laboratories of physicists Peter Philips, John Hasted, Harold Puthoff and Russell Targ, and electrical engineers Robert Jahn and Arthur Ellison (to name only a few researchers), recently observed mind-matter phenomena detected with ultra-sensitive instrumentation indicate that an energy link must be hypothesized to exist between "mind" and "matter," if parsimony is to be served.

The phenomena these scientists and John Upledger are talking about represent, in my estimation, different views of an energetic cosmos in which body, emotions, mind and spirit are all transformations or expressions of the same basic energy. Aurobindo, referring to the duality bind in which many matter-bound thinkers languish, suggested that if you are embarrassed by the word "spirit," then do not use it. Instead, refer to spirit as the "subtlest form of matter." If, however, you are not embarrassed by the word, matter can be thought of as the densest form of spirit.

Considering the "V-spread" technique as a recent addition to a tradition extending back several millenia, it seems that this method uses the old "energy" in a new way, new at least to Western medicine. Does this seem strange? Not to everyone. As pointed out many years ago by J.B. Rhine, perhaps the most significant application of psychokinetic research will be in medicine.

John Upledger provides a semi-traditional rationale for part of the "V-spread" data, when he suggests that electrophysiologic potentials of the therapist's hands might directly influence the skin and body of the patient. This makes use of classic bioelectric theory and possibilities, and is perhaps applicable in certain cases (at least it suggests new lines of research), but that explanation does not account for the condition in which the patient is fully clothed. "V-spread" phenomena are found even though the insulating effect of garments clearly block the flow of classic electricity. In my view, therefore, it is especially useful to consider the mind-body-energy theories from old China and India, to reconsider "chi" and "prana," and their affirmed (and fascinating) relation to imagery and volition.

For skeptics, the traditional way out of this data-based bind is to deny the existence of the data. But at the present stage of knowledge, this is a waste of time, money, opportunity and intellect. As Upledger says, *"This technique works."* And I would add, experience the phenomena yourself and then make an effort, if desired, to come up with a more adequate theory.

Upledger is fully aware, I know, that his mini-rationale for the "V-spread" phenomena is not fully inclusive, but as a medical researcher and clinician he is in a peculiar non-data type of bind. As he puts it, "some practitioners believed that they were directly funnelling divine healing power through their hands."

Upledger's problem: how to talk about an intervention method that works "as though under the control of your mind," how to separate fact from fiction, science from fantasy, knowledge from superstition—and move boldly into unknown territory in such a way that the elastic boundary of the medical frontier does not close up behind him, and he vanish from sight, his work relegated to the land of "quackish esoterica," to use his phrase.

Just a few more words before you begin this remarkable book. The *sensation* experienced by the therapist in using the "V-spread" technique *is* a "directing of energy." Some critics say that this sensation is "projection," limited to the mind of the therapist. But to this observer and experiencer, and seeker after rationales, Upledger and other therapists who are working in the many-leveled domain of mind-body are finding refreshing facts that support the idea of unity in medicine and yoga, body and mind, conscious and unconscious.

At the present state of knowledge and experience, perhaps it is best to be a monist, remain rational, be undogmatic, be flexible, become intuitive, and continuously seek out and make room for new facts. We must not be like the Soviet physicist we recently met who, when asked to discuss some of the new facts in the area of "body electricity," pounded his fist on the table and shouted, "In this area, there are no new facts." Other, more open-minded Soviet scientists, however, gave the energy a new name, "bioplasma," because of its apparent electric plasma-like properties, and started new research projects.

To start new research projects is what we should do with the "V-spread" or "direction of energy" technique, and with the medical milieu from which it emerges, craniosacral therapy. The main work has just begun. As Upledger says, this book contains a "considerable amount of observation and theory that has not yet withstood rigorous scientific testing."

ELMER GREEN, PH. D.

The Menninger Foundation
Topeka, Kansas
August 25, 1982

Preface

As in any new field of study, the craniosacral concept is changing rapidly. This book contains the most recent information available. Also included is a considerable amount of observation and theory that has not yet withstood rigorous scientific testing. We ask your indulgence in this matter. By continued clinical application and observation, the practitioner can begin to sort out the fact from the fantasy. Time will demonstrate the effectiveness of craniosacral therapy. On the other hand, we do not believe that low-risk, potentially high-benefit diagnostic and therapeutic techniques should be withheld from suffering patients while the slowly turning wheels of scientific method seek either to confirm or refute them. In other areas of health care where the risk to the patient is higher and the potential dangers more formidable, our position on this issue would be quite different.

Moreover, craniosacral therapy has the potential of providing dramatic help to a significant number of so-called "medical basket-cases," "crocks" and others for whom conventional medicine has proved ineffective. These are people who continue to suffer even though they have passed through the portals of some of the finest health care facilities in the world. Why? This is so because orthodox medicine has yet to recognize the existence of the craniosacral system and its pathophysiologic significance. Although the possibility of such a system was discussed over 50 years ago, its scientific basis was unclear. It therefore was unreasonable to seriously doubt the accepted dogma of the fused skull and to embrace instead the concept of dynamic activity involving skull bones, meningeal membranes, cerebrospinal fluid, the intracranial vascular system, the development of the brain, the movement of body fluids, the tonicity of muscles and the function of total body connective tissues as influenced by the craniosacral system.

As our research began to support the existence of a craniosacral system, we started to search for its significance. Many people suffer from dysfunctions and diseases of unknown etiology. When a new concept about a heretofore disregarded physiological system appeared, it was reasonable to search for cause and effect relationships between dysfunction of this system and the disease syndromes of obscure etiology. Based upon this rationale, we applied craniosacral therapy to the wide variety of health problems which are discussed in this book.

The craniosacral concept has been utilized by a small number of practitioners for several generations, without a complete understanding of how it works or why it has been successful. It was effective when applied by these few, but appeared so mysterious in its application and results that it became known to others as a form of faith healing. In fact, some practitioners believed that they were directly funneling divine healing power through their hands. This obviated the need for an understanding of the underlying anatomy and physiology. The work did not die because the results could not be denied. Thus, while some observers regarded it as medical quackery and others as divine healing, still others continued to be curious about the anatomical and physiological bases of the results observed in response to craniosacral therapy.

Our own interest in the craniosacral concept came about quite by chance. I (Upledger) first became involved during a surgical procedure in 1971. I was assisting a neurosurgeon in the removal of an extradural calcification from the posterior aspect of the dural tube in the midcervical region. Our goal was to remove the calcified plaque without incising or disrupting the integrity of the dura mater. My task was to hold the dural membrane still with two pairs of forceps while the neurosurgeon removed the plaque without cutting or damaging the underlying dural membrane. But the membrane would not hold still. I was embarrassed because I could not carry out such a simple task. The fully anesthetized patient was in a sitting position. I had no difficulty in reaching or seeing the operating field. There were no excuses.

It became apparent that the movement of the dural membrane was rhythmical at about 8 cycles per minute. This rhythmic activity was independent of the patient's breathing and cardiac rhythms. It was another physiological rhythm. It appeared to be an ebb and flow of the fluid which is contained within the dural membrane. Neither the neurosurgeon, the anesthesiologist, nor I had ever observed this phenomenon before. My curiosity was piqued. I could find no relevant information in the conventional medical or physiology literature.

The patient had been suffering from a dystrophy of the skin of both feet. He had been unable to walk because the skin on his feet continuously turned black, cracked and peeled off. It was very painful. Following the removal of the calcified plaque, his condition of about eighteen months duration improved. Three months after the operation, his feet appeared to be normal. The plaque itself was the result of a systemic echinococcus infection which had produced cystic formations in the liver and brain. Medical treatment for these problems was successful. The extradural plaque was a residual effect of the infection.

Ultimately, I became aware of a course in cranial osteopathy, the concepts of which seemed to fit with the observations described above during the surgical procedure. I used some of the techniques which were taught in the course with great success. There is no positive feedback like success, so I delved deeper into cranial osteopathy. In 1975, I left private practice and joined the Department of Biomechanics at the Michigan State University College of Osteopathic Medicine. I became part of an interdisciplinary research team. One of our tasks was to investigate cranial osteopathy.

During the course of our work, I heard a lecture by my co-author, Jon Vredevoogd. Jon is a designer and an architect. The essence of his lecture can be summarized by the following quotation:

Nature makes the best designs. Every design in nature is for a purpose and is the most efficient way to accomplish a task. We should study the way nature does things and try to emulate it, rather than clumsily and egotistically trying to invent our own. We cannot improve on natural design; we need only understand it.

I gave Jon a disarticulated human skull and challenged him to explain to me why nature designed this skull as it was, and to explain the function of the design of the various bones. For the last six years, Jon and I have been working together on these problems.

On a general level, this book is for the curious medical biologist or physiologist, or anyone who has an interest in the integrated mechanical and physiological functions of the human body. The craniosacral concept demystifies and provides a straightforward explanation for many observed but unexplained physiological phenomena and clinical syndromes.

On a more practical level, this book is for anyone who is a "body worker"; that is, anyone in a healing profession who uses their hands as diagnostic or therapeutic tools. Included are medical and osteopathic physicians, dentists, chiropractors, physical therapists, polarity therapists, movement therapists, psychotherapists, and many, many more. Most of the people in these professions have a good background in anatomy. In this book, we hope to help build upon that solid anatomical foundation an expanded concept of dynamic anatomical and physiological function.

We enthusiastically encourage readers to improve their palpatory skills. I (Upledger) am fascinated by the vistas which have opened for me since I began to develop my own palpatory skills. The fascination is illustrated by the comment of a Czechoslovakian neurologist who recently visited our university. He had heard of the craniosacral concept and wanted me to teach him to feel the rhythm. I laid supine upon the treatment table, gently placed his hands upon my head and instructed him to close his eyes and perceive. At first he felt the cardiovascular rhythm, then the breathing rhythm, and then very clearly the craniosacral rhythm. Spontaneously and theatrically, he stated, "Once you have found it, you'll never let it go."

I owe the writing of this book to all of my students who persisted in questioning and prodding me to verbalize and explain the things that my hands so often do automatically. Outstanding among these gentle prodders is the student who put together into syllabus form my lecture notes and published articles, Sister Anne Brooks, now an osteopathic physician.

I am deeply indebted to Stacy F. Howell, Ph.D. under whose tutelage I completed a three-year fellowship in Biochemistry at the Kirksville College of Osteopathic Medicine. Dr. Howell unceasingly attempted to teach me the difference between a technologist and a doctor of the philosophy of science. His influence turned me into a naturalist observer.

Louis Hasbrouck, D.O. and Anne Wales, D.O. were both inspirational during my first experience at a Cranial Academy seminar. Later on in my craniosacral development, Herbert C. Miller, D.O. helped me to further gain trust in my hands and intuition. I owe all of these people a great deal.

Ann Eschtruth and Laura Hayes managed to decipher my handwriting and thereby turn the manuscript into something readable. Charles Lincoln, D.O. (U.K.) was always there to proofread and discuss my presentation of the concepts and techniques. A prodigious amount of time was invested in the designing, typesetting, proofreading and keylining of this book. For their patient devotion to these tasks, Jon Vredevoogd and I particularly wish to thank Patricia O'Connor, Lilian Lai Bensky, Peggy Welker and Catherine Nelson. John O'Connor and Dan Bensky of Eastland Press did the final round of editing for which we are grateful.

My wife Dianne offered encouragement and support whenever I needed it. Without her, this book would not have been written.

Chapter 1
Introduction to the Craniosacral Concept

The craniosacral concept is a potent therapeutic vision grounded upon certain anatomical, physiological and therapeutic observations. To utilize craniosacral therapy in diagnosis and treatment requires a particular point of view: that of seeing the individual as an integrated totality.

Unfortunately, for teaching purposes we must initially separate anatomy and physiology from therapy and discuss various parts of the body as discrete topics. This artificial, linear approach to what in reality is an integrated whole necessitates a certain degree of repetition. Concepts and techniques introduced here are later modified, or viewed from different angles at other points in the text.

As a starting point, in Chapter 1 we will introduce the concept of craniosacral motion, also known as the cranial rhythmic impulse. This chapter, together with the anatomical and physiological definitions in Chapter 2, will serve as a foundation for the remainder of the book.

THE CRANIOSACRAL SYSTEM AND ITS RELATIONSHIP TO OTHER BODY SYSTEMS

The craniosacral system may be defined as a recently recognized, functioning physiological system. The anatomic parts of the craniosacral system are:

1. The meningeal membranes
2. The osseous structures to which the meningeal membranes attach
3. The other non-osseous connective tissue structures which are intimately related to meningeal membranes
4. The cerebrospinal fluid
5. All structures related to production, resorption and containment of the cerebrospinal fluid

The craniosacral system is intimately related to, influences, and is influenced by:

1. The nervous system
2. The musculoskeletal system
3. The vascular system
4. The lymphatic system

5

5.   The endocrine system
6.   The respiratory system

Abnormalities in the structure or function of any of these systems may influence the craniosacral system. Abnormalities in the structure or function of the craniosacral system will necessarily have profound, and frequently deleterious effects upon the development or function of the nervous system, especially the brain.

The craniosacral system provides the "internal milieu" for the development, growth and functional efficiency of the brain and spinal cord from the time of embryonic formation until death.

WHAT IS CRANIOSACRAL MOTION?

The craniosacral system is characterized by rhythmic, mobile activity which persists throughout life. This craniosacral motion occurs in man, other primates, canines, felines, and probably all or most other vertebrates. It is distinctly different from the physiological motions which are related to breathing, and different from cardiovascular activity as well. It may be the underlying mechanism of, or closely related to, the Traube-Herring phenomenon, which has been observed but not yet adequately explained. Craniosacral rhythmic motion can be palpated most readily on the head. With practice and the development of palpatory skills, however, it can be perceived anywhere on the body.

The normal rate of craniosacral rhythm in humans is between 6 and 12 cycles *per minute.* (This is not to be confused with Alpha rhythm from the brain, which is between 8 and 12 cycles *per second.*) In pathological circumstances, we have observed craniosacral rhythmic rates of less than 6 and more than 12 cycles per minute.

During the summer of 1979, one of your authors (Upledger) had the privilege of examining several long-term coma cases at the Loewenstein Institute for Neuropathology in Ra'-anana, Israel. We were specifically interested in craniosacral motion. In several cases, coma due to anoxia and intracranial lesions involving the brain most frequently resulted in a reduction of the cranial rhythm to as low as 3 or 4 cycles per minute. A few coma cases due to drug overdosage resulted in a cranial rhythm above 12 cycles per minute. These rhythms were palpated on the patient's head.

OBSERVATIONS OF CRANIOSACRAL MOTION

Hyperkinetic children have been observed to present with abnormally rapid craniosacral rhythmic rates, as have patients suffering from acute illnesses with fever. Moribund and brain-damaged patients will often present with abnormally low rhythmic rates. As the clinical conditions improve, the rhythmic rates move toward the normal range.

In non-pathological circumstances, the rate of the craniosacral rhythmic motion is quite stable. It does not fluctuate as do the rates of the cardiovascular and respiratory systems in response to exercise, emotion, rest, etc. Therefore, it appears to be a reliable criterion for the evaluation of pathological conditions.

Under reasonably normal circumstances this rhythmic activity appears at the sacrum as a gentle rocking motion about a transverse axis located approximately one inch anterior to the second sacral segment. The rocking motion of the sacrum correlates rhythmically to a broadening and narrowing of the transverse dimension of the head. As the head widens, the sacral apex moves in an anterior direction. This phase of motion is referred to as *flexion* of the craniosacral system. The counterpart of flexion is *extension*. During the extension phase, the head narrows in its transverse dimension. The sacral base moves anteriorly while the sacral apex moves posteriorly.

During the flexion phase of the craniosacral motion cycle, the whole body externally rotates and broadens. During the extension phase, the body internally rotates and seems to narrow slightly. A complete cycle of the craniosacral rhythmic motion is composed of one flexion and one extension phase. There is a *neutral zone* or relaxation between the end of one phase and the beginning of the next phase of each cycle. The neutral zone is perceived as a slight pause which follows upon the return from the extreme range of one phase, and before the physiological forces move into the opposite phase of motion (ILLUSTRATION 1-1-A).

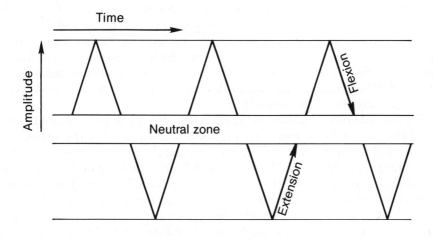

Illustration 1-1-A
Representation of Craniosacral Motion — Normal

Experienced clinicians are able to palpate the craniosacral motion anywhere on the body. Valuable diagnostic and prognostic information can be gained very quickly by palpating the craniosacral motion for rate, amplitude, symmetry and quality. This diagnostic potential was tested at the Loewenstein Institute when neurological patients were examined using the techniques of craniosacral rhythmic motion evaluation, and diagnoses were suggested without any other knowledge of the patient. By close examination for changes in craniosacral motion, we were able to accurately localize levels of spinal cord lesions which were responsible for paraplegia and quadriplegia in cases of poliomyelitis, Guillain-Barre syndrome, cord tumor and spinal cord severance due to trauma. We were also able to localize neurological problems in the cranium which were due to cerebral hemorrhage, thrombosis and tumor.

The craniosacral rhythm was observed to be between 20 and 30 cycles per minute in those parts of the body which were no longer under the influence of the higher centers of the central nervous system. Thus, by palpating to determine the spinal level of rhythmic motion change in the paravertebral musculature, the level of spinal cord lesion or injury can be determined. The cord function is interrupted about two segments above the palpable change in the paravertebral muscle rhythm.

Denervated muscles move rhythmically between 20 and 30 cycles per minute, whereas innervated muscles move physiologically in correspondence with the craniosacral rhythm. (6 to 12 cycles per minute is normal.)

Low amplitude of craniosacral rhythm indicates a low level of vitality in the patient; that is, the patient's resistance is low, and hence the susceptibility to disease is high.

Occasionally, the craniosacral rate, as palpated on the head, is twice normal and the amplitude is low; but the internal energy which drives the craniosacral system seems quite high. We interpret this finding as indicating that the boundary of the hydraulic system, which is the meningeal membranes of the craniosacral system, is rather restrictive and lacks accommodation to craniosacral motion. Therefore, the rate has doubled while the amplitude is reduced by approximately 50%. This condition maintains a normal distance of motion per minute (ILLUSTRATION 1-1-B). We

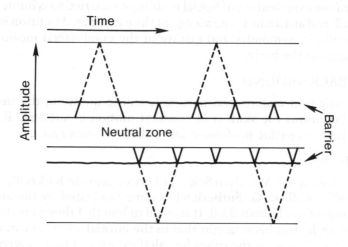

Illustration 1-1-B
Representation of Craniosacral Motion —
Effect of Barriers

often find this situation in cases of inflammatory problems which presently involve, or have in the past involved the meninges and/or the central nervous system. We also frequently find this clinical abnormality in autism. This may mean that autism is the result of a previous physiological problem which involved the meningeal membranes, and which rendered them less compliant.

Lack of symmetry in the craniosacral rhythmic motion throughout the body is an indicator which can be used to localize pathological problems of any type which cause loss of physiological motion, such as osteopathic lesion of the musculoskeletal system (somatic dysfunction), inflammatory responses, adhesions, trauma with cicatrix, surgical scars, vascular accidents, etc. While the asymmetry of motion will not indicate what the problem is, it will tell you where the problem is located. Once located, you must rely upon other diagnostic methods to determine the exact pathological nature of the problem. Restoration of symmetrical craniosacral motion to the area of restricted motion can be used as a prognostic tool. As the asymmetry is eliminated and normal physiological motion restored, you may confidently predict that the problem is being or has been resolved.

THE ROLE OF THE BODY FASCIA

One may consider the body fascia as a slightly mobile, continuous from head-to-toe, laminated sheath of connective tissue which invests in pockets (between lamina) all of the somatic and visceral structures of the human body. With this model in mind, it is apparent that any loss of mobility of this tissue in any specific area can be used as an aid in the location of the disease process which has caused that lack of mobility. By some means, probably via the nervous system, this fascial system is normally kept in constant motion in correspondence with the craniosacral rhythmic motion. By direct connections and common osseous anchorings, the extradural fascia and the meninges are interrelated and interdependent in terms of their motion. Therefore, the amount of diagnostic and prognostic information which can be obtained from the examination of fascial mobility or restriction is limited only by the palpatory skill and anatomical knowledge of the examiner. Attention is directed to the rate, amplitude, symmetry and quality of the craniosacral motion and its reflection throughout the body.

HISTORICAL BACKGROUND

While the origin of craniosacral motion is still in question, the theory that under normal conditions the skull is in constant motion is not new. It was first introduced to the osteopathic profession more than 50 years ago.

SUTHERLAND'S MODEL

While a student at the American School of Osteopathy in Kirksville, Missouri in the early 1900's, William G. Sutherland became fascinated by the anatomical design of the bones of the human skull. It seemed to him that they were designed to move, even though he had been taught that in the normal adult human the skull-bones are fused solidly one to the other by calcification and that movement was, therefore, impossible. The only exceptions to this condition of immobility in the human skull were said to be found in the tiny mobile ossicles of the ear and at the temporomandibular joints. The anatomists taught Sutherland, as many still teach today, that the skull serves protective and hematopoetic functions only.[1]

Possessing the deep conviction that all nature's designs are purposeful, Sutherland became convinced that the bones of the cranium must therefore move in relation to each other throughout normal life. Certainly, detailed study of the human skull and its sutures indicates the potential for interosseous cranial motion.

After Sutherland became more familiar with cranial motion by self-experimen-

---

[1] Italian anatomists in the early 1900s, however, taught that cranial suture ossification was pathological in the mature human adult. These teachings therefore contradict the British anatomists, who taught the doctrine of sutural ossification and cranial immobility as a normal condition. (*Anatomia Umana,* Vol 1, 1931, by Professor Guiseppe Sperino, p. 203.)

tation, he began experimenting on others by gently palpating their heads. Soon he was able to sense minute rhythmic motions of the crania of humans of various ages. An early correlative finding was the palpable sacral motion in synchrony with the motion of the cranium.

Sutherland accounted for the rhythmic synchrony of motion between the cranium and the sacrum on the basis of the continuity of the tubular spinal dura mater which firmly connects the occiput to the sacrum with few significantly restrictive osseous attachments between. He reasoned that motion of the occiput at the dural attachment of the foramen magnum must necessarily influence sacral physiological motion and vice versa, except under pathological, restrictive conditions.

He then developed a model which placed the sphenoid as the keystone of the osseous cranium. The sphenoid supplied the driving force which was transmitted to the rest of the cranium via its articular relationships with the occiput, temporals, parietals, frontal, ethmoid, vomer, palatines and zygomae. (There is also an inconstant articular relationship with the maxilla by the sphenoid.) From this model, it is obvious that a force which moves the sphenoid must necessarily cause motion in all the bones with which it articulates. Bones such as the mandible, with which the sphenoid has no direct articulation, are influenced indirectly by the sphenoid through the temporals and other bones. The sphenoid influences the maxillae by way of the vomer and the palatine bones. From a mechanical point of view, this model of interosseous relationships with the sphenoid as the driving force is quite plausible.

Some doubt has been cast upon the possibility of motion at the sphenobasilar joint in the adult human. However, motion at this joint is an essential part of Sutherland's functioning model. Early in embryonic life the sphenobasilar joint is a synchondrosis. It is located just posterior to the sella turcica and anterior to the foramen magnum, where the posterior projection of the sphenoid body joins the anterior projection of the occipital base. This thin band of cartilagenous material probably retains some degree of flexibility throughout life. Sutherland incorrectly described this joint as a symphysis. His illustrations of the joint as a symphysis make use of the characteristics of the symphysis to hypothesize abnormal shearing conditions between the sphenoid and occiput as well as torsions, sidebending and flexion-extension motion patterns.

The torsions, sidebending and flexion-extension motions can conceivably occur if some flexibility is retained between the sphenoid and occiput. The shearing relationship between the sphenoid and occiput, which Sutherland called a vertical or lateral strain is, however, somewhat more difficult to conceptualize as inherent in a joint which is not, in fact, a symphysis.

Histologically, the sphenobasilar joint is correctly named a synchondrosis. It does maintain some degree of flexibility throughout life. It is probably more correct to conceptualize anatomical distortions between the components of the spheno-basilar synchondrosis as secondary to cranial base suture dysfunctions and/or abnormal membrane tensions within the dura mater. Abnormal sphenobasilar relationships are probably not maintained by inherent primary distortion of the anatomical relationship between the sphenoid and the occiput. The dura mater is firmly attached to the bones of the cranial vault and base as periosteum and endosteum. Abnormal tensions placed upon the dural membranes are therefore transmitted to the various bones to which these membranes attach. This circumstance produces abnormal functional motion of these bones.

In Sutherland's model, the sphenoid was regarded as the driving force of the motion for the bones of the cranium. Inevitably, the question must be asked, "What is the driving force upon the sphenoid?" Sutherland suggested that the sphenoid moved in response to a circulatory fluctuation of the cerebrospinal fluid and its effect upon the intracranial membrane system. He saw the falx cerebri, the leaves of the tentorium cerebelli and the falx cerebelli as parts of a reciprocal tension membrane system which responds to the circulatory fluctuations of the cerebrospinal fluid by driving the sphenoid in its rhythmic pattern of motion at the cranial base. The origin of all this motion, Sutherland believed, was the rhythmic contraction and expansion of the ventricular system of the brain. He regarded the brain as the primary source of the force which drives the craniosacral system and produces motion.

This seems to be a phenomenal piece of insight and our research has largely supported this model. In general, modern technology is beginning to show that Dr. Sutherland's model is largely correct.

PRESSURESTAT MODEL

We find Dr. Sutherland's concept of a rhythmically contracting brain as the driving force behind the rhythmic rise and fall of cerebrospinal fluid pressure somewhat difficult to adopt. We do not believe that the tissue of the brain has the tensile strength to act as a hydraulic pump which rhythmically raises fluid pressure within this semi-closed hydraulic system. Second, although glial cells *in vitro* are seen to move rhythmically, their motion is perhaps one-tenth the rate that we observe in the craniosacral system. It would not seem possible to draw support from observations of glial cell movements for the concept of a rhythmically contracting brain as the basis for craniosacral system motion. It is true that the motion of individual cells *in vitro* may be much slower than those same cells *in vivo;* it may also be much faster. We cannot accept *in vitro* glial cell movement into evidence.

An alternative to the rhythmically contracting brain concept would be a pressurestat model. In this model one need only assume that cerebrospinal fluid production by the choroid plexuses within the ventricular system of the brain is significantly more rapid than is the resorption of cerebrospinal fluid back into the venous circulation by the arachnoid bodies. These arachnoid bodies are concentrated primarily in the intracranial venous sinus system. Probably the majority of resorption occurs in the sagittal venous sinus.

If production of cerebrospinal fluid is hypothetically twice as fast as resorption, when the production is turned on for a given period of time it will reach an upper threshhold of pressure. When that upper threshhold is reached, the production of cerebrospinal fluid is turned off by some homeostatic mechanism. The resorption of cerebrospinal fluid is constant throughout the production phase and after the production of fluid is shut off. Therefore, when fluid production is off, the fluid pressure will drop as a result of the constantly diminishing volume within the hydraulic system. When a lower threshhold of pressure is reached, the production of cerebrospinal fluid is again turned on and the cerebrospinal fluid pressure within the craniosacral system begins to rise again. In this manner, a rhythmic rise and fall of fluid pressure is achieved which, in turn, causes the rhythmic changes in the boundaries of the semi-closed hydraulic system.

CEREBROSPINAL FLUID PRESSURE CONTROL MECHANISMS

At this time, there appear to be at least two mechanisms:

1. Since we now know that cranial sutures constantly move in normal human adults and other primates, and since we have identified collagen and elastic fibers as well as vascular and nerve plexuses within the suture (APPENDIX A), it seems entirely possible that the suture contains a stretch reflex. When the suture is gapped open by intracranial fluid pressure to a specific dimension, an intrasutural stretch reflex is activated which telegraphs to the ventricular system of the brain to stop production of cerebrospinal fluid. When the suture is relieved of its stretch and begins to come together and ultimately to compress its contents somewhat (as intracranial fluid pressure is reduced), a message is sent to the brain to resume production of cerebrospinal fluid. This resumption of fluid production will therefore raise fluid pressure and reduce intrasutural compression.

    With this model in mind, we began to search for the telegraph system between the suture and the ventricular system of the brain. We have successfully traced single nerve axons in the monkey, from the sagittal suture centralward through the meningeal membranes to the wall of the third ventricle of the brain.[2] This histological work provides us with the structures necessary to support the conceptual model described.

2. In a description of the straight sinus found in *Gray's Anatomy* (39th BRITISH EDITION), there is mention of an arachnoid granulation body which projects into the floor of the straight sinus at its angle of union with the great cerebral vein. This body contains a sinusoidal plexus of blood vessels which become engorged and act as a ball-valve mechanism. This mechanism may then control the outflow from the great cerebral vein which, in turn, by increasing back pressure, effects the secretion of the cerebrospinal fluid by the choroid plexuses of the lateral ventricles. The drainage of these regions of the brain is from the internal cerebral vessels, which empty into the great cerebral vein.

We would hypothesize the presence of these structures as supportive of yet another mechanism whereby the production of cerebrospinal fluid is under homeostatic control. We suggest that it is this pressurestat mechanism which causes the ventricular system of the brain to dilate and contract rhythmically, rather than some intrinsic contractile power of the brain tissue itself. Observation of living human brain tissue *in situ* does show the rhythmic motion of the brain tissue. However, it seems more reasonable to conclude that the ventricular system of the brain is responding to changing cerebrospinal fluid pressure, rather than creating it by contraction.

Independently, E.A. Bunt, M.D., a South African neurosurgeon, has developed a similar model while researching in the area of idiopathic, normotensive hydrocephalopathy. Dr. Bunt has shown us serial tomogram X-rays taken through the lateral and third ventricles of the brain which show approximately a 50% area change during dilation and contraction of the lateral ventricles of the brain at a rhythm of 6 cycles per minute in a normal patient. Dr. Bunt believes that the pressurestat concept is viable.

---

[2]This work is in progress in conjunction with Dr. E.W. Retzlaff of the Michigan State University Department of Biomechanics.

BECKER'S MODEL

Still another model which might explain the origin of the craniosacral rhythmic motion was put forth by Frederick Becker, Ph.D., an anatomist and previously a colleague in the Department of Biomechanics at Michigan State University.

Dr. Becker hypothesized that the craniosacral rhythmic motion may result from the tonic response of the extradural muscles to the forces of gravity. These muscles might provide either (1) a stimulus input into the central nervous system which produces the cerebrospinal fluid pressure fluctuations, or (2) via fascial continuity, the voluntary muscles might act directly upon the dural membranes. (These membranes form the boundary of the cerebrospinal fluid hydraulic system.) Such an influence could cause a rhythmic rise and fall of hydraulic pressure within the system by rhythmically changing the tension upon these dural membranes.

However, our experience in examining neuropathological patients tends to refute this hypothesis. We have detected strong cranial rhythm at the heads of patients who have little or no skeletal muscle tone due to spinal cord injury with resultant quadriplegia. If craniosacral motion were dependent upon skeletal muscle tonus, we would expect a weakening of cranial motion amplitude. Further, denervated muscle and connective tissue seem to move rhythmically, 20 to 30 cycles per minute. If craniosacral rhythmic motion were dependent upon skeletal muscle tonus, it does not seem possible that the elevated rate in the skeletal muscles could exist in the quadriplegic, without seemingly influencing the cranial rhythm. In many quadriplegia cases, cranial rhythm of the head remains within normal limits, both in amplitude and in cycles per minute.

Chapter 2
The Craniosacral Concept:
Basic Terminology

Most readers of this text have a good background in anatomy and physiology. However, many terms and concepts used in craniosacral therapy are not emphasized in conventional anatomy and physiology courses. Other terms have specific meanings in craniosacral therapy which differ from those used in other fields of medicine. Thus, before embarking upon the main body of the text, in this chapter we will survey the most important anatomical, physiological and therapeutic terminology used in craniosacral therapy, as well as the language of anatomical position. Many of these terms will be discussed in greater detail in later chapters of the book.

THE CRANIOSACRAL SYSTEM

This is a recently recognized physiological system. It possesses its own physiological rhythmic activity. It has all the characteristics of a semi-closed hydraulic system. Functionally, it is intimately related to the central nervous system, the autonomic nervous system, the neuromusculoskeletal system, and the endocrine system. Its boundaries are formed by the meningeal membranes, most specifically the dura mater. The system's fluid intake is via the choroid plexus, which allows passage of fluid from the vascular system into the ventricular system of the brain. The choroid plexus is selective in its passage of solutes from blood into the craniosacral system. The fluid which passes through the choroid plexus is known as cerebrospinal fluid. Cerebrospinal fluid is returned into the venous system by the arachnoid villae. These villae are most concentrated in the sagittal venous sinus within the cranial vault, but are found in significant numbers throughout the intracranial venous drainage system.

A semi-closed hydraulic system is formed by the dura mater membrane and its contents. The dural membrane is essentially impermeable to the cerebrospinal fluid which it holds. Intake and outflow of fluid from the system is by means of specialized tissue structures (choroid plexuses and arachnoid villae) which are under homeostatic control. These intake and outflow mechanisms qualify the hydraulic system as semi-closed.

Homeostatic mechanisms are those self-correcting and self-balancing mechanisms which rely upon feedback loops. Biological systems are laden with homeostatic mechanisms which enable them to effect second-by-second adaptation to

14

constant changes in both internal and external environments. An example of a homeostatic mechanism in the human body is the production of thyroid hormone by the thyroid gland, which is under control of the thyroid stimulating hormone from the pituitary gland. The pituitary gland receives information about whether or not to release more thyroid stimulating hormone into the bloodstream from the level of thyroid hormone in the blood, which is constantly monitored by the pituitary gland. Blood sugar, body heat, blood pressure and a million other activities in the body are continuously regulated by homeostatic mechanisms.

As a hydraulic system, the boundaries of the craniosacral system, the dural membranes, are given shape by the fluid pressure within the system and by its more rigid aspects, the cranial bones to which the membrane is firmly and lavishly attached within the cranial vault. This design allows us to regard the cranial bones functionally as "hard places" in the dural membrane. These hard places are used as indicators in diagnosis and as handles in treatment.

The craniosacral semi-closed hydraulic system obeys the laws of fluid mechanics. The cerebrospinal fluid which fills the system is largely incompressible and therefore behaves like water. It is our belief that although the cerebrospinal fluid is moving within the system, the movement is of low velocity and without much force. Therefore, we suggest at this time that the cerebrospinal fluid obeys the laws of fluid mechanics as though it were static.

Since fluids present negligible shearing forces within their boundaries, the application of any force to the fluid surface is transmitted equally in all directions. Therefore, when we apply a pressure or force to an area of the boundary of the hydraulic system, the resultant force is transmitted equally via the cerebrospinal fluid to the remainder of the boundaries of the system. This characteristic makes the craniosacral system amenable to "shotgun" types of therapy.

We must also keep in mind that this hydraulic system includes the brain, which is more compressible than the cerebrospinal fluid. Severe pressure upon the external boundary of the system is transmitted through the relatively incompressible cerebrospinal fluid to the more compressible brain substance.

MEMBRANES

The membranes of the craniosacral system include the dura mater, the arachnoid membrane and the pia mater.

The *dura mater* is the external layer of the three membranes, named the meninges, which envelop the brain and spinal cord. It is a tough, relatively inelastic connective tissue which is fused with the internal aspect of the skull. It forms vertical sheets, the falxes cerebri and cerebelli, which separate the hemispheres of the cerebrum and the cerebellum respectively. It also forms the relatively horizontal sheets, the tentorium cerebelli, bilaterally, which separate the cerebrum from the cerebellum. It is the dura mater which contains the cerebrospinal fluid and thereby forms the craniosacral hydraulic system. This layer is also referred to as the dural membrane.

The *arachnoid membrane* is thin, delicate and vascularized. It is separated from the dura and pia mater by the subdural and subarachnoid spaces. The arachnoid membrane does not follow the convolutions of the brain. The spaces which separate the arachnoid membrane from the dura mater externally, and from the pia mater internally, are filled with fluid. This allows for a degree of independent motion between the three meningeal membranes.

The *pia mater* is the highly vascularized, delicate internal layer of the meningeal membranes. It follows all of the convolutions of the brain and spinal cord and delivers blood supply.

Since the three meningeal layers are capable of independent motion, one of the functions they serve is to allow the spine to rotate and bend without moving or stressing the spinal cord. In cases of arachnoiditis where this ability is lost due to inflammation and adhesion of the arachnoid to the other membranes, intolerable pain is produced during certain spinal movements.

DURAL MEMBRANE

This boundary of the craniosacral semi-closed hydraulic system has various bony (osseous) attachments. These attachments act as anchors by which dural membrane tensions are transmitted to connective tissues outside of the system. It is by virtue of these common bony moorings between the dura and the connective tissues that abnormal tension patterns cross the dural boundary. Conversely, and more easily discerned, is the fact that via these common anchorings the extra-craniosacral system connective tissues transmit tensions into the dural membrane system. By way of dural continuity, these tensions are transmitted to distant and very hard-to-predict regions of the meningeal membrane system.

Within the cranial vault the dura provides a layer of endosteum which is generously and firmly attached via periosteum to the bones of the cranial vault. Contrary to common belief, the bones of the cranial vault are in constant motion as they accommodate the ever changing fluid dynamics and dural membrane tensions within the craniosacral system. The sutures or joints where the cranial bones meet each other do *not* fuse under normal circumstances, no matter what age the individual has achieved. While this is contrary to traditional Anglo-American anatomical dogma, it is consistent with Mediterranean anatomical teachings. Our findings clearly demonstrate the capability for continued sutural mobility throughout life.

CRANIAL BASE

The cranial base is formed by the horizontal part of the frontal bone and the ethmoid bone's contribution as it penetrates the notch in the frontal bone (ILLUSTRATION 2-1). It includes the body of the sphenoid, the petrous parts of the temporal bones and the base and condylar parts of the occiput. This set of bony parts forms a floor for the cranial vault. The joint in the floor between the anterior occiput and the posterior sphenoid body is referred to as the sphenobasilar joint. It is a synchondrosis, which means that there is a tongue of somewhat flexible cartilage-nous bone between sphenoid and occiput. This flexible synchondrosis accommodates the flexion and extension activity of the cranial base which continues throughout life.

CORE LINK

This is the name applied to the dural membrane between the foramen magnum and the sacrum. The name itself suggests the function of this tube of membrane. The core link of spinal dural membrane is relatively free to move within the spinal canal. Therefore, under conditions of rest and with the spine in a relatively neutral

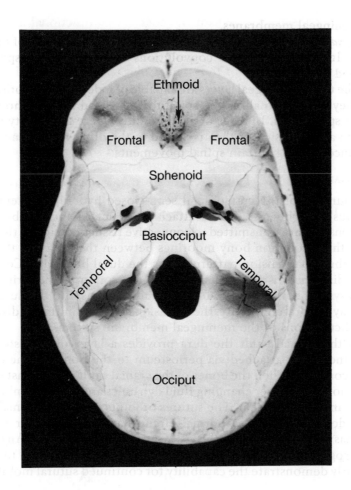

Illustration 2-1
Cranial Base

position, the occipital and sacral motions mime each other. Unless abnormal restriction to mobility is present within the core link, the membrane transmits tensions imposed upon one of these bones directly to the other.

SACROCOCCYGEAL COMPLEX

This refers to the functional unity of these two bones. The meningeal membranes enter the sacrum from above with the cauda equina. All three membranes blend together, and within the sacral canal there is firm bone attachment only at the level of the second segment. This is probably why the sacrum seems to rotate about an axis at this level as it conforms to the motion of the craniosacral system. In the sacral canal, the dura blends with the terminal aspect of the pia, the filum terminale. The filum terminale exits the sacral canal through the sacral hiatus, which is usually at the level of the fourth sacral segment. The membranes are now quite fibrous, tough and blended together. They merge with and thereby contribute to the periosteum of the coccyx. From a craniosacral therapy viewpoint, it is therefore advantageous to consider the sacrum and coccyx as a functional unit.

VENTRICULAR SYSTEM OF THE BRAIN

This system is composed of four ventricular spaces, two of which are lateral while the third and fourth are midline (ILLUSTRATION 2-2). The lateral ventricles are cavities within the cerebral hemispheres. The third is connected to them by the Foramen of Munro; the communication between the third and fourth ventricles is via the Aquaduct of Sylvius. The Foramena of Lushka and of Magendie connect the fourth ventricle of the brain with the subarachnoid space. Cerebrospinal fluid is formed by the choroid plexuses within this ventricular system. The fluid enters the pool of cerebrospinal fluid via the duct system. Atresia of the duct between the third and fourth ventricles with a resultant fluid back pressure is a common cause of congenital hydrocephalus.

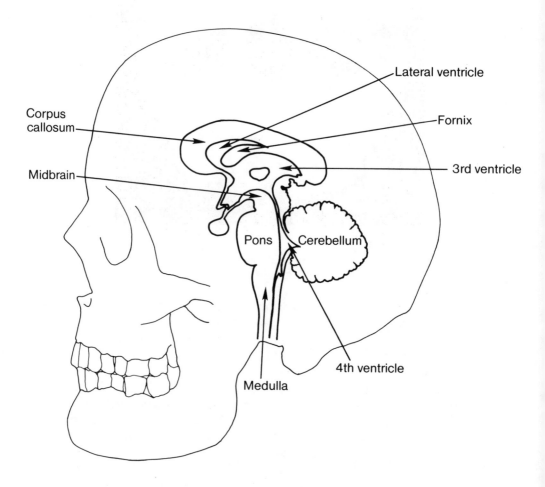

Illustration 2-2
Ventricles

MOTION

Motion has a special meaning to people who are involved in craniosacral therapy. In this work, craniosacral motion is that motion which the whole body performs rhythmically in response to the craniosacral system's activity. This motion is very subtle and short in range. We speak of the craniosacral motion as physiological because it is unconscious and involuntary; it is inherent in the individual's biological system. Those motions which are physiological and inherent are necessary for the continuation of life.

Non-physiological motion may refer to abnormal inherent motion which is the adaptational result of an obstacle or restriction interfering with normal, inherent physiological motion. It is a distorted motion pattern which is the result of restriction. Non-physiological motion is also sometimes used to describe extrinsically induced motion. However, this usage is less common and is not intended where the term appears in this book. Instead, we use the word *movement* for extrinsically induced motion. *Passive movement* is present when the therapist does the moving and the subject puts no effort into the movement. *Active movement* is, of course, the opposite and implies effort on the part of the subject.

A *restriction* is an impairment to normal physiological motion within the body. The inherent energy that causes physiological motion is present, but is fighting against the restriction. Usually, restrictions occur in the connective tissue or fascia. They can result from inflammation, adhesion, somatic dysfunction and neuroreflexes. When a restriction dissipates, it is called a *release*. A release is sensed as a softening of the obstacle or restriction against which the inherent physiological motion was fighting. The resistance melts and there is a palpable relaxation of the tissues. Release is always a therapeutically positive event.

The craniosacral system proceeds through cyclical flexion and extension at a rate of approximately 6 to 12 cycles per minute under normal circumstances. *Flexion* is an extreme range of motion during which the head becomes wider transversely and shorter in its anterior posterior dimension. During flexion, the whole body externally rotates and widens. After flexion, the physiological motion passes through a neutral or idling zone on its way into *extension,* during which phase the head narrows and elongates. The whole body internally rotates slightly. A complete cycle from flexion through neutral into extension, back through neutral and again into flexion requires about 6 seconds.

Once you tune into these motions, you can perceive your own body doing flexion-extension cycles as you stand or walk. After a time you will learn to tune yourself in and out to your own physiological body motion at will.

From the diagnostic, prognostic and therapeutic points of view, we are interested in a qualitative estimate of the strength of the inherent energy which is driving the physiological motion, the symmetry of the body motion response (both of the craniosacral system and of the extrinsic body connective tissues), and in the range and quality of each cyclical motion. Is it fighting against a resistance barrier?

A *resistance barrier* is a perceptible point during the course of a normal motion cycle at which the body motion either hesitates and exerts extra effort to pass, or is unable to pass at all. Restrictions to motion and motion barriers can be characterized as either rigid or elastic. *Rigid barriers* and restrictions represent bony problems where one bone cannot move in relation to another because they are jammed together. *Elastic barriers* and restrictions represent abnormal membrane tensions which prevent normal physiological motion. Abnormal membrane tensions will often permit the motion to continue, but increased energy is needed to make this occur. When you encounter a membrane problem during treatment, its restriction has an elastic "give" when you try to force gently and directly against it.

The whole body response to the craniosacral system is based upon the concept of fascial continuity throughout the body. The motion of the body is probably related to the effect of the fluctuation of the cerebrospinal fluid upon the nervous system, which in turn influences the tonus of the body tissues.

PALPATION

Palpation is typically defined as examination by touch. It is the development of this skill to which this book is largely dedicated. Palpation is an art which is grossly neglected in the health care professions. Even the "body workers" frequently use only one kind of palpation and thus develop but a small part of their potential as palpators.

Most of you have been taught to palpate or touch with your fingertips. This is supposed to be the preferred method because the fingertips are the most sensitive parts of the hand. We, however, would urge you to palpate with your whole hand, arm, stomach or whatever part of your body comes in contact with the patient's body. The idea is to "meld" the palpating part of your body with the body you are examining. As this melding occurs, the palpating part of your body does what the patient's body is doing. It becomes synchronized. Once melding and synchronization have occurred, use your proprioceptors to determine what the palpating part of your own body is doing. Your proprioceptors are those sensory receptors located in the muscles, tendons, and fascia that tell you where the parts of your body are without using your eyes.

The key to this type of palpation is to be as non-threatening and non-intrusive as possible. The objective is to have that part of your body which is examining and palpating a patient do exactly what your patient's body is doing, and would otherwise be doing even if you weren't there. We know it is impossible to be totally non-intrusive, but try. With gentle palpatory contact, after a short time the patient's body seems to relax and behave as though you were not touching it. You must be as passive as possible. Allow your palpating hand, arm or other part of your body to become synchronized with the patient's body. Make the boundary between yourself and the patient somewhere deeper in your body. For example, if you are palpating with the whole palmar surface of your hand on the patient's upper abdomen, rest your hand on the examination site very lightly. Soon your hand will begin moving with the patient's body. Now shift the line of demarcation between you and the patient to your wrist or your forearm. As this transition occurs, you have proprioceptors giving you information from your hand, wrist and forearm which seem to be located within the patient's body.

If you work with your eyes closed in a quiet state of concentration, there is a good chance that your hand will begin to sense the movement of peristalsis within the patient's upper digestive tract. It will receive information regarding the degree of pylorospasm present. Gall bladder and biliary duct system activity will become apparent, as will many other physiological phenomena which are occuring under your hand. The key to success in using this type of palpation is your quiet, non-intrusive melding with the patient.

There is one other requirement which should be mentioned. You must accept as real the information which your sensory receptors give you. As a beginner, accept what seems to be without critical evaluation. After you develop the palpatory skill to some degree, you will have plenty of time to critically appraise the information which comes into your brain through your senses.

TREATMENT TECHNIQUES

The techniques used in craniosacral therapy are usually non-intrusive and indirect. In certain situations you may resort to direct treatment techniques applied against resistance barriers, but only after the patient's body has demonstrated the need for the direct approach.

An *indirect technique,* as we define it, is one that releases a restriction or abnormal barrier to motion by encouraging motion in the direction of ease (which is usually opposite to the direction of the restriction). This is sort of an "unlatching" principle. Often, in order to open a latch we must first exaggerate the closure. The same is true of indirect cranial technique. The therapist follows the restricted structure to its limit in the direction toward which it moves with ease, i.e., the direction toward which it exhibits the greatest range of inherent motion. When the structure attempts to return from this extreme position, the therapist becomes immovable. You do *not* push against the structure or attempt to extend the limit of its easy range of motion. Rather, you simply refuse to move. It is the inherent motion of the structure as it attempts to return to neutral that pushes against you. As the inherent motion of the structure stops pushing against you it will travel farther in the direction of the easy range of motion, often called the "direction of ease." As this movement away from you occurs, follow it, take up the slack but without pushing. At the end of a cycle the motion will again move against you. Once more, the therapist becomes immovable. Repeat this procedure through several more cycles of inherent craniosacral motion. Ultimately, a tissue softening or release will occur. This is the therapeutic effect for which you have been waiting. The tissue has "unlatched" itself. Follow a few cycles and re-evaluate for ease of motion and symmetry.

As you perform this therapy, the pathways of motion may change. Our rule is to allow the structure to move along any new pathway it desires. Do not let it return toward neutral along the same pathway from whence it came. This procedure is what we mean by the indirect technique.

Direct technique is essentially the opposite of indirect technique. Once a barrier to normal physiological motion is identified, the therapist gently assists the restricted structure or membrane to pass through and thus break the abnormal restriction barrier.

In *motion testing,* which is a primary method used in the search for abnormal restriction barriers, the therapist induces the motion; as soon as the structure begins to move in the direction of urging, the therapist reverts to the role of passive monitor. The purpose is to see how far and with what degree of ease or restriction the structure moves in response to inducement. The purpose is *not* to see how far and through how many barriers the structure can be pushed. In the process of pushing you may never find the true underlying problem, which may be compounded by causing further injury or restriction barriers to develop.

We speak of the restoration of *autonomic flexibility* as a positive therapeutic effect of craniosacral therapy. Autonomic flexibility is a term used to describe an improvement in the ability of the autonomic nervous system to respond effectively to stress and challenge.

The autonomic nervous system maintains the vital functions and helps one survive without the need of conscious thought. It has two major divisions: the *sympathetic* and the *parasympathetic.* The sympathetic division causes the body to respond to danger, adversity, stress, anger and ecstacy by increasing heart rate, blood pressure, air exchange volume, blood flow to muscles and all the other things which are needed to spring into action. The parasympathetic division monitors body functions during times of rest, sleep, food digestion, elimination, etc., when the body is not ready to spring into action.

As stressful situations occur in daily life, the sympathetic system is activated over and over again. Frequently, it cannot discharge the accumulated stress because modern society does not allow sufficient opportunity for the body to spring into action so as to dissipate the energy generated by a stimulated sympathetic nervous system. Therefore, the level of tone or tonic activity of the sympathetic system increases day by day as we accumulate more energy from stressful stimuli than is dissipated. This increase in sympathetic nervous system tonus causes the heart to speed up, the blood pressure to rise, the stomach to tighten, the bowels to move toward spasticity and the blood flow to be diverted from vital organs to muscle. Left in this condition, the body would not survive very well. In order to counteract the condition of readiness for "fight or flight" instituted by the sympathetic hypertonus, the parasympathetic nervous system has to act more powerfully to slow the heart rate, lower the blood pressure, aid the digestive processes and reduce the spasticity of the bowels.

The stress stimuli keep coming in. The balance sheet shows more stress stimuli being received than are dissipated, so the sympathetic tonus continues to rise. The parasympathetic tonus must also rise in order to counteract the sympathetic system's effect. Finally, a point is reached at which the parasympathetic nervous system can no longer cope with nor effectively counteract the increased energy in the sympathetic system. The blood pressure rises, the heart rate increases, and one may develop spastic colitis and peptic ulcer or any number of other dysfunctions. We call these functional diseases. The autonomic nervous system has lost its flexibility. It can no longer deal effectively with the accumulated stressful energy within the sympathetic nervous system. The parasympathetic system has topped out.

A beneficial effect of many of the therapeutic techniques described in this book is the restoration of autonomic flexibility. Because the autonomic nervous system plays a large role in the homeostatic activity of the body, when autonomic flexibility is restored many homeostatic mechanisms are made more effective.

There are a number of other words and phrases which it may be useful to define here so that we can avoid misunderstanding later in the text.

Fascial continuity is a phrase which indicates that the human body fascia is continuous from the top of the head to the bottoms of the feet. We regard the total body fascia as laminated, with pockets, invaginations and tubes for the various organs and structures. It is largely oriented in a longitudinal direction and is free to glide on the order of millimeters when the body musculature is relaxed. You can travel from any part of the body to any other part via the fascia.

The term *cross-restricting diaphragms* suggests the conceptual framework in which we place these structures. We regard these diaphragms as transverse support systems for the longitudinally oriented fascial lamina. They are an integral part of the system and are essential to its functional integrity. Cross-restricting diaphragms represent areas of increased stress within the body fascial system; they are therefore frequent sites of fascial system dysfunction.

The term *neuromusculoskeletal system* is meant to indicate that any division between the nervous system, the muscle system and the skeletal system from a functional point of view is artificial. Therefore, we use the word neuromusculoskeletal to express the functional integration of these systems.

A *lesion* is an area of localized diseased or dysfunctional tissue. An *osteopathic lesion* is the term used to designate palpable paraspinal areas of tissue texture deviation toward either tightness or swollen bogginess. It implies a syndrome of dysfunction which includes vascular abnormality, muscular hypertonus, tenderness to palpation, spinal cord segmental facilitation, visceral dysfunction and autonomic dysfunction, all somewhat localized at the area of osteopathic lesion.

Somatic dysfunction is a term adopted by some of the osteopathic profession to replace osteopathic lesion. Proponents of the term somatic dysfunction believe it is more scientifically acceptable than "osteopathic lesion." Opponents argue that the osteopathic lesion complex or syndrome is much more than a somatic or body (meaning musculoskeletal) dysfunction.

The *internal milieu* is the environment inside the skin of the body, within which all of your molecules, cells and organs function. It includes everything from interstitial fluid viscosity to hydrogen ion concentration in the urine. It also includes physical parameters such as pressure, as within the cranial vault, and temperature.

In our discussion of brain dysfunctions we refer to several conditions which are discussed below:

Autism is a condition of unknown etiology. The autistic child is unsociable, preferring to interact with non-living things in the environment. The child is frequently self-abusing and will bite its hand and wrist or bang its head, etc. Autistic children seldom display emotion other than during destructive temper episodes. They usually will not make eye contact or display affection to other people, although we have befriended many autistic children. They often have seizure problems. They are of variable intelligence, and often display excellent motor coordination. Since the cause of autism is unknown, there is much disagreement about the diagnosis.

Hyperkinetic children are those with short attention spans, an inability to sit still, and who have been labeled as such by the "system." Our inclination was to regard this as a convenient diagnosis attached to difficult-to-handle children. However, as we describe in Chapter 15, many of these children have responded dramatically to craniosacral therapy. The suggestion from our experience is that the behavioral syndrome called hyperkinesis should be further subdivided into hyperkinesis due to craniosacral system dysfunction, hyperkinesis due to food and chemical intolerances, and hyperkinesis due to emotional and psychosocial causes.

Learning disabilities might be considered similarly to the description of hyperkinesis above. We have found a significant number of learning disabled children who have favorably responded to craniosacral therapy alone.

There are also several anatomical terms we have used which may require brief definition (ILLUSTRATION 2-3):

Anterior—toward the front of the body.
Posterior—toward the back of the body.
Cephalad—toward the head end of the body.
Caudad—toward the tail end of the body.
Pedad—toward the feet.
Lateral—toward the side of the body.
Medial—toward the center of the body.
Superior—above.
Inferior—below.

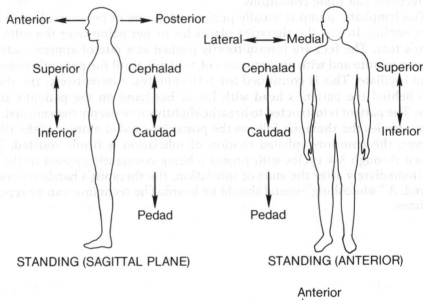

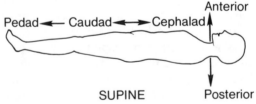

Illustration 2-3
Anatomical Directions

The following places on the skull are given special names:

Asterion—junction of the temporal, parietal, and occipital bones.
Bregma—junction of the coronal and sagittal sutures.
Inion—external occipital protuberance.
Lamda—junction of the occipitoparietal and sagittal sutures.
Pterion—junction of the frontal, parietal, sphenoid, and temporal bones.

Viscera—an organ which is not a muscle or bone. The liver, heart, lungs, etc., are viscera.

Adnexa—the connective tissues intimately related to a viscera.

Thenar eminence—the thick, fatty, muscular part of the palm of the hand on the thumb side. The hypothenar eminence is on the side of the fifth finger.

Internal rotation—the inward rotation of the extremities. E.g., the feet pigeon-toe inward, etc.

External rotation—the opposite of internal rotation.

Lymphatic pump—any treatment technique which assists the movement of lymphatic fluid through the body. The rationale for the use of the lymphatic pump technique is to enhance the removal of toxic waste substances from the body, and to improve the circulation of antibodies. This technique is recommended as treatment for infections and toxic conditions.

The lymphatic pump is usually performed in one of two ways, both with the patient supine. In one the therapist places his or her palms over the soles of the patient's feet. The feet are intermittently pushed at a rate of approximately 180 times per minute and with an excursion of 5-10 cm. until the patient's abdomen is seen to oscillate. This is continued for 5-10 minutes. Alternatively, the therapist stands behind the patient's head with his or her hand on the patient's anterior thorax. The patient is instructed to breathe slightly more deeply than normal. As the patient exhales the therapist follows the posterior-caudad motion of the rib cage. However, the anterior-cephalad motion of inhalation is firmly resisted. This is repeated through 3-4 cycles with pressure being constantly applied to the chest. Then immediately after the start of inhalation, the therapist's hands are suddenly removed. A "whooshing" sound should be heard. The technique can be repeated 2 or 3 times.

Chapter 3
Craniosacral Motion: Palpatory Skills

Most of you have spent years studying the sciences and have learned to rely heavily upon your rational, reasoning mind. You probably have been convinced that the information which your hands can give you is unreliable. You may consider facts to be reliable only when they are printed on a computer sheet, projected on a screen or read from the indicator of an electronic device. In order to use your hands and begin to develop them as reliable instruments for diagnosis and treatment, you must learn to trust them and the information they can give you.

Learning to trust your hands is not an easy task. You must learn to shut off your conscious, critical mind while you palpate for subtle changes in the body you are examining. You must adopt an empirical attitude so that you may temporarily accept *without question* those perceptions which come into your brain from your hands. Although this attitude is unpalatable to most scientists, it is recommended that you give it a short trial. After you have developed your palpatory skill, you can criticize what you have felt with your hands. If you criticize before you learn to palpate, you will never learn to use your hands effectively as the highly sensitive diagnostic and therapeutic instruments which, in fact, they are.

Recently, brain function has been conveniently divided into left and right hemispheric activities. This division may be simplistic, but is useful for the purpose of developing a conceptual model upon which we can base an understandable explanation.

Consider the left side of your brain as being the rational, thinking and critical side; the right side, the creative, fantasizing, imaginative and intuitive side. The educational process to which we have all been subjected, especially in the sciences, has supported the development of the left side of the brain. The right side of the brain has been neglected except in art, music and other creative activities. Often, creative studies are regarded as being of less value than the sciences. As a result, the left side of the brain has grown to be hyper-critical, self-centered, omniscient, intimidating and almost autonomous. On the other hand, the right brain hemisphere is quiet, retiring, shy, fearful and perhaps immature. This untapped right hemisphere may carry a wealth of intuitive insight which has been largely untapped, because when an idea begins to emerge from the right side of the brain into the consciousness, the left side of the brain immediately begins to tell you why that idea is silly and irrational.

In order to develop the palpatory skills and to begin to perceive the physiological motions of the craniosacral system, it is necessary to shut off the input from your left brain for a while. Allow the skills to develop without listening to the message from your left brain consciousness which insists that what you are feeling isn't really there, that it is your imagination. Ignore this criticism. Let your right brain have a chance to develop and gain confidence. The talents and information which are suppressed in your right brain may astound you. Your right brain has probably been intimidated for so long that it has become extremely shy. Therefore, the first right brain messages which you consciously perceive may be very weak, tentative and fleeting. Nurture them, draw them out, be kind and gentle with your intuition. It will develop quickly if it is given a chance. Once you have followed your perceptions and sensations for a while, as an empiricist rather than a scientist, and after your palpatory skills and right brain have gained in development and confidence, you will have plenty of time to critically consider the information gathered from your senses. We do not mean to suggest that you totally arrest the activity of your left hemisphere. Rather, we want to give it a rest so that the remainder of you has a chance to develop.

Therefore, we make this plea in the beginning: *accept what you sense as real.* Do not rationally try to understand it. Give yourself a chance to learn. The risk when playing the game of "I trust my hands" is minimal to the loser. The potential payoff for those who succeed is great, much greater than you can perhaps imagine right now. Remember that the potential of humankind is limited only by its own concept of that limitation. Relax and let it happen.

We usually begin training people to palpate the craniosacral rhythm by starting with the more obvious motions of the human body. One of these motions with which you should already be familiar is the cardiovascular pulse. Take your time. Be comfortable. If you are not comfortable, the stimulus input from your own tense muscles and discomforts will create an input noise level which will interfere with your perception.

With the subject lying comfortably supine, palpate the radial pulses. Feel the obvious peak of the pulsation. Tune in also to the rise and fall of the pressure gradient. How long is diastole? What is the quality of the rise of pulse pressure after diastole? Is it sharp, gradual, smooth? How broad is the pressure peak? Is the pressure descent rapid, gradual, smooth or stepped? Memorize the feel of the subject's pulse so that you can reproduce it in your mind after you have broken actual physical contact with the subject's body. You can often sing a song after you have heard it a few times; similarly, you should be able to mentally reproduce your palpatory perception of the pulse after you have broken contact.

Now palpate the carotid pulse wave of the subject. Commit its characteristics to memory just as you did the radial pulse. Compare the memory of the radial pulse wave morphology with that of the carotid pulse wave morphology.

Now palpate both radial and carotid pulse waves simultaneously. Compare them. Are the sloping rises similar? Are the peaks the same? You are now learning to compare the characteristics of one pulse with another. If you are aware of subtle differences, don't worry about why or why not those differences exist. For the time being they exist.

Try to remember the characteristics of the pulses of your subject. Then

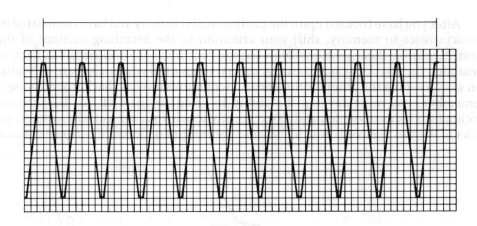

Illustration 3-1
Diagrammatic Representation of Pulse Wave
Morphology: Cardiac, Respiratory or Craniosacral

compare them with another subject's pulses. It sometimes helps to draw a graphic representation of the pulse wave morphology to begin to make the connection between palpation and visualization of what you feel (ILLUSTRATION 3-1). In the beginning, you may be more comfortable at visualizing than you are at palpating, because you have been trained this way. Your palpatory perception may seem too intangible to be trusted.

After you have concentrated upon the body pulses at the radial and carotid regions, simply lay your hands over the thorax of the subject and palpate the cardiovascular activity (ILLUSTRATION 3-2).

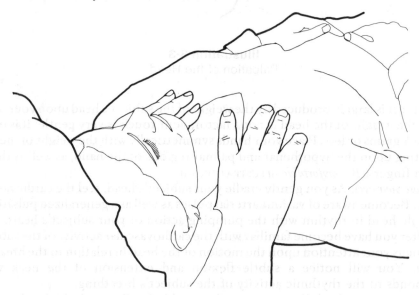

Illustration 3-2
Palpation of Thorax

After you have focused upon the cardiovascular activity and have committed its characteristics to memory, shift your attention to the breathing motions of the chest. Memorize those motions. Now change your focus to cardiovascular, back to breathing, then back to cardiovascular several times until you can palpate only what you wish, keeping the other motions at an unconscious level as "background noise." Remember, you must develop the ability to bring any part of that background motion into focus upon demand. Next, gently touch your subject's head (ILLUSTRATION 3-3). We use the word "touch" because the amount of pressure between you and

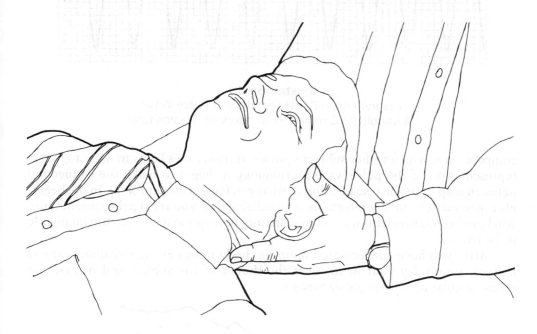

Illustration 3-3
Palpation of the Head

your subject is largely produced by the weight of the subject's head upon your hands. Where the weight of the head is not a factor, your touch is very gentle: it is on the order of 5 grams or less. Place your hands symmetrically with the weight of the occiput resting upon the hypothenar and palmar regions of the hand, as well as the 4th and 5th fingers. *Be comfortable* (ILLUSTRATION 3-4).

Close your eyes. As you gently cradle your subject's head, feel the cardiovascular activity. Become aware of various arterial pulses as well as a generalized pulsation of the whole head in rhythm with the pumping action of your subject's heart.

After you have become familiar with the cardiovascular activity of the subject's head, focus your attention upon the motion of the head in relation to the breathing activity. You will notice a subtle flexion and extension of the neck which corresponds to the rhythmic activity of the subject's breathing.

Keep your eyes closed. Once you are thoroughly familiar with the head motions corresponding to the subject's cardiovascular and breathing activities, discard them both from your conscious awareness. Become aware of other motions which were

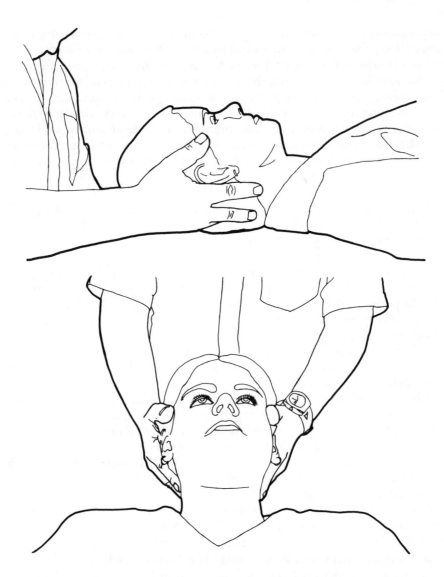

Illustration 3-4
Position of Your Hands When Palpating
Craniosacral Motion at the Occiput

unknown to you. Let your hands move with your subject's head as though the hands and the head are welded or soldered together. Use your whole hand to palpate, not just the fingers. Feel what your hands are doing by becoming aware of the messages from the proprioceptors in your arms. As you continue this melding together of your hands with your subject's head *with your eyes closed,* it will begin to seem as though your hands are making larger and larger motions. Open your eyes and you will see that your hands are hardly moving at all, according to your visual perception. When this happens, you are beginning to magnify your palpatory and proprioceptive senses.

As you continue your exploration into the realm of palpatory input, you will become aware that the subject's head begins to broaden and narrow slowly and rhythmically, about 6 to 12 cycles per minute. As the occiput broadens, its base seems to move anteriorly, arcing about a transverse axis of motion approximately 2 inches anterior to inion, the posterior occipital protuberance. This broadening motion, as it arcs anteriorly, is the flexion phase of the motion cycle of the craniosacral system. After the occiput ends the flexion phase of motion and returns to a neutral, relaxed position for an instant, it begins to move into the extension phase of the craniosacral system motion cycle. This feels like a narrowing of the transverse dimension of the occiput, with an arcing motion the reverse of that perceived in flexion.

With your hands in the same position, you can palpate some of the temporal mastoid regions and some of the posterior regions of the parietal bones. During the extension phase of craniosacral motion, the transverse dimension of these bones narrows somewhat.

Additionally, you can now begin to notice the symmetry of the flexion and extension motion phases as they proceed through their cycles. The ideal condition is one of perfectly symmetrical motion. This perfect symmetry is seldom found unless the subject has been successfully treated using craniosacral techniques prior to your examination.

You should also become aware that the occiput, the temporals and the parietals are moving independently of each other. The suture is the structure that allows for this independent motion.

Allow your hands to remain in place for a few minutes. Keep your eyes closed and remain relaxed. Let your imagination run wild. You have probably been taught that the kinds of motions you are feeling do not exist; or if they did exist, they would be impossible to perceive with instruments as crude as the human hands.

If this is the case, what are you feeling? Is it really your imagination? There is plenty of time to decide that later. First, give your senses a chance to develop and gain confidence. It will happen very quickly.

After you have palpated (or imagined that you have palpated) the subtle and gentle motions of the craniosacral system on this subject, examine other subjects. Repeat the procedures. Learn to distinguish among the various physiological motions in one subject, and then among those in other subjects.

As you gain experience, you will begin to note individual differences from person to person; your brain will begin to store information about norms of perceived physiological motions.

Once you have successfully experienced the palpatory perceptions created by focusing upon the cardiovascular motions, the breathing motions and the motions of the craniosacral system on one or more subjects, the question of whether you are feeling the subject's physiological motions or your own arises. In order to answer this question, you must practice upon yourself and become thoroughly familiar with the "feel" of your own body rhythms.

Sit down. Touch your head lightly with your hands. Become aware of the cardiovascular, breathing, and craniosacral systems' physiological motions in your own head. Familiarize yourself with these motions. Once you know your own motions, you will not be confused about which palpatory sensations are coming from the patient and which are coming from your own body. If you spend time

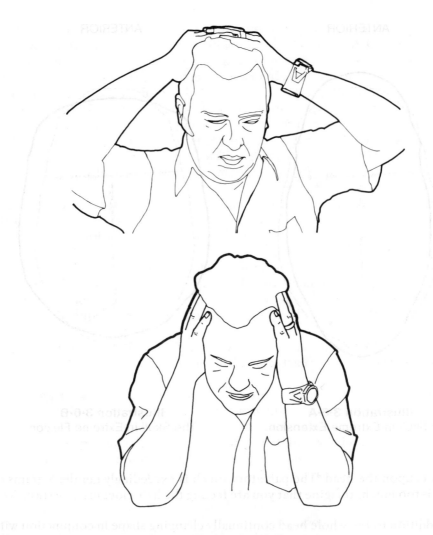

Illustration 3-5
Position of Hands for Self-Examination

doing, you will gain the experience necessary to enable you to palpate with confidence (ILLUSTRATION 3-5).

After you are comfortable and confident that you have experienced cardio-vascular, breathing and craniosacral system motion on several subjects' heads, and after you are able to shift your focus from one physiological motion to another, you are ready to move to other parts of the head and body.

It was indicated above that the flexion phase of craniosacral motion is, in general, a broadening of the posterior portions of the head. The extension phase is a slight narrowing. When describing the head as a whole, flexion seems to be a transverse widening of the whole head as it shortens in its anterior-posterior dimension. Extension is just the opposite, i.e., a transverse narrowing accompanied by an anterior-posterior lengthening. These changes can be palpated by various hand

ANTERIOR ANTERIOR

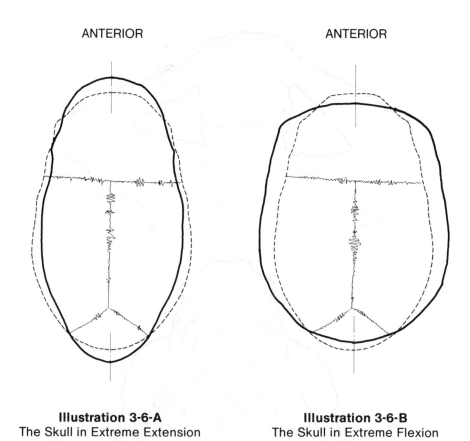

Illustration 3-6-A
The Skull in Extreme Extension

Illustration 3-6-B
The Skull in Extreme Flexion

placements upon the head. The palpatory touch is exceedingly gentle: 5 grams of pressure is too much. Imagine that you are feeling the hair move (ILLUSTRATIONS 3-6-A and 3-6-B).

In addition to the whole head continually changing shape in conjunction with the rhythmic movement of the craniosacral system, the whole body also moves physiologically and involuntarily in conjunction with the craniosacral rhythm.

During the flexion phase of craniosacral motion, the whole body seems to externally rotate slightly and widen. During the extension phase, the body seems to internally rotate and narrow slightly. These motions can be palpated easily at the feet and ankles, thighs, pelvis, thorax, arms, neck and other parts of the body. The key to the discovery of this type of body motion is in the gentleness of your touch. If your contact with the subject's body elicits any tissue-guarding response, you will inhibit the very motion which you are trying to perceive. If you, the examiner, are not relaxed and comfortable, *your own tension will inhibit your ability to perceive.*

Rest your hands gently upon the subject's body. Meld your hands with that body, and perceive proprioceptively the movements of your own hands.

The next area of craniosacral system motion with which you should become familiar is the sacrum, which is attached to the caudal end of the dural tube.

In order to palpate sacral motion, the sacrum sits in your hand so that the subject's sacral apex rests in the palm of your hand. The sacral spine should lie

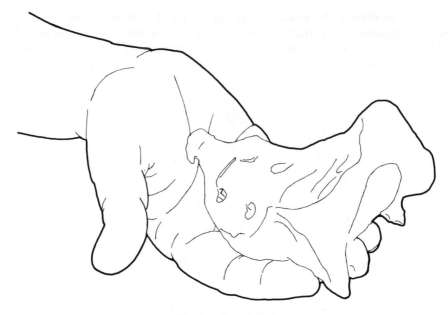

Illustration 3-7-A
Palpation of Sacrum

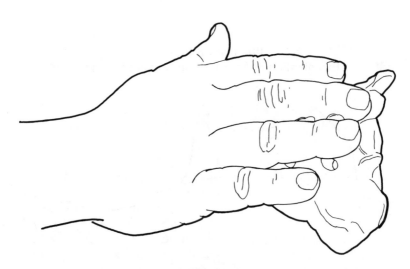

Illustration 3-7-B
Sacral Spines Between Third and Fourth Fingers

between your third and fourth fingers. Your fingertips will usually extend cephalad beyond the subject's sacral base to the level of the 4th or 5th lumbar vertebrae (ILLUSTRATIONS 3-7-A and 3-7-B).

As the craniosacral system moves into the flexion phase of its motion, the sacral apex moves anteriorly. During the extension phase, the sacral apex moves posteriorly. These motions are subtle and may be in perfect synchrony with the craniosacral motion of the head or may lag a second or two, depending upon the quality and quantity of restrictions which may be affecting free sacral mobility.

The subject can be in either the supine, lateral recumbent or prone position for examination of sacral motion (ILLUSTRATIONS 3-8-A, 3-8-B and 3-8-C). In learning to palpate

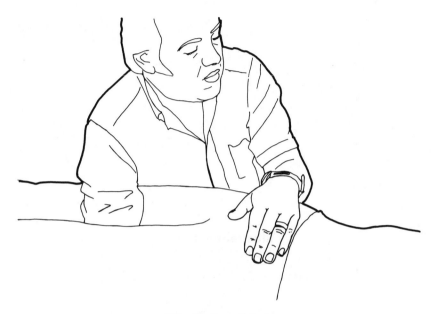

Illustration 3-8-A
Examination of Sacrum with Subject Supine

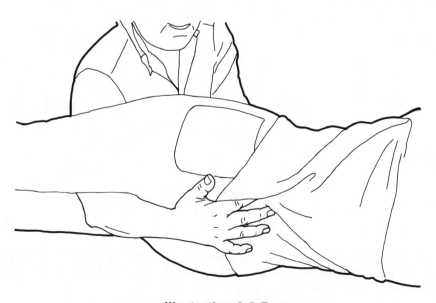

Illustration 3-8-B
Examination of Sacrum with Subject
in Lateral Recumbent Position

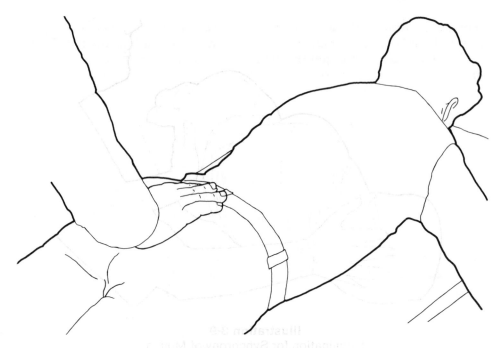

Illustration 3-8-C
Examination of Sacrum with Subject Prone

sacral motion, you should practice all three subject positions and develop a facility with their uses. Usually, novice examiners complain of numbness of the hand under the sacrum when the subject is supine. However, this pressure paresthesia does not reduce proprioception; as a matter of fact, it enhances proprioceptive sensitivity somewhat by removing tactile noise. When the sacrum of the subject is supine on your hand, lean heavily upon your elbow, close your eyes and let your hand meld with the sacrum. Feel what your hand is doing.

Another helpful technique for developing familiarity with sacral motion is to palpate for the synchrony of motion between the sacrum and the occiput. This can be done by having one examiner palpate the occiput, while another palpates the sacrum, each examiner indicating verbally to the other when flexion and extension phases begin and end. It can also be achieved by placing one of your hands on the sacrum and the other hand on the occiput of the subject so that you can monitor flexion and extension motions at both ends of the dural tube simultaneously.

Simultaneous palpation of the sacrum and occiput by one examiner can be easily performed with the patient in the lateral recumbent position (ILLUSTRATION 3-9). In this position, the patient must have a proper pillow beneath the head so that the neck is not crimped to one side. Crimping or sidebending of the neck may interfere with the synchrony of movement between the occiput and sacrum. This interference can be demonstrated by having the subject severely sidebend the head as you palpate the craniosacral motions at the occiput and sacrum.

With some experience, using living bodies as learning aids, you will begin to notice significant differences in range of motion, symmetry of motion and energy

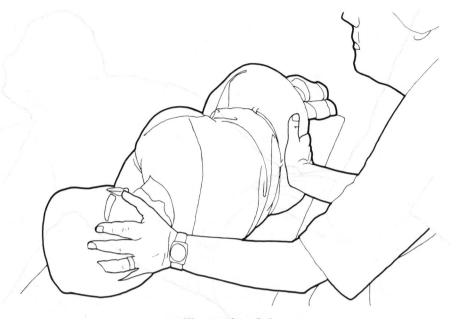

Illustration 3-9
Examination for Synchrony of Motion
Between Occiput and Sacrum

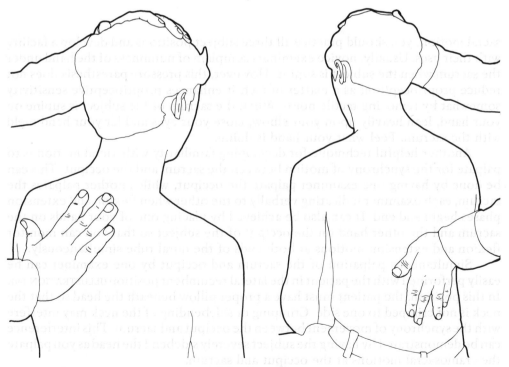

Illustration 3-10
Palpation of Paravertebral Musculature

which drives the motion from one subject to another. Collect this data in your brain's memory stores. Store information about what is normal so that you will become aware of variations from the norm. Ultimately, these variations will take on diagnostic and pathophysiologic meaning.

The paravertebral musculature is another area of palpation which can be diagnostically useful (ILLUSTRATION 3-10). With the subject sitting or lying prone, palpate the craniosacral motion in the paravertebral regions from the occiput to the sacrum. Keep the spinous processes between your fingers. Changes in craniosacral rhythm of the paravertebral regions can be used diagnostically to locate nerve root impingement and spinal cord lesion. Denervated muscle presents a physiological motion between 20 and 30 cycles per minute (APPENDIX B). This information can be used in the differential diagnosis between the pain of somatic dysfunction and nerve root compression.

As with any skill, the development of palpatory sensitivity requires practice. The experience gathered from practice time where small groups of practitioners work together with a non-critical approach is the most productive.

To reiterate, do not let your intellect obstruct the development of your palpatory skills. Develop familiarity with this extended use of your hands. After you know on a "gut level" what your hands can do, you will then have plenty of time to be intellectually critical. Give your "right brain" a chance to demonstrate its ability without having your "left brain" continually harping about "What is this?" or "Is this possible?" *Learn by doing.*

Chapter 4
Techniques for Modification of Craniosacral Rhythm

Thus far you have palpated physiological motions and rhythms, being careful not to interfere with their normal activities. Your purpose has been to study and learn from the body in its natural resting, yet dynamic state. You have learned that the practiced touch of the examiner (perhaps better named the "discoverer") should offer only security to the subject. There should be no threat to which the subject's body might respond by guarding, either consciously or unconsciously.

Now you should become familiar with and experience the use of techniques which will modify craniosacral system rhythmic activity. Your purposes are discovery, diagnosis, treatment and prognosis.

Compared with the palpation you have learned thus far, the techniques which modify craniosacral motion may seem rather invasive. However, compared with the manipulative techniques ordinarily used by physicians and therapists, these techniques are still exceedingly gentle. We coax the craniosacral system; we do *not* brutalize it, shock it, or even scare it. Approach it as you would a timid child or an animal whose trust you wish to gain. Do not force the craniosacral system to make non-physiological motions. Rather, the goal is simply to prevent it from returning from extreme positions along its usual pathway, and to encourage it to find a new route. Such coaxed discovery of new routes will introduce added mobility into the system and its library of motions.

One of the easiest ways to learn about the gentle modification of craniosacral system motion begins with the feet. As you cradle the heels in your hands, "tune in" to the external rotation (the flexion phase of craniosacral motion), the return to neutral, the excursion into internal rotation (craniosacral extension) and so on, as the rhythm repeats itself (ILLUSTRATION 4-1).

As you discover this motion, answer these questions. Does the motion seem symmetrical? Do the feet rotate externally or internally with more facility? As an example, assume that the left foot rotates externally further than the right, and that neither foot rotates internally as easily or as far as it does externally. In order to change this less-than-perfect situation, follow each foot to the extreme range of motion to which it moves with the greatest ease. In our example, this would mean that you follow both feet into external rotation. When each foot has moved as far into external rotation as it will go (in this case, the left foot rotates externally further

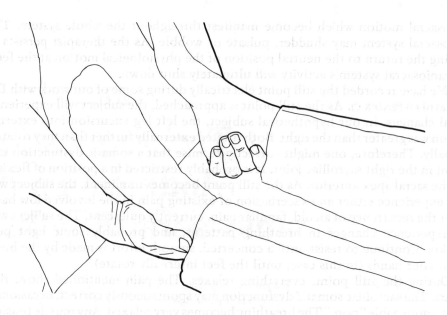

Illustration 4-1
Palpating Craniosacral Rhythm at the Feet

than the right), resist the return to neutral by making your hands immovable. Do not push further into external rotation; simply resist the return to neutral by the feet from their extreme positions of external rotation.

As the return to neutral is resisted or prevented by applying gentle force at the subject's feet, another examiner monitoring the head will feel a subtle resistance to the cranial bones' attempted return to neutral, and thence into the extension phase of craniosacral motion. *The return to neutral and the move into extension will occur on the head, but with less facility.* This perceptible change at the head is due to the resistance you have caused by manipulating the subject's feet. As the craniosacral system again returns to its flexion phase, you will notice further movement into external rotation at either one or both feet.

Follow this external rotation closely. Carefully take up the slack, just as you would keep a fishing line slightly taut when reeling in a fish, or as you would keep the front bumper of your automobile snug against the rear bumper of a car you are pushing. When the external rotation reaches the limit of its new range of motion and attempts to return to a neutral position, the hands of the therapist again become immovable. The rest of the craniosacral system will reluctantly return to neutral. Then, against the new and increased resistance, it will proceed into its extension phase. This occurrence can be witnessed by an examiner monitoring the activity at the subject's head.

Each time the feet rotate externally a little further, carefully take up the slack and resist internal rotation. After some repetition (the number will differ, usually between 5 and 20), the total craniosacral system motion will "shut down," i.e., become perfectly still. This is called the *still point.*

The still point has been induced by the therapist's resistance to the physiological motion at the subject's feet. It is usually heralded by gross irregularities of the craniosacral motion which become manifest throughout the whole system. The craniosacral system may shudder, pulsate or wobble. As the therapist persists in resisting the return to the neutral position of the physiological motion at the feet, the craniosacral system's activity will ultimately shut down.

We have recorded the still point electrically during some of our work with Dr. Zvi Karni (APPENDIX C). As the still point is approached, the subject will experience several changes. In our hypothetical subject, the left leg excursion into external rotation was greater than the right. Both rotated externally further than they rotated internally. Therefore, one might correctly surmise that a somatic dysfunction was present in the right sacroiliac joint. It is probably restricted in a position of flexion with the sacral apex anterior. As the still point becomes imminent, the subject will likely experience either an exacerbation of existing pain in the involved low back area or the recurrence of an old, familiar pain, currently quiescent. The subject will also experience changes in breathing patterns, and probably some light perspiration. Continue to resist until a concerted, smooth effort is made by the body against your hands (in this case, until the feet internally rotate).

During the still point, everything relaxes. The pain mentioned above disappears. The sacroiliac somatic dysfunction may spontaneously correct, occasionally with a noticeable "pop." The breathing becomes very relaxed. Any muscle tension seems to melt away.

The still point may last a few seconds to a few minutes. When it is over, the craniosacral system will resume its motion, usually with a better symmetry and a larger amplitude.

After you have induced the still point, you should only monitor. Notice changes in the quality and range of motion at the feet. If the excursions into internal and external rotations are now restored to equality, and left-right symmetry of motion is improved, nothing further is required. If, in your judgment, the motion is not satisfactory, you may repeat the procedure to another still point. Each repetition will bring the abnormality closer to the norm and benefit the patient.

We have never done more than ten still point repetitions during the same treatment session. However we know of no side-effect, other than extreme relaxation and sleepiness, which will occur. *The still point is contraindicated in cases of intracranial hemorrhage and aneurysm, where changes in intracranial fluid pressure might prove detrimental to the patient.*

With practice, the technique described for induction of a still point using the feet can be applied anywhere on the body. It is a question of determining the direction of greatest ease and range of physiological craniosacral motion. Follow this motion to its physiological end point, and resist its return. Take up the slack with each ensuing cycle until a still point of craniosacral system function is reached. After the still point is ended and improved craniosacral system activity is resumed, the therapist monitors and evaluates the new physiological motion patterns.

The still point is most often induced from the head and sacrum. Techniques applied to these anatomical parts are usually somewhat more rapidly effective than when applied to other parts of the body. The goal is simply to modify the activity of the craniosacral system.

THE CV-4 TECHNIQUE

The still point achieved by application of the technique to the subject's occiput is traditionally called a "CV-4" technique. CV-4 means compression of the 4th ventricle. In this case, 4th ventricle refers to the ventricle of the brain. Dr. Sutherland, the originator of this technique (SUTHERLAND 1939), believed that he was compressing the 4th ventricle of the brain and thus affecting all of the vital nerve centers located in and about the walls of this ventricle (ILLUSTRATION 4-2).

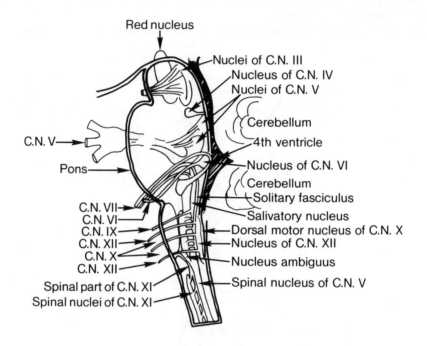

Illustration 4-2
4th Ventricle and Related Structures

The occipital squama provide an accommodation to changing intracranial fluid pressures. The CV-4 technique significantly reduces the ability of these squama to accommodate. The intracranial hydraulic fluid pressure is therefore increased and redirected along all other available pathways when the motion of the occipital squama is extrinsically restricted. Thus, the CV-4 technique promotes fluid movement and hence, exchange. The enhancement of fluid movement is always beneficial except in cases of intracranial hemorrhage when clot formation is enhanced by stasis, and in cases of cerebral aneurysm where changing intracranial pressures could produce leaking or rupture.

The CV-4 technique affects diaphragm activity and autonomic control of respiration, and seems to relax the sympathetic nervous system tonus to a significant degree. I have often used this technique to reduce chronic sympathetic hypertonus in stressed patients. Autonomic functional improvement is *always expected* as a result of still point induction.

Clinically, this technique is beneficial in cases where a lymphatic pump technique is indicated (MAGOUN 1978). It has significantly lowered fever by as much as 4°F in

30-60 minutes. It relaxes all connective tissues of the body and therefore benefits acute and chronic musculoskeletal lesions. It is effective in degenerative arthritic processes, in both cerebral and pulmonary congestion, in regulating labor and as a means of reducing dependent edema.

The CV-4 technique is, quite simply, an excellent "shotgun" technique for a multitude of problems in that it enhances tissue and fluid motion and restores flexibility of autonomic response.

As the therapist, cup your hands so that the thumbs make a "V" (ILLUSTRATION 4-3).

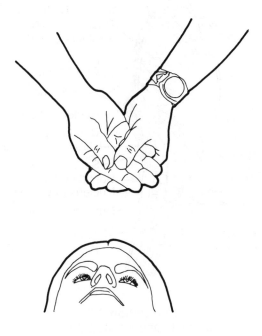

Illustration 4-3
Hand Position for Occipital CV-4

The apex of the "V," formed by the thumbs, should be level with the spines of the second or third cervical vertebra. The thenar eminences are applied to the occipital squama medial to, and *totally avoiding* the occipitomastoid sutures (ILLUSTRATIONS 4-4-A and 4-4-B). As the subject's occiput narrows in the extension phase of the craniosacral system cycle, this movement is followed by the thenar eminences. As the subject's occiput attempts to widen during the flexion phase of the cranial cycle, you should resist this widening. *Your hands become immovable. You do not squeeze.* As extension phase narrowing of the subject's occiput recurs, take up the slack by following the narrowing of the subject's occiput. The occipital broadening of the flexion phase of craniosacral system motion is again resisted. This procedure is repeated until the cranial rhythm becomes reduced and disorganized, then ultimately stops, temporarily but completely.

When this stop occurs in the cranial rhythm, the still point has been induced. The still point will continue for a variable number of seconds or minutes. The subject's respiration will change, and light perspiration will often appear on the forehead. A noticeable relaxation of the body will occur.

Within a few minutes, you will notice that the subject's occiput once again attempts to broaden into the flexion phase of the craniosacral system's rhythmic cycle. When you feel a concerted strong motion bilaterally, stop your resistance. Follow this broadening and evaluate for amplitude and symmetry of craniosacral motion.

A still point can also be induced anywhere on the subject's head by applying the same principles of following the motion to its extreme extension and resisting the return to neutral until the rhythmic activity temporarily ceases.

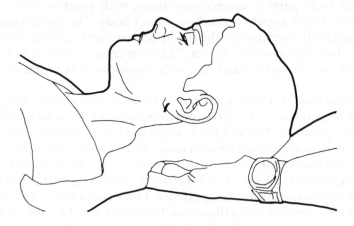

Illustration 4-4-A
CV-4 Hand Position

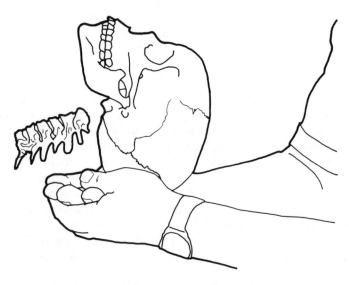

Illustration 4-4-B
CV-4 Relationship to Bony Structures

SACRAL STILL POINT INDUCTION

When inducing a still point through the sacrum, the therapist's hand is applied to the sacrum. Follow the sacral motion into either the flexion or extension phase, whichever seems to present the greater excursion. Resist the attempt by the patient's sacrum to return to neutral through several cycles until the inherent motion of the craniosacral system ceases. The still point has been induced.

Several factors might be considered in selecting where on a patient's body the still point should be induced. Selection may be based upon convenience when, e.g., the therapist is already holding the sacrum or the feet and does not wish to disturb the patient's body by changing position. It may also be based upon a desire to monitor the effect of the induced still point upon a given body part. Manual contact with painful body parts is unnecessary since, with practice, still points may be induced from almost anywhere on the patient's body. The motion may be palpated in a restricted body region when the therapist desires to evaluate the effect of a still point upon the restriction in that area. The most convenient method of monitoring this effect is to have your hand or hands upon the area in question during the procedure.

The induction of a still point from the body extremities when, e.g., one is attempting to evaluate and treat an uncooperative child, is an excellent means of obtaining cooperation. The still point experience is a pleasant one for the patient. The child soon learns to associate your touch with the pleasant experience of the still point. Cooperation ensues from this association and the stage is set for a mutually beneficial therapeutic process. It is beneficial to the therapist, both in terms of satisfaction and also as an education experience. Once cooperation and trust have been achieved, more specific and efficacious treatment can be used. We particularly recommend this approach in developing a cooperative rapport with autistic children.

Chapter 5
Release of Transverse Restrictions Which Impair Fascial Mobility

The majority of the fascial planes of the human body are arranged in the longitudinal rather than the transverse direction. A small amount of gliding motion is characteristic of these fascial structures. This gliding mobility is therefore more apparent in the longitudinal direction than in the transverse.

Anatomically, there are specific structural divisions which, when hypertonic or imbalanced in their tonicity, act as areas of functional restriction to this natural longitudinal glide of the body's fascial sheets. These structural/functional divisions are located wherever there is a predominance of connective tissues which are orientated transversely across the body. They can easily impair the free longitudinal glide of the majority of the fascial lamina.

RESPIRATORY DIAPHRAGM

The most apparent of these potentially restricting transverse structures is the respiratory diaphragm (ILLUSTRATION 5-1). This diaphragm divides the human body into the thoracic and abdominal cavities. It is essentially a musculofibrous septum. The periphery of the respiratory diaphragm is the muscular part which arises from the internal aspects of the xiphoid process of the sternum, from the lower six cartilages and ribs, from the aponeurotic lumbocostal arches, and via its crura from the upper three lumbar vertebrae and their intervertebral fibrocartilages. The peripherally arranged muscle of this diaphragm inserts into its central tendon.

The respiratory diaphragm affords passage to the structures which traverse between the thoracic and abdominal cavities. These structures include the esophagus, the aorta, the vena cava, the azygos and hemiazygos veins, the thoracic duct, esophygeal blood vessels, the internal mammary artery, the vagus nerves, branches of the phrenic nerves and the greater and lesser splanchnic nerves. The sympathetic nerve trunks usually pass through the medial lumbocostal arches, which also afford passage to the quadratus lumborum muscles. Keep in mind that the fibers of the pericardium penetrate this diaphragm from above, and are contributory to the inferior diaphragmatic fascia.

The right crus of the diaphragm arises from the anterior longitudinal ligament of the vertebral column, from the anterior surfaces of the bodies of lumbar vertebrae 1, 2 and 3, and from their intervertebral fibrocartilages.

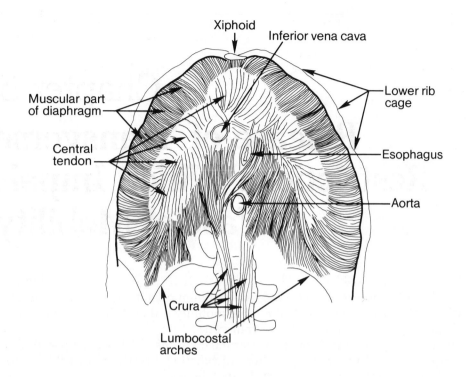

Illustration 5-1
Respiratory Diaphragm — Inferior Oblique View

The left crus is smaller and attaches to the corresponding parts of the upper two lumbar vertebrae and the anterior longitudinal ligament. Fibers of the two crura extend anteriorly and medially where they cross to form the aortic hiatus. They then complete a "figure 8" to form the esophygeal hiatus.

When the muscle of the respiratory diaphragm contracts, it pulls the central tendon downward, thus reducing the intrathoracic pressure and increasing intra-thoracic volume. At the same time it increases intra-abdominal pressure and reduces intra-abdominal volume. A contraction of the respiratory diaphragm also exerts an inferiorly directed traction upon the pericardium which is transmitted via fascial continuity through the carotid sheath to the base of the skull. Hence, patients with chronic diaphragmatic hypertonicity frequently manifest less than optimal cranio-sacral system mobility.

The diaphragm is innervated by branches of the ventral primary divisions of thoracic nerves 9 through 12 and by the phrenic nerve, which arises primarily from the 4th cervical nerve but which may also receive contributions from the 3rd and 5th cervical nerves.

An abnormal state of hypertonus or contracture of the respiratory diaphragm may occur unilaterally or bilaterally. It may occur from problems associated with any one or all of the lower four thoracic nerves on one or both sides. It may occur as a result of problems along the course of one or both of the phrenic nerves or from one or both sides of the cervical region at the levels of the 3rd, 4th and/or 5th segments. It may occur from inflammation of the pleura which spreads to the diaphragm, from pericarditis and from inflammation of the hepato-biliary system and other related abdominal viscera.

Dysfunction of the diaphragm may also occur secondary to somatic dysfunction which involves the lower six ribs, the sternum and xiphoid process, the upper three lumbar vertebrae, the psoas major muscle, the quadratus lumborum and/or the fasciae related to any of the structures named above. It may also occur secondary to inflammation of any of the structures which pass through it, such as the aorta, the esophagus or the vena cava.

The significant point is that abnormal hypertonus of the diaphragm is a common secondary finding in a vast number of conditions. Frequently, after the primary condition is cleared, the diaphragm autonomously maintains and continues the asymmetrical tension patterns and abnormal hypertonus created within it. The dysfunctioning diaphragm then interferes not only with proper breathing activity but also with craniosacral system function and freedom of fascial mobility. The patient is thus somewhat devitalized. This reduced level of health sets the scene for recurrent illnesses, vague complaints of fatigue, migratory pains, the accumulation of toxic wastes due to reduced fluid mobility and gaseous exchanges, depression and general malaise.

The above scenario provides some of the basis for our contention that with all craniosacral system dysfunctions, special diagnostic and therapeutic attention should be paid to the naturally occurring cross-restrictions of the human body.

The technique for releasing abnormal tension in the respiratory diaphragm is quite simple (ILLUSTRATION 5-2). The patient lies supine upon the treatment table. The

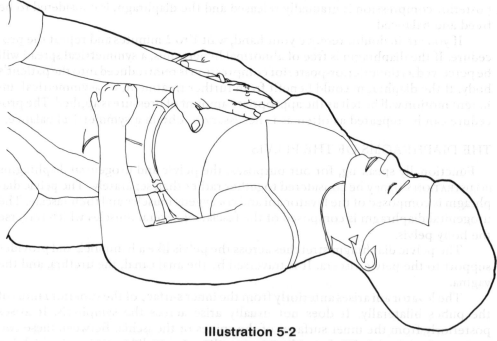

Illustration 5-2
Hand Position for Release of Respiratory Diaphragm

therapist sits comfortably next to the patient. Place one of your hands under the thoracolumbar region of the patient so that the spines of the 12th thoracic and the upper three lumbar vertebrae are in the palm of your hand. Your other hand, placed anteriorly, should cover the epigastrium, the xiphoid process and the anterior inferior costal margins.

While using one hand under the patient as a rather firm and immovable foundation, apply pressure from anterior to posterior with the anteriorly placed hand. Begin the pressure very lightly, then *slowly* increase it until you feel a motion within the patient. When you perceive this motion, follow it in any direction which it tends to go. Maintain the anterior-posterior compression with just enough force to cause this inherent motion to occur and continue.

The inherent motion which you perceive may be predominant in either the posterior or the anterior regions of the patient's body, or it may appear to be uniform throughout the body. You may palpate it as a shear, a torsion, a rotation or any combination of these. Any other possibilities which represent the releasing of hypertonic tissues may occur.

When you consider the directional orientation of the muscle fibers of the diaphragm, it becomes apparent how various restrictions and distortions of tissue motion can occur. Not only are all transverse angles represented by these fibers, but the variation of angle from almost longitudinal to transverse is great. This circumstance provides a three-dimensional potential for the restriction of normal mobility. Additionally, these angles change as respiratory effort and other variables change the level of the diaphragm between the thoracic and abdominal cavities.

As the tissues between your hands begin to relax, a new balance will be achieved within the patient's body. This new condition will be heralded by a softening of the tissues which is readily perceptible. Once that softening occurs, the anterior-posterior compression is gradually released and the diaphragm is considered to be freed and balanced.

If you are in doubt, remove your hand, wait 1 to 2 minutes and repeat the procedure. If the diaphragm is free of abnormal hypertonus, a symmetrical spread will be perceived as the anterior-posterior compression is reintroduced into the patient's body. If the diaphragm could benefit from further treatment, an asymmetrical, inherent motion will be felt as the appropriate amount of pressure is applied. The procedure can be repeated as often as is necessary to obtain a symmetrical balance.

THE DIAPHRAGMS OF THE PELVIS

Functionally speaking, for our purposes, the pelvic and urogenital diaphragms (ILLUSTRATION 5-3) may be considered together rather than separately. The pelvic diaphragm is composed of the levator ani and coccygeus muscles and their fasciae. The urogenital diaphragm is composed of the fasciae of several muscles which traverse the bony pelvis.

The pelvic diaphragm stretches across the pelvis like a hammock and provides support to the pelvic viscera. It is traversed by the anal canal, the urethra, and the vagina.

The levator ani arises anteriorly from the inner surface of the superior ramus of the pubes bilaterally. It does not usually arise across the symphysis. It arises posteriorly from the inner surfaces of the spines of the ischia. Between these two regions of origin, it arises from the arcus tendinus musculi levatoris ani, which is a

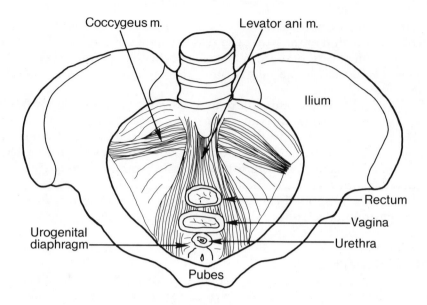

Illustration 5-3
Pelvic Diaphragms

thickened band of obturator fascia attached to the pubic bone and the spine of the ischium. The muscle fibers run medially and posteriorly and insert into the lower two coccygeal segments, the anococcygeal raphe, the external anal sphincter and the central tendinous point of the perineum. It is innervated by branches of the pudendal plexus derived from the 3rd, 4th and 5th sacral segments.

The levator ani acts to support and raise the pelvic floor. It resists increasing intra-abdominal pressure. It draws the anus upward and constricts it. It is respons-

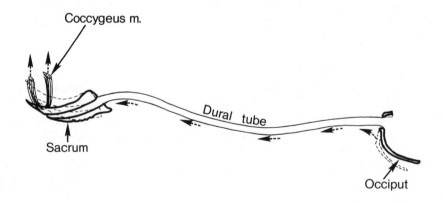

Illustration 5-4
Coccygeal Hypertonus Inducing Flexion of the
Craniosacral System

ible in large part for vaginal tonus.

The coccygeus is mixed muscle and tendon fiber. It arises from the ischial spine and the sacrotuberous ligament, and inserts into the sacrococcygeal junction. It is innervated by branches from the pudendal plexus derived from the 4th and 5th sacral segments. The coccygeus acts to draw the coccyx and sacral apex anteriorly, thus inducing an element of flexion into the craniosacral system (ILLUSTRATION 5-4).

The urogenital diaphragm is composed of two layers of fascia, the deep layer and the superficial layer. The deep layer spans the distance between the ischiopubic rami. It represents the fascial layers of the transversus perineal muscles, the levator ani muscles and the supra anal fascia. It is attached to the symphysis pubis anteriorly, and to the perineal body posteriorly. Laterally, it is continuous with the obturator fascia and attaches to the ischiopubic rami. It affords passage to the urethra and the vagina, and blends with their walls as they pass through.

The superficial layer of the urogenital diaphragm attaches laterally to the ischiopubic rami from the arcuate pubic ligaments to the ischial tuberosities. It too affords passage to the urethra and the vagina and blends with their walls.

Because of the intimate interconnections among these structures through common anchoring points and muscle attachments, any fragmentation of treatment or analysis would be illusory.

Because of the powerful influence of the pelvic diaphragms, not only upon sacrococcygeal mobility but also upon longitudinal fascial mobility and the delivery of

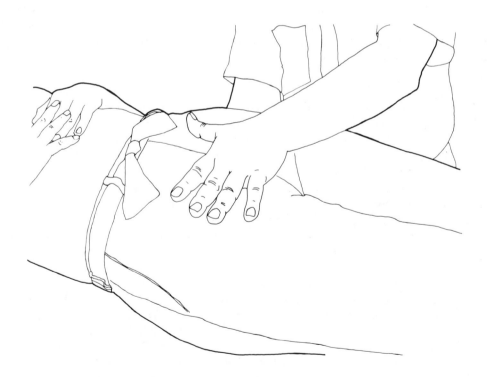

Illustration 5-5
Hand Position for Release of Pelvic Diaphragms

fluid through these transverse structures, it is imperative that hypertonus and tension imbalances be successfully treated before we can expect free craniosacral system and fascial mobility.

The technique for releasing the pelvic diaphragms is quite similar to the technique used for releasing abnormal tonus of the respiratory diaphragm. The position of the therapist's hands is, of course, different (ILLUSTRATION 5-5).

Place one of your hands under the supine patient and hold the sacral body so that the spine runs across your palm. Your hand acts as a foundation which offers firm resistance once you begin the anterior-posterior compression.

Place your other hand upon the patient so that the hypothenar eminence covers the pubes and the rest of the hand covers the suprapubic region.

Begin to apply a compressive force with the anteriorly placed hand against the patient's pubes and suprapubic area. The hand under the patient offers firm resistance. As the compressive force is gradually increased, it will reach an effective level at which point a normally symmetrical pelvic diaphragm will allow a laterally symmetrical spread of the tissues. If abnormal tonus of the pelvic tissues exists, an inherent motion between your hands will begin to show as a shear, torsion or rotation. All of these motions should be followed without resistance, but the therapist should maintain the minimal compressive force required to continue the self-correcting activity of the patient's pelvis. When the softening sensation of release of abnormal tonus is perceived, the treatment is finished. If in doubt, repeat the technique to determine the normalcy of response to the anterior-posterior compressive force which you have induced. This technique can be repeated as often as necessary to obtain the desired result. Release of the pelvic diaphragm will often immediately enhance the amplitude and balance of the cranial motion, as the sacrococcygeal complex is mobilized.

THORACIC INLET

Another area of potential transverse restriction which frequently causes reduction of longitudinal fascial motion and craniosacral system mobility is the region of the cervico-thoracic junction and/or the thoracic inlet. We refer to this anatomical complex as the "inlet" because of the blood and lymph channels which pass through it as they return their fluids into the thoracic cavity from the head. If the return of fluid from the cranial vault to the thoracic cavity is even slightly inhibited by abnormal tissue hypertonus at the thoracic inlet, cranial motion is correspondingly impaired by fluid congestion within the vault.

The bony structures which are involved in the thoracic inlet include the vertebrae of the cervicothoracic junction, the upper ribs, the clavicles, the acromion processes of the scapulae and the upper sternum.

The fasciae of the neck are continuous with the fasciae of the thorax. The subcutaneous fasciae of the neck contain the fibers of the platysma muscles. They are separated from the deep cervical fasciae by a distinct cleft which allows mobility. The superficial cervical fasciae are continuous over the clavicles with the superficial fasciae of the pectoral and deltoid regions anteriorly. Posteriorly, they are continuous with the tela of the back of the neck, which is tough and fibrous. The tela adheres to the deep fascia in this region. The deep cervical fasciae make connections between the head and thorax. They also contribute greatly to the fasciae of the upper limbs.

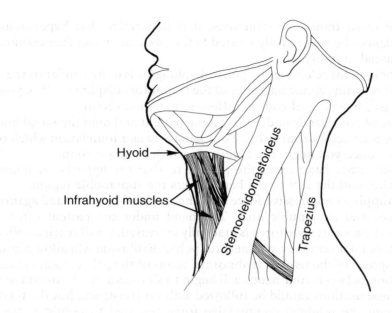

Illustration 5-6
Neck Muscles Which Attach
to the Thoracic Inlet from Above

At the thoracic inlet, the oblique courses of the sternocleidomastoid and trapezius muscles and their fasciae cause them to exert great influences upon the functional mobility of the bony structures of the thoracic inlet, as well as upon fluid flow and fascial mobility. The infrahyoid muscles and their fasciae also have great potential for interfering with the normal mobility of these regions (ILLUSTRATION 5-6).

The investing layers of the cervical fasciae in the infrahyoid regions offer perfect examples of the concept of fascial sheets splitting into lamina to form pockets for the investment of muscles and other structures. In this region the fasciae are continuous across the midline. They form pockets which invest the sternocleidomastoid and trapezius muscles. These fasciae then fuse between the muscles into single sheets. These fasciae are also continuous with the investing fasciae of the pectoral and deltoid muscles. They attach at the superior nuchal line, the spinous process of the 7th cervical vertebra, the ligamentum nuchae, the hyoid, the achromia, the clavicles and the manubrium sterni. Since these fascial laminae form the investing fasciae of numerous muscles (and yet are truly parts of a single fascial sheet), contraction or hypertonus of any one or a number of these muscles affects the fasciae in such a way as to result in an imbalanced, hypertonic and restricted condition of the thoracic inlet. The external and anterior jugular veins are actually imbedded in the superficial layers of these investing fasciae. Thus, an increase in fascial tension due to muscle hypertonus may increase venous back pressure into the head.

Prevertebral fascia is the name given to the anterior portions of the vertebral fasciae which invest the vertebral column and all of its muscles. These fasciae are continuous from skull to coccyx. They are continuous with the fasciae of the levator scapulae and the splenius muscles. They extend over the scalene muscles and are continuous with the fasciae of the thoracic walls. Deep fibers of the prevertebral fasciae form conical fibrous domes bilaterally which arch over the apices of the lung as Sibson's fasciae. These fasciae attach firmly to the transverse processes of the 7th cervical vertebra and to the medial borders of the first ribs. They merge with the carotid sheaths and are continuous with the endothoracic fasciae. They form the axillary sheaths which cover the subclavian arteries and veins (as their names change to axillary artery and vein) and the brachial nerve plexuses as they move into the axillary region.

The complexity of the anatomy through the thoracic inlet can be quite literally mind-boggling to anyone other than a devout anatomist. Suffice it to say that the potential for reduction of fluid flow, restriction of fascial mobility and osseous somatic dysfunction or restricted motion at the thoracic inlet is immense. Restriction of the thoracic inlet can greatly interfere with free mobility of the craniosacral system by several mechanisms. It must be made as freely mobile as possible in order to allow for maximum efficiency of the craniosacral system.

The technique used to mobilize the thoracic inlet incorporates techniques similar to those used for the respiratory and pelvic diaphragms. These techniques of fascial release are best (but not necessarily) preceded by a general cervicothoracic thrust to enhance osseous mobility of this region.

The general cervicothoracic thrust is not aimed at any specific osseous restriction but is intended to mobilize the intervertebral articulations as well as the upper ribs. It stretches the fasciae and by some mechanism, probably neural, reduces general cervical muscle tonus (APPENDIX D).

First, sidebend the patient's cervicothoracic junction over the fulcrum provided by your hand. Sidebend to the extreme range of motion. (Use gentle to moderate force in the sidebending procedure.) Do not intentionally introduce flexion or extension of the neck at this point (ILLUSTRATION 5-7).

When the sidebending has proceeded to the extreme range of motion, ask the patient to take a deep breath and hold as long as possible. When exhalation occurs, the sidebending will go a little further. After this breathing exercise has been performed a few times until it produces no further movement into sidebending upon exhalation, rotate the head in the opposite direction while keeping it sidebent. Continue to use only gentle to moderate force (ILLUSTRATION 5-8).

When the rotation has been carried as far as it will go, repeat the breathing procedure described for sidebending to see if further rotation will occur. When you have reached the maximum of rotational movement, gently but very quickly thrust the neck into a little further rotation. Usually, multiple "pops" will occur as the articulations of the thoracic inlet are mobilized. Repeat the procedure in the opposite direction. (Never use more than 2 or 3 pounds of force.) Other specific cervical corrections can then be made if indicated.

To mobilize and then balance the transverse restrictions of the thoracic inlet, place one of your hands under the supine patient. The spinous processes of the 7th cervical and the upper few thoracic vertebrae should lie across your palm. Place your other hand upon the anterior superior thoracic wall so that the sternoclavicular joints, the suprasternal notch and the upper costochondral regions are covered. The hand under the patient acts as a firm, supporting foundation, while the hand on the

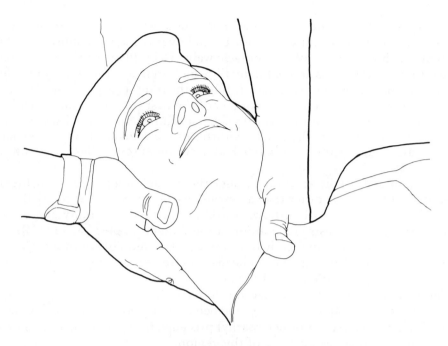

Illustration 5-7
Introduction of Sidebending of the Lower
Neck on the Upper Thoracic Spine

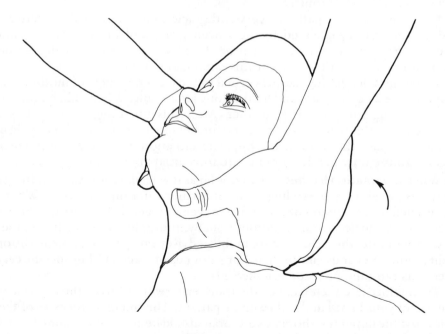

Illustration 5-8
Addition of Rotation of the Lower Neck on the Upper
Thoracic Spine While Maintaining Sidebending

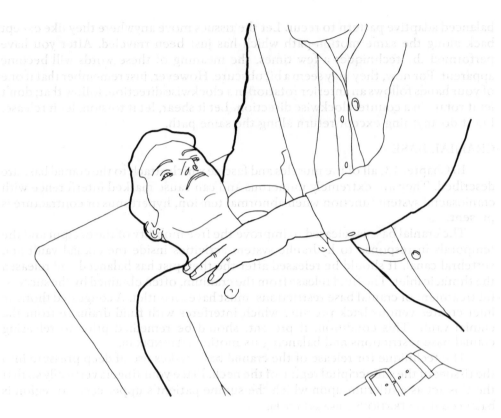

Illustration 5-9
Hand Position for Release of Thoracic Inlet

anterior surface begins an anterior-posterior compressive force. The amount of force is slowly increased until, under normal circumstances, the thoracic inlet releases and spreads laterally in a symmetrical manner on both sides (ILLUSTRATION 5-9).

If shearing, torsioning or rotational inherent motions are perceived between your hands, these motions should be followed. Hold just enough compressive force to cause the motions to continue until a release is achieved. The need for further treatment can be determined by repeating the procedure and evaluating the motion to see if symmetry is present.

In applying the techniques for the three transverse restrictions described above, the abnormal motion should be followed while the compressive force is maintained at the minimal level required to cause continuation of the abnormal motion. This means that the force used is constantly being adjusted according to the body's response to your pressure. Too much force will cause a defensive body tissue contraction. This will obliterate the inherent balancing motion which is the therapeutic effect you are trying to induce. *Too much force is self-defeating.*

When following abnormal motion to achieve a point of balance so that release of tissue tonus will occur, there is one other rule to keep in mind: *do not let the motion return in the same direction from which it came.* Otherwise, you simply are allowing the imbalanced adaptive pattern to recur. Let the tissues move anywhere they like except back along the same motion-path which has just been traveled. After you have performed the techniques a few times, the meaning of these words will become apparent. For now, they may seem a bit obscure. However, just remember that if one of your hands follows an anterior rotation in a clockwise direction, follow that; don't let it rotate in a counterclockwise direction. Let it shear, let it torsion, let it release. Let it do anything except return along the same path.

CRANIAL BASE

In Chapter 13, all of the muscles and fasciae which attach to the cranial base are described. They are extremely numerous and can cause marked interference with craniosacral system function when abnormal tension, hypertonus or contracture is present.

The cranial base is released to improve the free mobility of the occiput and the temporals in response to hydraulic system activities inside the cranial vault and vertebral canal. It should be released after the therapist has balanced and released the thoracic inlet. The fluid release from the cranium, often obtained by the successful treatment of cranial base restrictions, must have an outlet. A congested thoracic inlet creates venous back pressure which interferes with fluid drainage from the cranial vault. This condition, if present, should be remedied prior to releasing cranial base restrictions and balancing its motion (APPENDIX D).

The technique for release of the cranial base makes use of deep pressure into the tissues of the suboccipital region of the neck. Place your fingers vertically so that the tips act as a fulcrum upon which the supine patient's upper cervical region is balanced (ILLUSTRATIONS 5-10-A and 5-10-B).

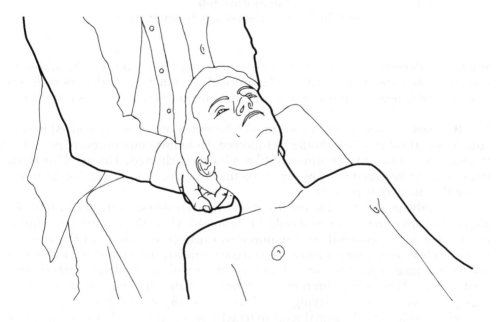

Illustration 5-10-A
Release of Cranial Base

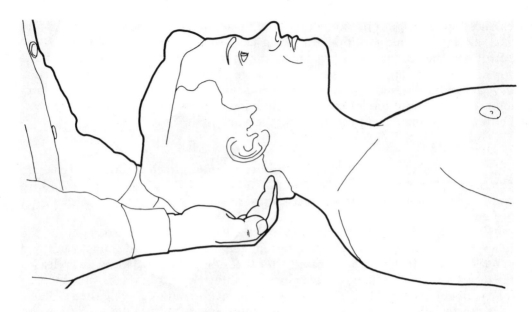

Illustration 5-10-B
Release of Cranial Base

The pads of your fingers should maintain contact with the occiput. The head of the patient should be poised above the palms of your hands.

The therapeutic force is supplied only by the weight of the patient's head. As the tissues of the suboccipital region begin to relax due to fingertip pressure, the patient's head will begin to settle into the palms of your hands. Continue the pressure at the suboccipital region in a straight anterior direction. Maintain fingerpad contact with the occiput. Don't let the tissues move your fingers in an inferior or caudad direction.

Ultimately, as the tissues relax, you will feel the firmness of the posterior arch of the atlas. Slowly the atlas will begin to disengage from the occiput. This occurrence is signaled by a "floating" sensation. As it floats, follow and "balance" it. Once it seems free from the occiput, support the atlas anteriorly with the tips of your ring fingers. Move the occiput gently and minutely in a posterior direction with the tips of your middle fingers. This procedure further disengages the occiput from the atlas and decompresses the occipital condylar region.

This technique not only mobilizes the cranial base but also releases the tissues around the jugular foramena. This enhances fluid drainage via the jugular veins from the cranial vault, thus reducing intracranial fluid congestion. The reduction of intracranial fluid congestion will further contribute to craniosacral system mobility.

The glossopharyngeal, the vagus, and the accessory cranial nerves pass through the jugular foramena (ILLUSTRATION 5-11). Release of any compromise of these foramena often has a beneficial effect on the function of these nerves.

OTHER TRANSVERSE RESTRICTIONS

Any joint is a potential cross-restriction to the free, gliding movement of longitudinally oriented fascia. This includes the hips, knees, ankles, shoulders,

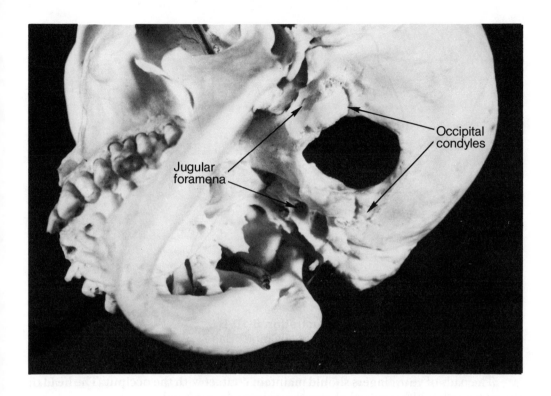

Illustration 5-11
Structures at the Cranial Base Which Are Favorably
Influenced by Release of the Cranial Base

elbows, wrists and even the fingers and toes.

Restriction in any of these regions drags upon the fascia which, in turn, to some degree impairs the free motion of the craniosacral system. Treatment is predicated upon locating the neutral position of the joint and holding until the tissues release. In osteopathic circles, this technique is commonly known as *position and hold* functional technique (APPENDIX E).

Chapter 6
Dysfunctions of the Craniosacral Dural Membrane System: Diagnosis and Treatment

In our opinion, the most frequent, clinically significant cause of craniosacral system dysfunction is abnormal tension in the dural membrane system. The dural membrane is a tough, fibrous connective tissue. Its elasto-collagenous bundles are interlaced and appear disorganized. The dural membrane is made up of two layers which are tightly adherent except where the venous sinuses are formed between them (RHODIN 1974).

When the dural membrane is subjected to abnormal tension in a certain direction over a considerable period of time, the fibers within the membrane seem to organize and align themselves with the direction of tension. Dissection of human cadavers displays these abnormally organized arrangements. Study of the fiber orientation patterns may disclose the direction of principal tensions to which these membranes were subjected during life (ILLUSTRATION 6-1).

We have dissected both human and primate cadavers in a manner which preserves the *in vivo* geometry of the dural membranes—specifically the falx cerebri, the tentorium cerebelli and the falx cerebelli—and have frequently found abnormal fibrous changes which suggest the directions of principal tension in the membrane (ILLUSTRATIONS 6-2-A and 6-2-B).

For purposes of craniosacral diagnosis and treatment, and to begin to appreciate the significance of the dural membrane system, you might consider the bones of the cranial vault simply as hard places in the dural membrane.

In the full-term infant skull, there is considerable distance between the edges of the various cranial vault bones. As we age, the spaces diminish in size but do not, under normal circumstances, disappear. Throughout life, under normal circumstances the sutures between cranial vault bones do *not* fuse or ossify completely. Sutural mobility, small though it may be, is always maintained (RETZLAFF 1978) (ILLUSTRATIONS 6-3-A and 6-3-B).

Once you accept the idea that the cranial vault bones are merely hard places in the dural membrane, the techniques of diagnosis and treatment of abnormal dural tensions become much more tenable, and the required skills much easier to master.

60

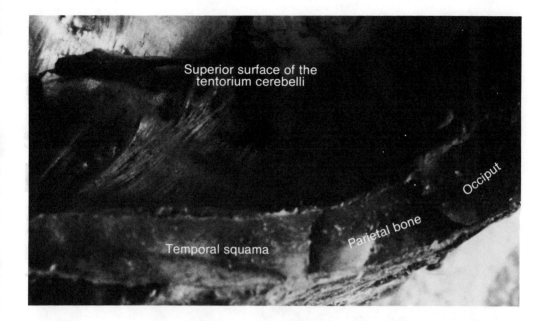

Illustration 6-1
Fiber Orientation of Human Dural Membrane

Toward this end, think of the cranial bones and the sacrum and coccyx as levers which can be used to evaluate and treat dural membrane abnormalities.

Following is a brief review of the functional anatomy of the dural membrane structure.

The two layers of the dural membrane are tightly attached except where venous sinuses are formed. The outer layer is attached to the inner surface of the bones which form the cranial vault.

At the sinuses the dura separates away from itself and from the bone (ILLUSTRATION 6-4). It affords space for the collection of blood and then adheres to the dura from the opposite side of the sinus to form either a falx or the tentorium. It is this endosteal contribution of dural membrane to cranial vault bone which enables you to use these bones of the cranial vault as levers to diagnose and treat the intracranial membranes. The dural membrane forms the functional, if not the strict morphological boundary of the hydraulic system. The cerebrospinal fluid is the hydraulic part of the system (ILLUSTRATION 6-5).

Remember, it is within the dural boundaries of this hydraulic system that the central nervous system must develop and function.

Understanding the geometry of the dural membranes where they are not attached to bone offers the key to successful diagnosis and treatment of the cranio-sacral system (ILLUSTRATION 6-6).

The two falxes—cerebri and cerebelli—furnish the vertical component of the non-osseous-attached intracranial dural membrane system. The two leaves of the cerebellar tent furnish the component of this system which may be functionally considered as horizontal. (There is some deviation from the horizontal at certain

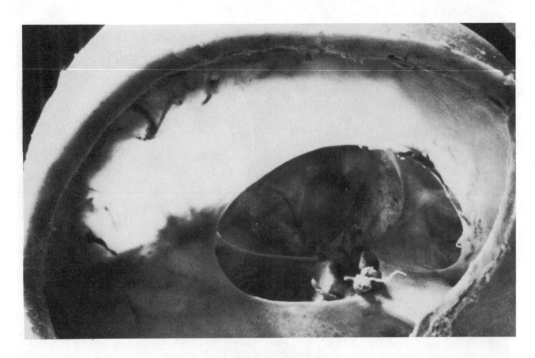

Illustration 6-2-A
Human Dural Membrane

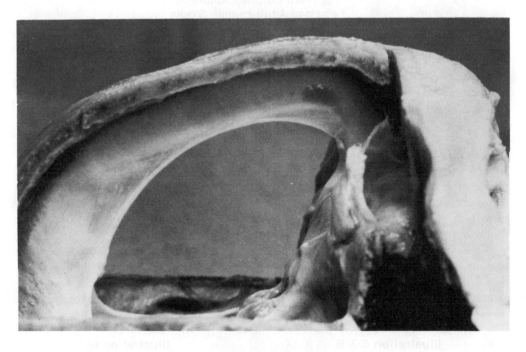

Illustration 6-2-B
Primate Dural Membrane

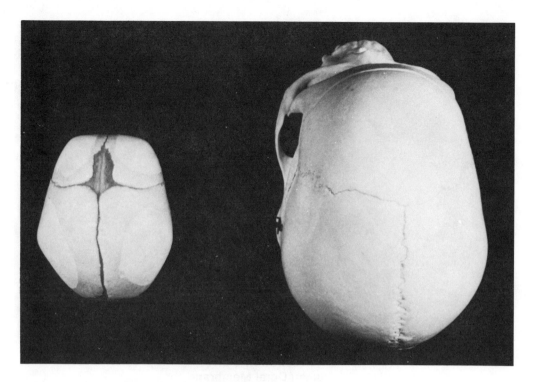

Illustration 6-3-A
Apparent Sutural Closure in
Fetal and Adult Human Skulls

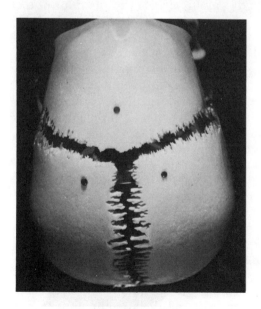

Illustration 6-3-B
"Exploded" Adult Human Skull
Demonstrating Non-Closure of Sutures

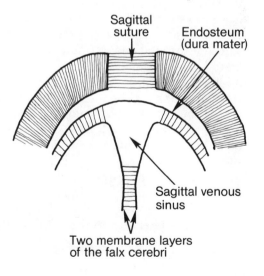

Illustration 6-4
Intracranial Venous Sinus

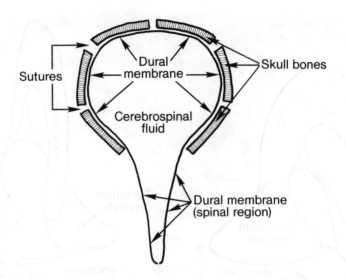

Illustration 6-5
Semi-Closed Hydraulic System of the
Cerebrospinal Fluid and Dural Membrane

anatomical regions of the tentorium cerebelli.)

Dr. Sutherland spoke of this system as a "reciprocal tension membrane system." This is indeed the case (SUTHERLAND 1939) (MAGOUN 1966).

The anterior-inferior extreme of the falx cerebri attaches to the floor of the cranial vault at the crista galli of the ethmoid bone and to the ethmoid notch of the frontal bone (ILLUSTRATION 6-7).

The attachment then follows the midline superiorly inside of the cranial vault along the internal aspect of the metopic suture, under bregma, underneath the sagittal suture and under lambda to the internal occipital protuberance. It forms the sagittal venous sinus as it passes along the internal surface of the midline of the superior aspect of the cranial vault. The inferior and free border of the falx cerebri affords passage for the inferior venous sinus (ILLUSTRATION 6-8).

At the extreme posterior attachment of the falx cerebri to the internal occipital protuberance, its layers separate laterally to form the superior layer of the leaves of the tentorium cerebelli. The inferior layers of the leaves of the tentorium cerebelli come together medially to form the other vertical component of the reciprocal membrane system, the falx cerebelli.

There is a roughly quadrangular space where these membranes join. This space is the straight venous sinus which runs anteriorly and superiorly from the internal occipital protuberance to the union of the free borders of the falx cerebri and the two leaves of the tentorium cerebelli (ILLUSTRATION 6-9).

The falx cerebelli extends inferiorly down the internal midline of the occiput from the inferior leaves of the tentorium cerebelli and the straight sinus to the foramen magnum. At the foramen magnum, it contributes to the very strong and dense fibrous ring which encircles this opening in the occiput (ILLUSTRATION 6-10).

It is quite easy now to conceptualize the functional continuity between the

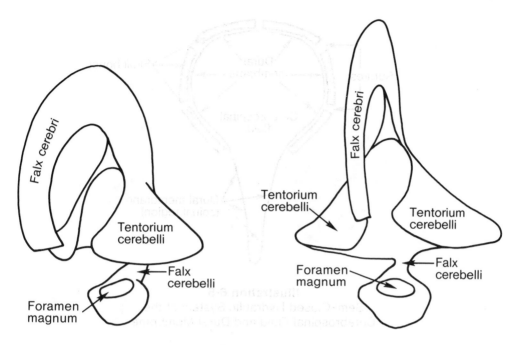

Illustration 6-6
Dural Membranes

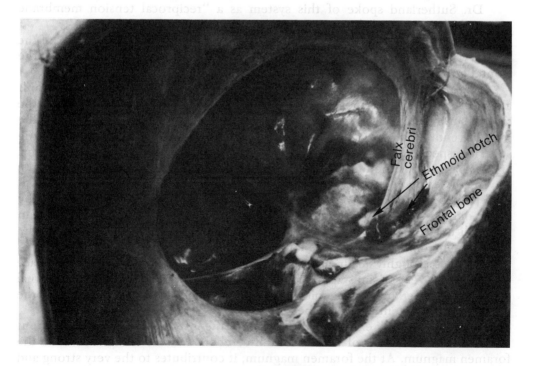

Illustration 6-7
Anterior-Inferior Attachment of the Falx Cerebri

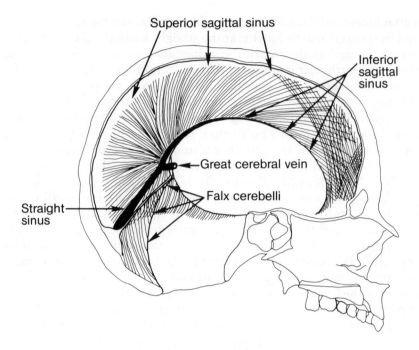

Illustration 6-8
Venous Sinuses within Falx Cerebri

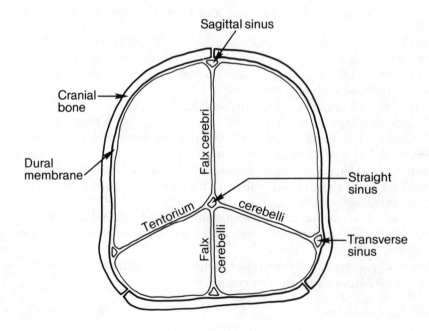

Illustration 6-9
Formation of the Straight Venous Sinus

anterior attachments of the falx cerebri at the glabella, and the frontal and ethmoid bones, and the posterior attachments at the straight sinus and the internal occipital protuberance, as well as the inferior attachments around the foramen magnum. Moving one step further, it is apparent that via dural tube continuity, the foramen magnum and the sacrum and coccyx are functionally connected in this *vertical* system. Hence, you can influence the ethmoid by use of the sacrum and coccyx, and you can influence the sacrum and coccyx by using the frontal bone (ILLUSTRATION 6-11).

Carrying the concept just a bit further, you can use the vertical falx and dural tube system to influence the straight sinus system which, in turn, exerts an influence upon the leaves of the tentorium cerebelli. And, of course, the converse is true: you can use the cerebellar tent to influence the vertical dural membrane system.

It is necessary to understand that ordinarily there are no "small-motion" restricting attachments of the dural tube within the spinal canal between the foramen magnum and the attachment to the inner wall of the sacral canal, except at the second and third cervical vertebrae. This allows some movement of the dural tube within the canal. Therefore, tension at either the inferior or superior ends of this dural tube may be transmitted to the other end.

A review of the functional anatomy of the leaves of the tentorium cerebelli will now complete the picture of the intracranial reciprocal membrane system.

The superior layers of the leaves of the tentorium cerebelli are continuous with the two layers of the falx cerebri as they separate to form the two superior walls of the straight venous sinus. From the straight sinus anteriorly, the superior layers of the leaves of the tentorium cerebelli form a free border called the incisura tentorii; the cerebral peduncles pass through this opening.

The inferior layers of the leaves of the tentorium cerebelli are continuous with the inferior walls of the straight sinus and then with the two layers of the falx cerebelli.

The layers of the tentorium cerebelli are largely adherent to each other after they leave the straight sinus to extend laterally. The inferior layers attach anteriorly to the posterior clinoid processes, and the superior layers attach to the anterior clinoid processes of the sphenoid bone.

Lateral to the clinoid attachments, both leaves of the tentorium cerebelli attach to the petrous ridges of the temporal bones. Here the tentorium encloses the superior petrosal sinuses. Moving posteriorly, the attachment is to the mastoid portions of the temporal bones, then to the posterior and inferior angle of the parietal bones and finally, moving posteriorly and medially, the attachment is to the transverse ridges of the occiput where it affords passage to the transverse venous sinuses (ILLUSTRATION 6-12).

It is now apparent that there is within the cranial vault and the vertebral canal a continuous membrane system through which tensions can be passed in a multitude of directions.

Essentially, there are three axes or dimensions to consider (ILLUSTRATIONS 6-13, 6-14-A and 6-14-B). Anatomically, these axes are:

1.   Anterior-posterior
     a. glabella to internal occipital protuberance
     b. sphenoidal clinoid processes and petrous temporal ridges to occipital internal ridges and straight sinus

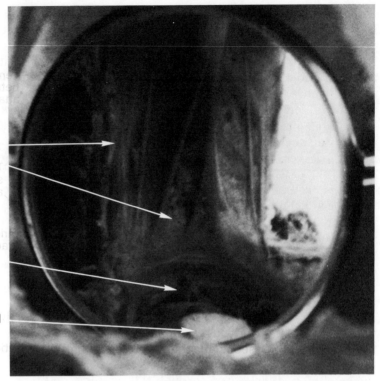

Fibers of the falx
cerebelli

Dural fibrous ring
around the foramen
magnum

Cut end of spinal cord

Illustration 6-10
Dural Ring Around Foramen Magnum

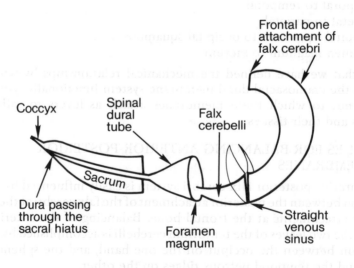

Illustration 6-11
Dural Membrane Continuity

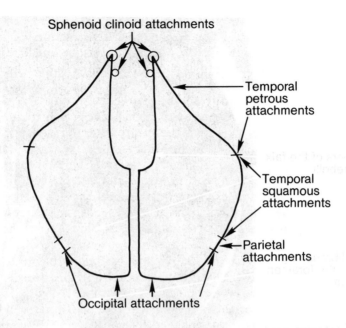

Illustration 6-12
Osseous Attachments to the Tentorium Cerebelli

2. Superior-inferior
   a. sagittal suture to foramen magnum, and to cribriform plate and notch of ethmoid-frontal bone complex
   b. foramen magnum to sacrum and coccyx
3. Horizontal or transverse
   a. temporal to temporal
   b. parietal to parietal
   c. occipital squamous to occipital squamous
   d. foramen magnum to sacrum

Now that we have defined the mechanical relationships by which you can understand the craniosacral dural membrane system functionally, you can simply use the bones to which these membranes attach as levers to influence these membranes and their tissues.

TECHNIQUES FOR BALANCING ANTERIOR-POSTERIOR DURAL MEMBRANES

The anterior-posterior falx cerebri system is easily influenced by placing very light traction between the posterior attachment of the falx cerebri at the occiput and its anterior attachments at the frontal bone. Balancing of the anterior-posterior tensions of the two leaves of the tentorium cerebelli is accomplished by placing very light traction between the occiput on the one hand, and the sphenoidal clinoid processes and the temporal petrous ridges on the other.

A frontal lift with traction is the technique most useful to diagnose and treat tension in the anterior-posterior direction of the falx cerebri. The traction is light and straight anterior. The weight of the contents of the cranium is enough to maintain the occiput in position on the table. The traction you apply to the frontal bone should not disturb the resting position of the occiput. The frontal bone is best grasped by the middle or ring fingers along the lateral ridges which form the anterior borders of the temporal fossae. The rest of the contact is with the palms and thumbs anterior to the coronal suture and bregma (ILLUSTRATIONS 6-15-A and 6-15-B).

Sutural restrictions will present firm resistance to the traction; the frontal bone may not move anteriorly because the sutures do not disengage. This resistance, if present, will be met first. After the sutures are disengaged (you may have to use direction of energy techniques which are described below), you are ready to evaluate membrane tension. Excess tension in the falx cerebri will be experienced as an elastic form of restriction, not firm and immovable as is the sutural restriction. The further you lift the frontal, the more you will sense a tendency toward elastic recoil upon the bone. Specific areas of restriction can be localized with practice; that is, the recoil tendency may be strongest over glabella or above a bregma.

Occasionally, you may sense an elastic restriction to your traction in the lateral aspect of the frontal bone. This probably means that the endosteal membrane which passes under the suture is restricted.

In conditions of normal membrane tension, the frontal will lift easily and seem to float once the sutures are disengaged. The head shape will change as you lift. You will sense a floating, plastic quality rather than an elastic recoiling quality.

When either sutural or membranous restriction is encountered, a correction can usually be made by patiently maintaining your traction. Seconds to minutes may be required to make the correction. The patient can be asked to take a few deep breaths and hold them as long as possible. These breathing maneuvers will often facilitate release of the restriction. The breathing maneuvers are usually more effective with sutural restrictions than they are with membrane tension problems.

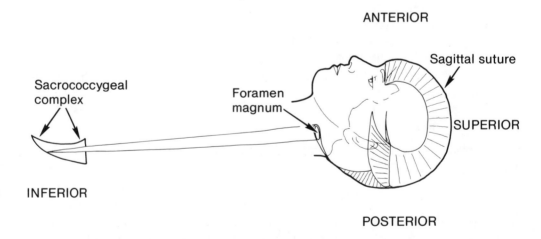

Illustration 6-13
Anterior-Posterior and Superior-Inferior Axes
of the Dural Membrane System

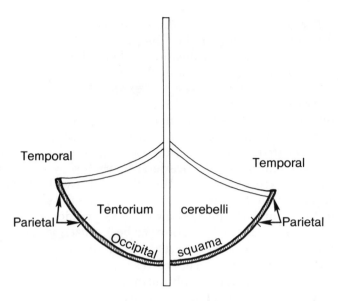

Illustration 6-14-A
Intracranial Horizontal Membrane System

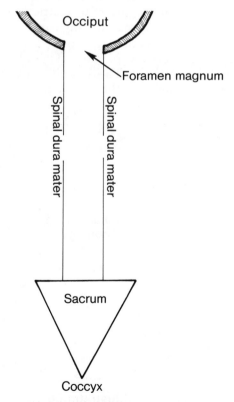

Illustration 6-14-B
Spinal Horizontal Membrane System

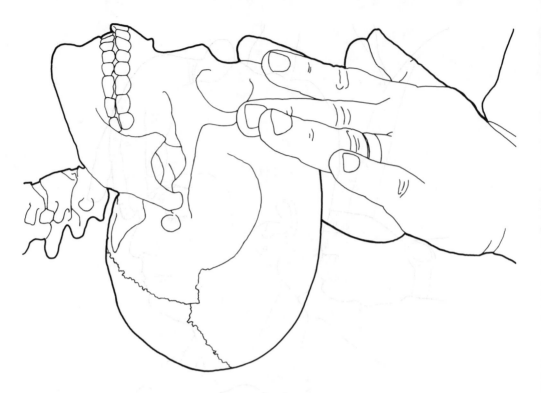

Illustration 6-15-A
Frontal Lift and Traction — Hand Position on Skull

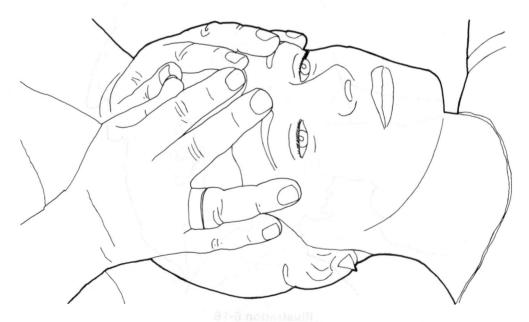

Illustration 6-15-B
Frontal Lift and Traction — Hand Position on Subject

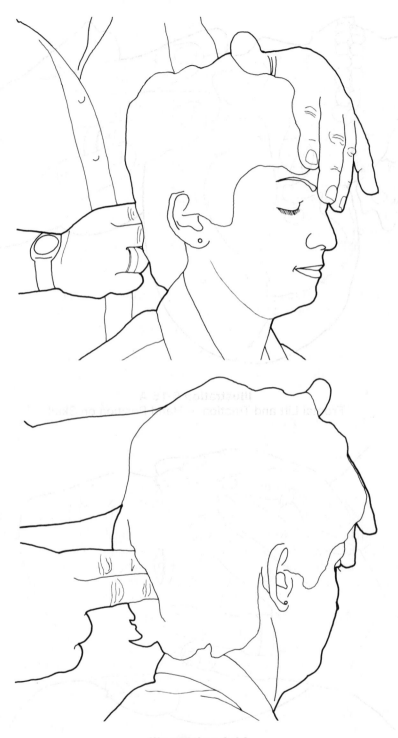

Illustration 6-16
Finger Placement for Direction of Energy Release
of Falx Cerebri

Another technique which we have found most useful in releasing falx cerebri restrictions is the direction of energy, or "V-spread" as it has been called. This technique consists of placing two fingers of one hand on either side of a restriction site, and one to all fingers of the other hand on a spot opposite to or linked with the restriction site. Pretend that your hands are electrodes and that you are passing energy back and forth between them until a palpable softening and therapeutic pulse are perceived at the site of restriction.

Applying this technique to the release of falx cerebri restrictions, simply place two fingers of one hand longitudinally on both sides of what you know to be the internal frontal attachment of the falx cerebri. The fingertips should be down over the nasal bones, and the bases of the fingers up near the coronal suture. About one-half inch of space between these two fingers is adequate (ILLUSTRATION 6-16). Place one finger of the other hand on the posterior occipital protuberance or immediately below it, but on the midline. Pretend your hands are electrodes and that you are sending electrical energy from the finger on the back of the patient's head through the falx cerebri to the anteriorly placed fingers. Usually within 1 or 2 minutes, you will feel a rapid pulsating activity (60±10 per minute) in the frontal region; there may be a tendency toward some twisting and turning, as though the falx is relieving itself of some torsional tension patterns. Follow but do not impede these motions. Ultimately, the frontal bone will seem to float freely in an anterior direction. When this occurs, your treatment is finished.

The same direction of energy technique can be used to alleviate subcoronal membranous restrictions. Simply place a finger inside the patient's mouth. Place two fingers of the other hand approximately one-half inch apart and parallel to the affected part of the suture. Point the sending finger, which is in the mouth, at the restriction. Then wait for the release to occur. The release will be heralded by a similar pulsating activity before it occurs (ILLUSTRATION 6-17) (APPENDIX D).

Evaluation and treatment techniques for anterior-posterior tentorium cerebelli restrictions make use of the clinoid attachments of the tentorium cerebelli and the generous posterior attachments to the internal occipital ridges. The great wings of the sphenoid, of which the exterior aspects are approximately 2 cm. posterior to the lateral canthus of the eye, are used as the contact points to apply an anterior lifting decompression traction between the sphenoid and the occiput. The occiput is gently cradled in the hands while the thumbs are applied to the tissue overlying the great wings of the sphenoid. Do not squeeze hard. The skin is attached on its deep side to connective tissue which ultimately attaches to the external surface of these wings. All you need do is maintain a non-sliding contact between your thumbs and the surface of the patient's skin. Take up the slack of the soft tissues and you will be indirectly applying traction or force upon the bone (ILLUSTRATION 6-18).

As you lift the sphenoid into decompression anteriorly, you will first meet rigid bony restrictions if they are present. They must be specifically treated if they do not spontaneously correct during the lifting of the sphenoid. The presence of osseous or sutural restrictions will always obscure the presence of membrane tension imbalances and must be treated before successful, reliable treatment of membrane restrictions can be carried out. In these cases, the V-spread techniques may be useful. Other specific techniques are described in Chapter 7.

In this technique, you are not only suspending the occiput from the sphenoid and thus correcting many sphenobasilar joint problems, you are also mobilizing the

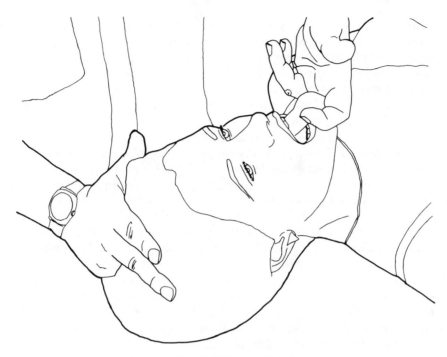

Illustration 6-17
Finger Placement for Direction of Energy Release
of Subcoronal or Coronal Restrictions

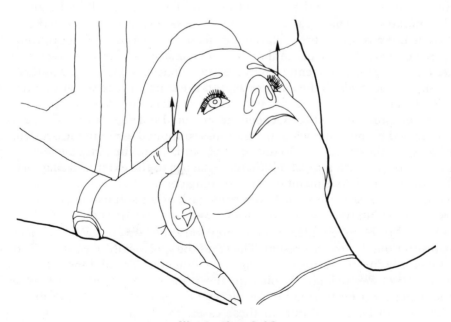

Illustration 6-18
Hand Position for Decompression
of Sphenoid

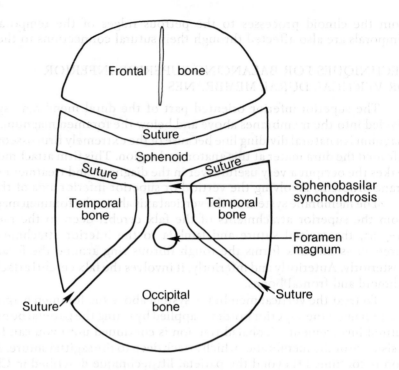

Illustration 6-19
Diagrammatic Representation of the Cranial Base

sutures of the cranial base (ILLUSTRATION 6-19). Those sutures are between the occiput and the temporals, and between the temporals and the sphenoid. Once the mobilization or decompression of the cranial base is accomplished, simply by suspending the sphenoid and waiting patiently for corrections, the membranes of the tentorium cerebelli can be evaluated. Remember, abnormal membranous restrictions offer elastic resistance.

The occiput will feel like a puppet suspended by strings from the sphenoid as first the bony or sutural, and later the membranous restrictions correct. You may need to wait 5 to 10 minutes for all the corrections to occur. They *will* occur if you wait. The weight of the intracranial contents is enough to stretch the membranes and to decompress the cranial base.

Bony cranial base compression is frequently accompanied by compression of the occipital condyles and the lumbosacral junction. Techniques for treating these conditions are described later in this chapter, and in Chapter 10.

The lifting of the sphenoid, after osseous and sutural decompression is achieved, will stretch the free border of the tentorium cerebelli. The induced tension is also transmitted through the straight venous sinus and has an emptying effect upon the blood within this structure, much as though you were "milking" the sinus.

The attachments of the tentorium cerebelli upon the petrous ridges of the temporal bones also lend themselves to use in the anterior-posterior stretching of these membranes. As the sphenoid is lifted, a traction is imposed via the membranes from the clinoid processes to the petrous ridges of the temporal bones. The temporals are also affected through their sutural connections to the sphenoid.

TECHNIQUES FOR BALANCING SUPERIOR-INFERIOR OR VERTICAL DURAL MEMBRANES

The superior-inferior oriented part of the dural membrane system may be divided into the membranes above and below the foramen magnum. The foramen magnum is a natural dividing line because of the extremely firm osseous attachment afforded the dura mater at this anatomical region. This firm attachment of the dura makes the occiput a very useful lever in the diagnosis and treatment of dural membrane problems involving the vertical or superior-inferior axis of the system.

The membrane system on the vertical axis above the foramen magnum extends from the superior attachments of the falx cerebri deep to the metopic suture, bregma, the sagittal suture and lambda to the inferior attachment of the falx cerebelli as this falx forms the tough fibrous ring around the foramen magnum posteriorly. Anteriorly and inferiorly, it involves the falx cerebri attachments to the ethmoid and frontal bones.

To treat the vertical membrane system above the foramen magnum, cephalad traction upon the superior border is applied by lifting the parietal bones free of their sutural involvement. Cephalad traction is continued until you can feel the elastic resistance of the membranes which attach deep to the sagittal suture. As gentle traction is continued (beyond the parietal lift technique described in Chapter 9), the membrane release travels through the falx cerebri and through the straight sinus. At this point in the treatment procedure, a horizontal balancing activity often becomes apparent; allow any untwisting and/or lateral balancing to occur while you continue your gentle cephalad traction. This untwisting or torsional correction represents the relief of abnormal tension patterns within the falx cerebri and the straight sinus. The lateral or horizontal balancing which occurs is largely due to the posterior-inferior attachments of the parietal bones to the cerebellar tent leaves (ILLUSTRATION 6-20).

Simply work with these factors until they seem to be balanced. After the tension patterns have been worked out of the falx cerebri and the straight sinus, and after any interfering imbalances of the tentorium cerebelli have been alleviated, the force of the traction is transmitted into the falx cerebelli and ultimately down to the foramen magnum. When the falx cerebelli releases, the patient will feel a sense of release and the parietal bones will seem to float even further in a cephalad direction.

Keep in mind that membrane releases are possible only after the sutures of the parietal bones have been mobilized. The technique that releases the vertical membrane systems is traction using the parietal bones as levers after a successful parietal lift has been performed (APPENDIX D).

Releasing the dural membrane tube between the foramen magnum and the sacrococcygeal complex requires that the cranial base, the thoracic inlet, the respiratory diaphragms and the pelvic diaphragm be released first. Spinal osteopathic somatic dysfunctions will interfere with the free mobility of the spinal dural tube and should therefore also be corrected.

With some experience, you will be able to discern with confidence whether or not restrictions from these diaphragms, the thoracic inlet, the cranial base or osteopathic somatic dysfunctions do indeed exist by simply examining the mobility of the dural tube. An excellent means of developing this skill is to evaluate the

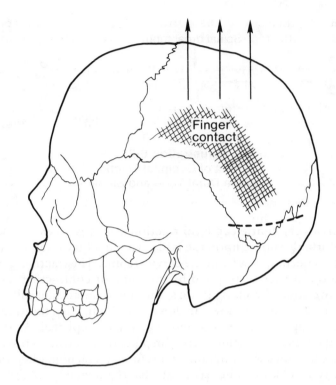

Illustration 6-20
Parietal Lift with Traction

mobility of the dural tube first. Then examine spinal motion, the paravertebral muscles, the cranial base, the thoracic inlet and the diaphragms for restriction. When restrictions are found, reexamine the mobility of the spinal dural tube; try to perceive the effect which these restrictions have on dural tube mobility. Then correct the extradural restrictions one at a time. After each correction, reexamine the mobility of the dural tube and note the effect which your correction or release of restriction has had upon its mobility.

At first, the achievement of this skill may seem impossible; however, as you learn to trust your hands and perceptions, you will find that you can achieve the impossible. Don't reason it out: just let it happen. With experience, you will begin to distinguish the feel of one kind of restriction from another. Another useful exercise is to work in pairs, with one therapist monitoring the dural tube and the other locating and correcting restrictions during the monitoring process. By practicing in this manner, the monitor will experience exactly how the corrections feel in the craniosacral mechanism.

The evaluation and treatment of dural tube mobility can be performed at both the occiput and the sacrococcygeal complex. At the occiput, you must first release the soft tissues at the cranial base and disengage the occipital condyles from the atlas. These techniques are described in Chapter 5 (release of the diaphragms) and 10 (occipital condyles).

After the occipital condyles are freed from the articular surfaces of the atlas, the

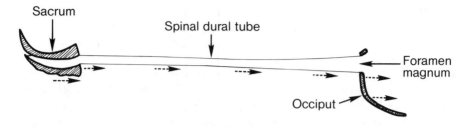

Illustration 6-21
Effect of Occipital Traction
on the Dural Tube and Sacrum

therapist begins a very gentle cephalad traction (ILLUSTRATION 6-21). The patient, of course, is comfortably supine upon the table. The first bit of traction will cause the occiput to further decompress from the cervical spine. The traction must be light so as *not* to cause the tissues to respond by guarding or contracting. Gradually, the occiput will move toward you. As it does, the spinal dural tube will begin to glide cephalad with it. Try to feel how far down the dural tube the traction force is reaching as the occiput continues to move gradually cephalad. As the dural tube gently follows the foramen magnum, you can perceive just when a restriction is met. If you know how far down the dural tube your force is reaching when the restriction presents itself, you will know where (i.e., at what segmental level) the restriction to dural tube mobility is located. Visualize, imagine and practice: you will be amazed at how rapidly you can develop this skill. Don't think critically or become anxious about it in the beginning. After all, what is the risk if the examination does not yield correct impressions at first? On the other hand, once you begin to get some correct impressions, your skills will develop rapidly.

Often, when you note a restriction to the free gliding of the dural tube, it can be corrected by continuing the same traction for a few minutes. Otherwise, a particular technique may be required for a particular restriction. Post-operative adhesions affecting the mobility of the dural tube may be successfully treated by multiple repetitions of the CV-4 technique. Gradually, increased fluid pressure seems to break down the adhesions. The CV-4 in these cases can be performed daily. Either the patient or a family member can be taught to apply the technique (APPENDIX F).

From the sacrococcygeal end of the dural tube, the technique is essentially the same. First, the sacrum and coccyx must be free to move in relationship to their adnexa and articulations. Commonly, the coccyx is restricted in an anterior position and may require gentle mobilization by placing a finger in the anal canal to release the coccyx posteriorly. Sacroiliac and lumbosacral joint dysfunctions are also common. Traditional techniques to mobilize the sacroiliac joint are usually satisfactory (MITCHELL 1979). The common lumbosacral compression ordinarily requires a decompression technique which can be applied in combination with the examination (CHAPTER 8). Another frequent cause of sacral immobility is hypertonus of the piriformis muscle (CHAPTER 8). This condition must also be resolved before good sacral motion, and hence free dural tube motion, can be obtained.

Decompression of the lumbosacral junction is performed with the patient supine and the therapist's arm placed between the patient's legs. Rest the sacrum so that the apex is in the palm of your hand, and the sacral spine is between your third and fourth fingers. Your fingertips should be placed just above the sacral base. Place your other hand under the patient's lumbar spine so that you are stabilizing the spines of the 5th lumbar and above. Now lightly apply traction in a caudad direction upon the sacrum while you hold the lumbar spines stable (ILLUSTRATION 6-22).

First, disengage or decompress L-5 and S-1. The sacrum will then attempt to float caudad and anterior at the apex. If the sacroiliac joints seem to impede the progress of the sacral floating, have the patient apply light medial pressure upon the anterior superior iliac spines with his or her hands. This pressure will tend to disengage the sacroiliacs posteriorly (ILLUSTRATION 6-23).

As the lumbosacral and sacroiliac joints disengage, the sacrum will begin to drift caudad in response to your *very gentle,* urging traction. As this phenomenon occurs, it will carry the dural tube with it via the cauda equina. Try to perceive how far up the dural tube your force is working. When you meet a restriction to the glide of the dural tube within the bony vertebral canal, you will then have an idea of where the restriction is.

When two therapists are working together, one on the occiput and one on the sacrum, the dural tube can be gently glided in one direction and then the other. The traction on one end can always be felt by the therapist on the other end.

Remember: the traction is light but steady. Do not elicit a tissue guarding response. A little force over a long period of time has just as much effect as a larger force over a short period of time. The difference is that the gentle force does not elicit resistance in the body, whereas the greater force does elicit such resistance against which the therapist must then work—usually without success.

TECHNIQUES FOR BALANCING HORIZONTAL DURAL MEMBRANES

The horizontally oriented structures of the membrane system may be divided into four parts: (1) temporal to temporal; (2) parietal to parietal; (3) occipital squamous to occipital squamous; and (4) foramen magnum to sacrum.

The temporal to temporal influence upon the two leaves of the tentorium cerebelli utilizes the generous and extensive attachments of the periphery of the tentoria to the petrous ridges of the temporal bones and to the internal aspects of the mastoid processes (ILLUSTRATION 6-24). At the medial regions of the petrous attachments, bear in mind that the anterior medial-most portions of the tentoria cerebelli are attached to the clinoid processes of the sphenoid. This arrangement creates a direct non-osseous functional connection between the sphenoid and the temporal bones. We alluded to this contact earlier in the chapter in the course of discussing the anterior-posterior oriented structures of the intracranial dural membrane system. When the sphenoid is used to create traction in the membranes anteriorly, the effect is also felt in the temporal petrous regions as an anterior force.

In the evaluation and treatment of the horizontal or transverse balance of the leaves of the tentorium cerebelli, the first technique utilizes the temporomandibular joint technique described in Chapter 12 (ILLUSTRATION 6-25). This technique is carried beyond its effect upon the temporomandibular joints and the temporoparietal sutures (APPENDIX G).

The cephalad traction upon the mandible first compresses the temporomandibular joints bilaterally, then affects the temporoparietal sutures by moving

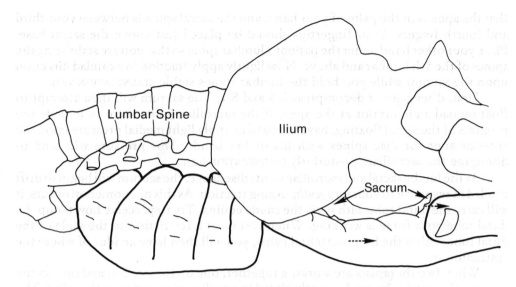

Illustration 6-22
Hand Position for Decompression
of the Lumbo-Sacral Junction

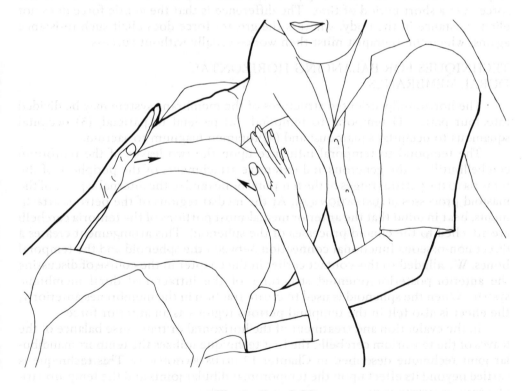

Illustration 6-23
Patient Assistance in the Disengagement
of the Sacrum from the Ilia

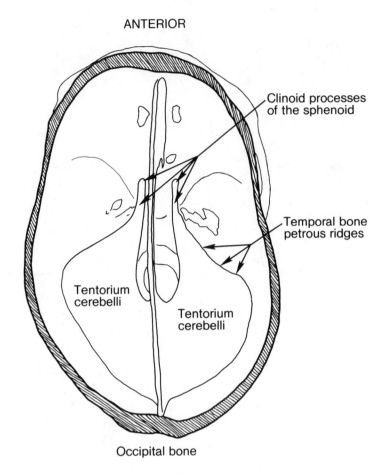

Illustration 6-24
Attachments of the Tentorium Cerebelli

the temporal squama cephalad. This force also causes the temporal squama in their superior boundaries to spread laterally. A nonphysiological shear is induced at the suture. The parietals are moved cephalad. The falx cerebri is now tractioned cephalad as a secondary functional parietal lift is induced by the temporoparietal sutural shear. As the falx cerebri resists the upward traction, the parietals are called into external rotation around the axes (ILLUSTRATION 6-26).

When you have reached this point, the mandible and temporals will begin to wobble side-to-side as you gradually achieve a horizontal balance among the leaves of the tentorium cerebelli, the temporal bones, the lateral components of the parietal bones and ultimately the falx cerebri as it affects and is affected by its attachment at the straight sinus. A closed circle is now formed with the leaves of the tentorium cerebelli.

If the traction is gently continued long enough, information about the balance of the occiput, the foramen magnum, the dural tube and the sacrum and coccyx may be obtained.

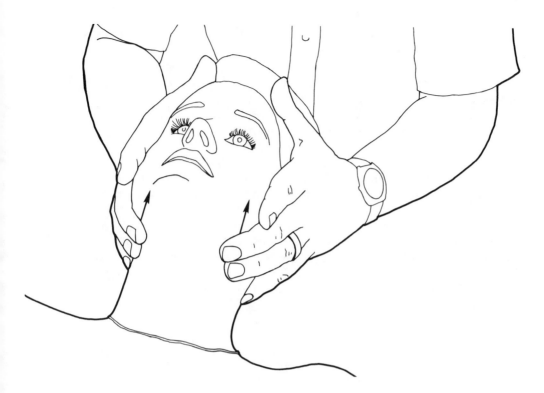

Illustration 6-25
Hand Position for Cephalad Mandibular Traction

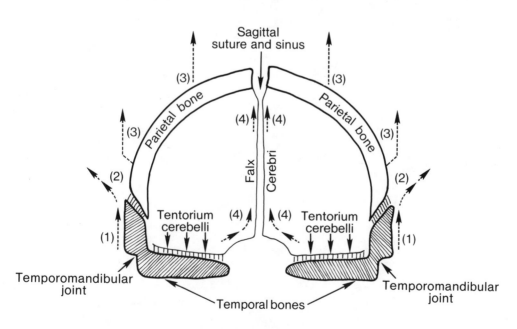

Illustration 6-26
Effects of Mandibular Traction

The membrane-balancing activity seems to begin closest to the therapist after osseous restrictions have been resolved. First the tent is elevated; this will move fluid about the intracranial space, from the spaces above the tentorium to the spaces below it. After the tentorium is balanced horizontally, the effect of the falx cerebri and the falx cerebelli can be perceived. Then the presence of the foramen magnum and finally the dural tube in its lateral aspects all the way to the sacrum can be felt. Close your eyes as you gently continue this traction until you can feel the whole membrane system balanced.

After balance has been achieved using cephalad traction on the mandible, we next use caudad traction over the angles of the mandible (ILLUSTRATION 6-27). Use enough pressure with your fingers placed on the patient's skin to prevent sliding. Your fingers should not move relative to the skin. The skin over the angle of the mandible is moved caudad. The underside of the skin is rooted to the bone surface of the mandible. Once the slack has been taken up, the traction on the skin will be transmitted to the mandible. The palms of your hands should gently rest over the patient's temporal squamous regions to monitor subsequent activity.

The caudad traction causes the temporomandibular joints to disengage. This will usually occur rather easily because the earlier stages of this technique have

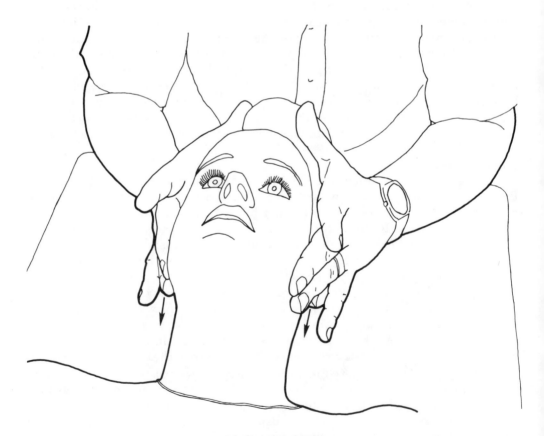

Illustration 6-27
Hand Position for Caudad Mandibular Traction

affected these joints and thus prepared the way for articular mobilization. The disengagement of the temporomandibular joints can be readily palpated by resting your hand gently on the side of the patient's head.

The mandible will usually then begin to sway side-to-side as it achieves a new and improved balance with the temporals. As traction is gently continued, the temporoparietal sutures begin to disengage. Then the lateral aspects of the temporal bones begin to move slightly caudad. At this point, the temporal bones will often begin to sway side-to-side, forming a parallelogram first in one direction, then in the opposite direction.

As the temporoparietal sutures disengage, the side-to-side swinging of the temporal squama continues as the temporal bones move caudad. This change in placement lowers the leaves of the tentorium cerebelli and imposes traction first upon the straight sinus and then upon the falx cerebri.

The supratentorial intracranial compartment is enlarged, and new fluid is sucked into the space by negative pressure. All of this can be perceived if you will listen carefully to your hands. As the fluid redistributes itself, a new horizontal balance of the mechanisms is achieved and the side-to-side swinging of the mandible and temporals will stop. The whole mechanism seems then to settle into a new and balanced pattern of reduced membrane tension.

The technique for balancing the leaves of the tentorium cerebelli between the parietal bones is very similar to the technique described for the temporals. However, the finger contact of the therapist is upon the parietal bones, and specific attention is given to raising the posterior inferior portions of these bones since this is where the tentorium cerebelli attaches to them. Using this technique, the parietal bones must be free of osseous and sutural restriction for the membranes to become effectively balanced. We cannot honestly cite, in our own experience, a single instance when our first choice has been to use the parietal contact to balance the tentorium cerebelli horizontally. You should, however, be aware of the technique in case the need arises in your own experience. This technique does favorably affect the transverse sinuses.

Balancing the tentorium cerebelli by use of the occipital squama is based upon the attachment of those membranes to the internal occipital ridge. Usually the occiput has been subjected to undue tension by extracranial force, such as cervical muscle hypertonus. In turn, the occiput places imbalanced tension upon the tentorium cerebelli. However, in a significant number of cases, imbalanced tension upon one or the other sides of the tentorium from within causes recurrent extracranial occipital somatic dysfunctions.

The occiput must first be freed of all abnormal tensions placed upon it by extrinsic muscles. It must be floated free from any restriction with the atlas (CHAPTER 10). The lambdoidal and occipitomastoid sutures must also be free to move. These sutures include not only those located in the external vault, but also those in the cranial base. Once these restrictions have been alleviated, the occiput is used much like a steering wheel to achieve the position of optimum balance in relationship to the attachments of the leaves of the tentorium cerebelli and the two falxes as they attach to the internal surface of the occiput.

In order to achieve this balance, we usually place the occiput in the palm of one hand and place the other hand either under the neck or over the bregma area of the head. Motion is encouraged between the two hands to achieve a relaxed balance.

The horizontal or transverse balance between the foramen magnum and the sacrum is achieved with both hands simultaneously, as though you were operating two pulleys connected by a belt. To equalize tension in both pulleys, you must cope with the belt tension as well as the separate tensions imposed upon each of the pulleys by their respective loads.

It is suggested that you place one hand under the occiput and the other hand under the sacrum. The patient is supine, lying on your hands. The occiput is one pulley; the sacrum is the other. The drive belt is the lateral ring formed by the dural tube (ILLUSTRATIONS 6-28 and 6-29).

You must then induce a rotational motion in either end and perceive the effect on the other end. As you induce rotations in both directions and upon both pulleys, the system will seem to loosen up. As the loosening occurs, you will notice a quicker and more complete transmission of the rotational force induced at one end to the other end of the system.

You should also be able to notice if external loads are restricting the free motion of either the sacrum or the occiput. These must be treated. Ultimately, when

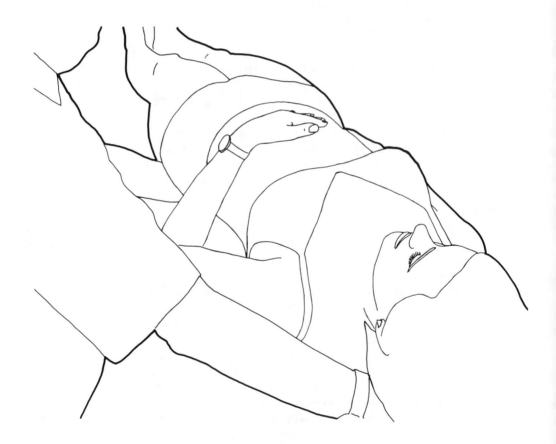

Illustration 6-28
Hand Position for Balancing of Sacrum
and Occiput with Patient Supine

free movement has been established for both occiput (foramen magnum) and sacrum, and when the message is transmitted without distortion from one end of the system to the other, the whole system will seem to settle into a position of very relaxed balance. The treatment is thus completed.

We hope that it is now apparent to you that diagnosis and treatment of the craniosacral system and its related systems require total integration of all possible approaches. Fragmentation is artificial. Yet, for purposes of explanation and understanding, we have had to separate and analyze. We have tried to make these separations along natural boundaries. Keep in mind, however, that in this type of hands-on work, one technique leads to another, and the progression of events is always dictated by the second-to-second and minute-to-minute patient responses to your ministrations.

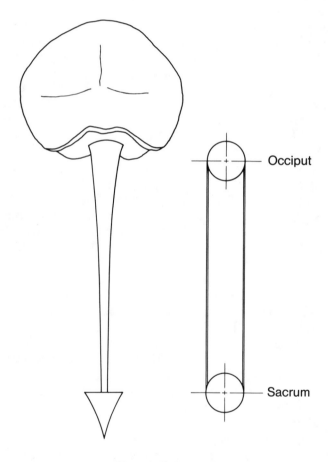

Illustration 6-29
Occiput and Sacrum as Pulleys

Chapter 7
Dysfunctions of the Cranial Base

The superior surface of the cranial base serves as the floor of the home in which the human brain develops and lives. It is the quality of the physiological and functional environment of the brain's habitat which can most be influenced by treatment directed at the craniosacral system. The floor of the cranial cavity is a frequent source of craniosacral system dysfunction. Under normal circumstances, this floor moves minutely yet freely and rhythmically in response to, and in accommodation of the rise and fall of cerebrospinal fluid pressure.

The osseous components of the cranial base are the frontal, ethmoid, sphenoid, temporal, and occipital bones (ILLUSTRATION 7-1).

In common with most floors in modern homes, the cranial cavity floor has a durable, flexible and long-wearing covering. This covering is dura mater. It is continuous up the sides of the cranial cavity and forms its interior ceiling cover. The same dura mater floor covering duplicates upon itself to form partitions: the falx cerebelli, which arises from the occiput; the falx cerebri, which arises from both the occipital and the frontal bone contributions to this floor; and the tentorium cerebelli, which arises from the occiput, the posterior inferior portions of the parietal bones and the temporal bones. It forms a second-story floor for the brain's residence. The dural membrane also attaches to all four clinoid processes of the sphenoid bone. Through the foramen magnum, the dural covering of the floor of the cranial cavity is continuous with the spinal dural tube (ILLUSTRATION 7-2).

This brief description of the dural floor covering and its continuities indicates the powerful functional interrelationships among the cranial base, the calvarium and the spinal dural tube with its attachments. Because of its firm osseous attachments, the dural floor covering contributes significantly to holding this floor together. However, it still allows for small but free movements with some flexibility.

The dural membrane which adheres to the whole interior of the cranial cavity affords passage to the various venous sinuses: the sagittal sinuses, the transverse sinuses, the occipital sinus, the petrous sinuses, and the straight sinus. The dural membrane transmits tension from any source through itself in a direction dictated by its geometry and its attachments (ILLUSTRATION 7-3). It is therefore not difficult to imagine abnormal membrane tensions interfering with normal cranial bone motion and with free blood flow through this venous sinus system. Interference with venous

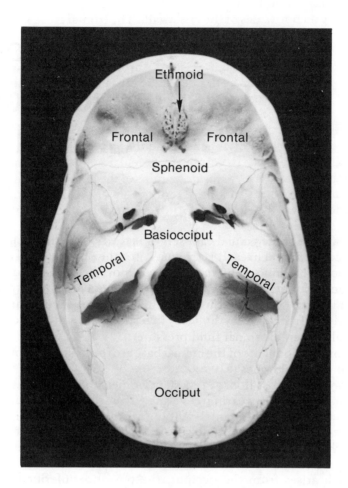

Illustration 7-1
Cranial Base

sinus drainage may result in increased intracranial venous back pressure, which will then reduce normal fresh blood delivery to the brain. It may also raise cerebrospinal fluid pressure slightly but significantly and thereby interfere with the normal movement of this vital fluid through the ventricular system of the brain and through the various subdural spaces.

THE CRANIAL BASE FOSSAE: ANATOMY

The floor of the cranial cavity forms the anterior, middle and posterior cranial fossae.

The floor of the anterior cranial fossa is formed by the orbital plates of the frontal bone, the cribriform plate of the ethmoid bone and the lesser wings and anterior body of the sphenoid bone. Its posterior boundary is the posterior borders of the lesser wings and the anterior margin of the chiasmatic groove of the sphenoid.

The frontal fossa is traversed by the frontoethmoidal and frontosphenoidal sutures. Its lateral parts support the frontal lobes of the brain. The median portion is the roof of the nasal cavity on both sides of the crista galli. The frontal crest, which ends at the foramen cecum, offers attachment to the falx cerebri and a groove for the superior sagittal sinus, which is afforded passage by this falx. Usually, a vein passes from the nasal cavity to the superior sagittal sinus through the foramen cecum. The cribriform plates are located on both sides of the crista galli; these plates support the olfactory bulb and afford passage to the olfactory and nasociliary nerves (ILLUSTRATION 7-4).

The middle cranial fossa traverses the cranial base between the temporal squama, the greater wings of the sphenoid and the sphenoidal angles of the parietal bones bilaterally. These bony structures form its lateral boundaries. The anterior boundaries of this fossa are the posterior margins of the lesser wings of the sphenoid, the anterior clinoid processes and the anterior ridge of the chiasmatic groove. The posterior boundaries are the superior portion of the petrous ridges of the temporal bones and the dorsum sellae.

The middle cranial fossa contains the chiasmatic groove, which stretches between the optic foramena anteriorly and the tuberculum sellae posteriorly. Posterior to the optic foramen, bilaterally, are the anterior clinoid processes which give attachment to the inferior layers of the tentorium cerebelli. Immediately posterior to the tuberculum sellae is the sella turcica, in which the pituitary

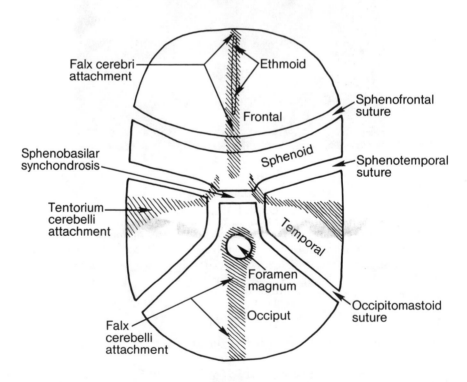

Illustration 7-2
Floor of Cranial Cavity with Osseous Attachments of
the Two Falxes and Tentorium Cerebelli

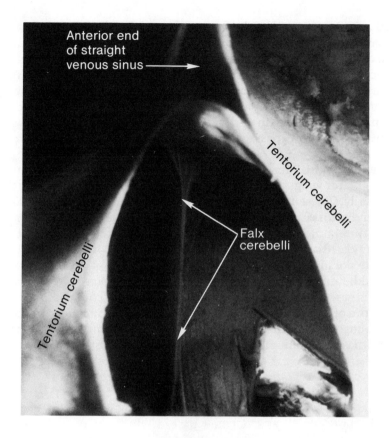

Illustration 7-3
Fibrous Changes in Dura

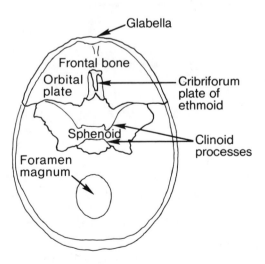

Illustration 7-4
Frontal Fossa

(hypophysis) gland is located. The posterior boundary of the hypophyseal fossa, as the entire depression is called, is the dorsum sellae. The dorsum sellae is a quadrilateral plate of bone oriented more or less vertically, the superior lateral angles of which are the posterior clinoid processes. These processes offer attachment for the superior layers of the tentorium cerebelli. Below each posterior clinoid process is the notch for the abducent nerve (C.N. VI). Alongside the sella turcica, bilaterally, are the carotid grooves which extend from the foramena lacerum to the medial sides of the anterior clinoid processes. The foramen lacerum passes the great superficial petrosal nerve. This foramen is actually a fibrocartilagenous opening between the great wing of the sphenoid and the petrous part of the temporal bone (ILLUSTRATION 7-5).

Research has shown that the great superficial petrosal nerve has significant effect upon the arterial blood supply to the occipital lobes of the brain (OWMAN and EDVINSSON 1977). Therefore, dysfunction between the sphenoid and temporal bones which interferes with the normal dynamic anatomy of the foramen lacerum may interfere with occipital lobe circulation and, thereby, its function.

The deep lateral regions of the middle cranial fossa are known as the temporal fossae. They support the temporal lobes of the brain. They are grooved for the passage of the anterior and posterior branches of the middle meningeal arteries and veins. The recurrent branches of the mandibular branch of the trigeminal nerve (C.N. V) and the middle meningeal artery pass through the foramen spinosum. Also located in these fossae are the superior orbital fissures which are between the greater and lesser sphenoid wings and the orbital plates of the frontal bone. These fissures afford passage to the oculomotor nerve (C.N. III), trochlear nerve (C.N.IV), opthalmic branch of the trigeminal nerve (C.N. V) and the abducent nerve (C.N. VI) as well as the opthalmic veins. Cranial base dysfunction involving the superior orbital fissure can (and often does) result in motor disturbances and venous engorgement of the eye.

Also located in the temporal fossae, bilaterally, are the foramen rotundum, which affords passage to the maxillary division of the trigeminal nerve (C.N. V); the foramen ovale, which affords passage to the mandibular division of the trigeminal nerve (C.N. V), the meningeal artery and the emissary vein; the foramen spinosum, which affords passage to recurrent branches of the mandibular division of the trigeminal nerve (C.N. V) and the middle meningeal artery; the foramen lacerum, which affords passage to the great superficial petrosal nerve; and the internal carotid artery with its sympathetic nerve plexus which passes across the superior part of the foramen lacerum. The foramen lacerum is filled with fibrocartilage which is pierced by a small nerve from the pterygoid canal and by a small meningeal branch from the ascending pharyngeal artery. The orifice of the carotid canal is located in the temporal bone over the roof of the tympanic cavity.

The posterior cranial fossa is larger and deeper than the anterior and middle fossae. It is bounded by the dorsum sellae, the sphenoid, the occiput, the petrous and mastoid parts of the temporal bone and the posterior inferior parts of the parietal bones. It is crossed by the occipitomastoid and the parietomastoid sutures. It houses the cerebellum, the pons and the medulla oblongata. It is separated from the middle cranial fossa by the dorsum sella and by the petrous ridges of the temporal bones. The tentorium cerebelli and its venous sinuses form the roof of the posterior cranial fossa. It is partially divided in its median plane by the falx cerebelli

(ILLUSTRATION 7-6).

In the center, located in the occiput, is the foramen magnum. On either side of the foramen magnum are the hypoglossal canals, which are situated in rough tubercles. The foramen magnum affords passage to the inferior medulla (as it becomes the spinal cord), the meningeal membranes (the dura is firmly attached to occipital bone at the foramen magnum), the spinal accessory nerve (C.N. XI), the

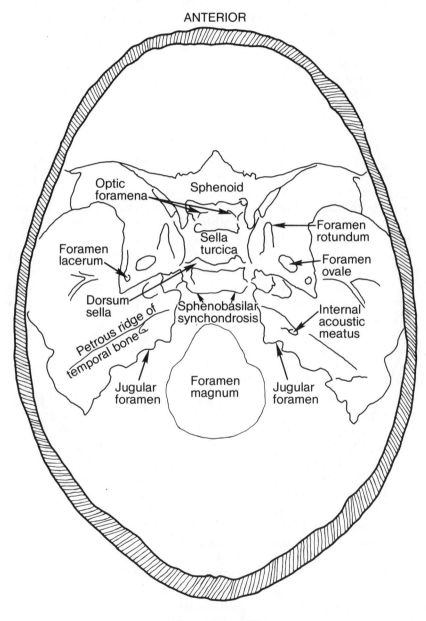

ANTERIOR

Optic foramena

Sphenoid

Foramen rotundum

Sella turcica

Foramen lacerum

Foramen ovale

Dorsum sella

Sphenobasilar synchondrosis

Internal acoustic meatus

Petrous ridge of temporal bone

Jugular foramen

Foramen magnum

Jugular foramen

Illustration 7-5
Middle Cranial Fossa

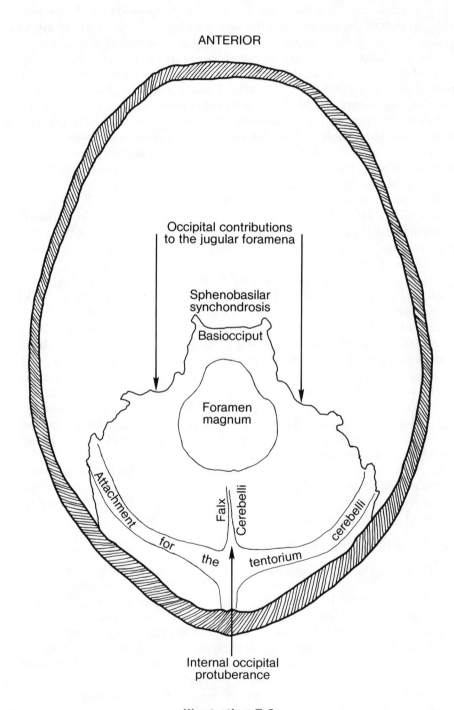

Illustration 7-6
Posterior Cranial Fossa

vertebral arteries, the hypoglossal nerve (C.N. XII) and the posterior meningeal arteries.

Anterior to the foramen magnum is the sphenobasilar synchondrosis, where the basilar part of the occiput and the posterior body of the sphenoid are joined by cartilage. The medulla oblongata rests over this sphenooccipital union.

The jugular foramena are between the petrous temporal bones and lateral aspects of the occipital base. These foramena are located just lateral to the externally placed occipital condyles. They afford passage to the glossopharyngeal nerve (C.N. IX), vagus nerve (C.N. X), and spinal accessory nerve (C.N. XI). They also transmit inferior petrosal and transverse venous sinuses which drain directly into the jugular veins. Meningeal vessels also pass through these foramena.

In dysfunction of the craniosacral system, the jugular foramena are extremely important. Tissue change in the regions of these foramena can result from cervical muscle hypertonus, somatic dysfunction of the occipital condyles, cranial base dysfunction and tension transmitted to the foramen magnum via the dural tube from below or above via the falx cerebelli and/or the tentorium cerebelli. Interference with normal function of the jugular foramena results in intracranial fluid congestion due to venous back pressure, and symptoms resultant to dysfunction of cranial nerves IX, X, XI and XII (APPENDIX D).

Also located in the posterior cranial fossa superior to the jugular foramena are the internal acoustic meati through which pass the facial nerve (C.N. VII), the acoustic nerves and the internal auditory arteries.

The internal occipital crest divides the inferior occipital fossae, which support the cerebellar hemispheres. This crest is the attachment for the falx cerebelli, which separates the cerebellar hemispheres and houses the occipital venous sinus. Tension upon this falx can interfere with the free passage of venous blood through this sinus.

The occiput also forms deep grooves for the transverse venous sinuses where the tentorium cerebelli attaches. These grooves are the posterior boundaries of the posterior fossae. The transverse venous sinuses drain through the jugular foramena. Thus, tension upon the tentorium cerebelli can further interfere with good venous drainage from within the cranial vault.

From this brief review of the pertinent anatomy, it should be apparent that dysfunction of the membranes or osseous structures of the craniosacral system may, and frequently does have far-reaching and often seemingly bizarre effects upon the function of the nervous, venous and endocrine systems.

CRANIAL BASE DYSFUNCTION

Originally, Dr. Sutherland held that cranial base dysfunctions were predominantly osseous in nature. This conceptual model works both in diagnosis and treatment and is presented herein as the traditional concept of cranial base and, more specifically, of sphenobasilar joint dysfunction (SUTHERLAND 1939).

However, as noted in Chapter 2, the sphenobasilar joint is a synchondrosis, not a symphysis. This means that motion at the joint, especially shearing motion, is more limited than that proposed by Dr. Sutherland (ILLUSTRATION 7-7). We believe that motion distortion of the cranial base is usually caused by abnormal soft tissue or dural membrane tensions which are transmitted to their osseous anchorings. Another significant cause may be suture immobility. These abnormal membrane and soft tissue tensions and sutural restrictions result in distortions of the normal

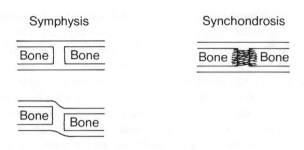

Illustration 7-7
Comparison of Movements Possible at a
Symphysis and Synchondrosis

motion which we have come to expect from the bones involved in the function (or dysfunction) of the craniosacral system. The further away from the sphenobasilar joint external forces on either of the bones act, the greater is the leverage exerted by them. Therefore, we would suggest that contracture of the trapezius muscle, for example, will cause a more pronounced distortion of cranial base motion via the occiput and temporal bones than will a contracture of the splenius capitis muscle, which attaches more closely to the sphenobasilar synchondrosis.

This difference of opinion between your authors and traditional cranial teachings becomes clinically significant when the physician is searching for the causes underlying craniosacral system dysfunction. Correction of osseous dysfunction is often temporary. The dysfunction continues to recur until the physician identifies and successfully treats the cause of abnormal soft tissue or dural membrane tensions. This cause may ultimately be found in the abdominal cavity, in an extremity or elsewhere in the patient. We cannot and should not attempt to limit the scope of our investigation to the confines of the craniosacral system alone.

We believe that it is a rare circumstance when the sphenobasilar synchondrosis motion aberration is of primary etiologic nature. Rather, we prefer to think of the cranial base as a unit which demonstrates motion dysfunctions secondary to sutural immobility, abnormal dural membrane tensions or other soft tissue tensions. The tensions are exerted upon significant osseous anchorings from both within and without the cranial vault and the spinal vertebral canal. Cranial base dysfunctions can also result from abnormal craniosacral system fluid dynamics and other, as yet unidentified causes.

EXAMINATION TECHNIQUES FOR THE CRANIAL BASE: VAULT HOLDS

We use three different hand positions to evaluate the quality and geometry of cranial base motion. The first two of these "vault holds," as they have traditionally been called, were described by Dr. Sutherland (MAGOUN 1966). The third is a modification which one of the authors has found to be most useful in view of the particular size and sensitivities of his hands. We suggest that the student of craniosacral system technique develop skill in the use of all three of these vault holds, and then develop a modification which is personally most satisfactory. We believe it is essential that you develop several workable approaches to each problem. Understanding of the total dysfunction is crucial. The therapy can then be designed or improvised individually for each patient. The most frequent and serious errors are committed when the patient's problem is forced to conform to a preconceived model of the therapist.

In the first vault hold (ILLUSTRATION 7-8), your index fingers are gently applied to the areas overlying the external surfaces of the great wings of the sphenoid, bilaterally. Your fifth fingers rest bilaterally in contact with the occipital squama approximately one-half inch medial to the occipitomastoid suture and slightly above the superior nuchal line. Some slight differences in the placement of these fingers may result if the therapist has small hands, or if the patient's head is relatively large in size. This will not interfere with the proprioceptive cues that can be perceived, however.

The third and fourth (middle and ring) fingers of your hands are *not* in direct contact with the head and do not participate in gathering information during the examination. Likewise, the thumbs do not contact the patient's head, but only touch each other. The thumbs serve to provide proprioceptive and kinesthetic cues about the quality and symmetry of motion of the therapist's hands. Movements in one direction are compared with reciprocal movements in the opposite direction.

The patient is positioned comfortably and usually supine on the examining table. You are seated behind the patient's head with your forearms resting comfortably on the table. Usually, resting your elbows on the table improves proprioception and is more comfortable for the therapist. *Comfort for both yourself and your patient is essential.* When you are tense, you receive stimulus input from your own body which becomes noise and interferes with perceiving the more subtle inputs from the patient. A tense, uncomfortable patient presents an increased tonus of body soft tissues. This circumstance dampens the gentle inherent motions originating in the craniosacral system which you are trying to evaluate. Although the evaluation can be performed with a tense patient, it requires a higher level of expertise on the part of the therapist. And even a very experienced therapist may not perceive a true picture under adverse circumstances.

The second vault hold was also described by Dr. Sutherland (ILLUSTRATION 7-9). Usually, patient and therapist are positioned as above. Your hands are placed so that the patient's occiput is held in one of your hands. Your other hand is placed so that the thumb overlies the area of one great wing of the sphenoid and the fifth finger overlies the opposite great wing.

Some would advise against allowing the remainder of your hand to rest upon the patient's head. However, we have experienced no difficulty when there is gentle contact between the frontal bone and the palm of the hand. In fact, with practice, much information can be obtained simultaneously about both frontal and sphenoidal bone motion when this contact is made. We suggest that both methods be explored.

The third vault hold (ILLUSTRATION 7-10) is a modification which evolved quite naturally for one of your authors (Upledger). It provides the maximum amount of information about the whole craniosacral system in the shortest amount of time. In the application of this vault hold, the patient is supine and the therapist is comfortably seated at the patient's head. Your fingers and thumbs are "fanned out" so that the fifth fingers are in contact with the patient's occipital squama. The fourth fingers are in contact with the occiput, just posterior to the occipitomastoid sutures. The third fingers are applied to the mastoid processes of the temporal bones with the

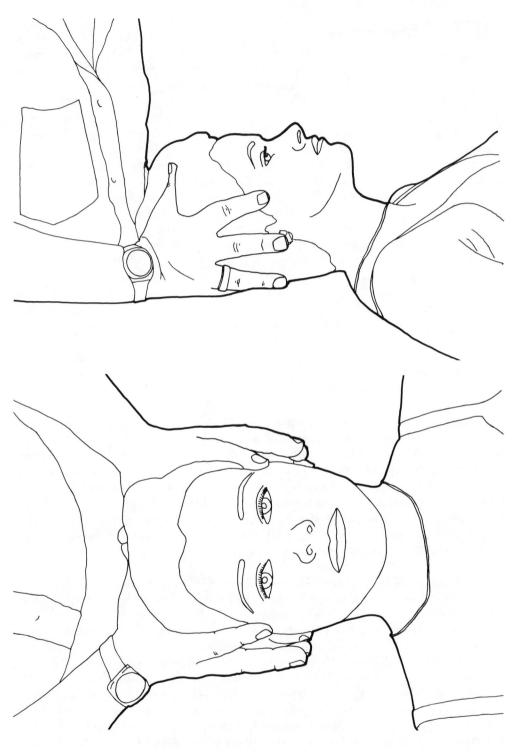

Illustration 7-8
First Vault Hold

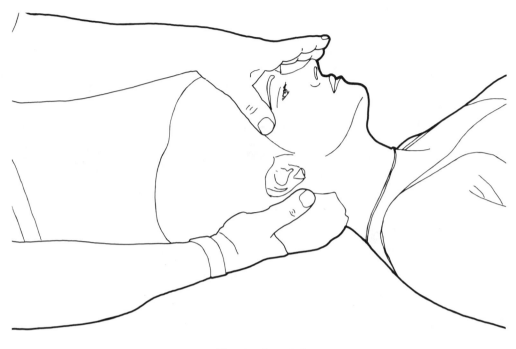

Illustration 7-9
Second Vault Hold

fingertips running inferiorly over the mastoid tips. Neither your fourth or third fingers actually overlay the occipitomastoid sutures. These fingers parallel the suture on both sides. The patient's external ear pinna is straddled by the space between your third and index fingers. The index fingers are allowed to rest anterior to the ear so that their tips approximately overlay the temporomandibular joints bilaterally, depending, of course, upon head size and finger length. Your thumbs are placed over the region of the great sphenoid wings, while your palms are allowed to gently rest over the temporal squama, the temporoparietal sutures and the parietal bones. I (Upledger) have found this hand application most convenient and flexible because:

1. I can examine for classical sphenobasilar joint dysfunctions (described below) by attending to my fingerpads upon the occipital squama and my thumbpads over the great wings of the sphenoid.
2. If I attend to my third and fourth fingers, I can evaluate occipitomastoid suture motion, gain a sense of the activity at the jugular foramen, and evaluate temporal bone motion by attending to the activity of the mastoid processes, mastoid tips and, very often, the transverse processes of the atlas.
3. My index fingers transmit information related to the temporomandibular joints, the anterior temporal bone, the zygomatic processes and the mandible.
4. My thumbs, of course, are in a position to evaluate sphenoid activity.
5. The finger bases and palms of the hands provide input about the temporal squama, the movements of the parietal bones, the activity of the sutures which intersect at pterion and asterion, the coronal suture, the temporoparietal

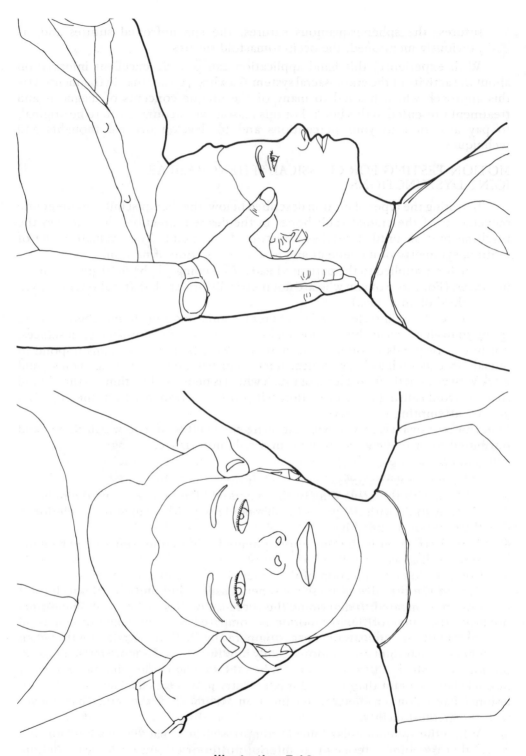

Illustration 7-10
Third Vault Hold

sutures, the sphenosquamous sutures, the sphenofrontal sutures and, as previously mentioned, the occipitomastoid sutures.

With experience, this hand application can provide excellent information about the activity of the craniosacral system as a whole, rather than in fragments. It is this approach which has led to many of the unique concepts of diagnosis and treatment presented in this book. For this reason, we encourage you to be original, to pay attention to your perceptions and to develop original thoughts and techniques.

MOTION TESTING FOR CLASSICAL SPHENOBASILAR JOINT DYSFUNCTIONS

In testing the types of motion described below, the therapist initiates the gentle movements of the cranial vault bones in the desired direction, then *monitors* the resulting motion until it reaches a restricted end point. You evaluate range of motion, symmetry of movement and ease or restriction of motion.

The force applied to the patient's head is exceedingly light, 5-10 grams in most instances. (For those of you who are not metrically oriented, that is about one-sixth to one-third of an ounce.)

Greater force interferes with inherent cranial motion. Remember, you are trying to evaluate what this craniosacral system does under normal circumstances, not how it responds to outside interference. Most biological systems respond to outside threats such as heavy touch, traction or pain, by contracting. You should work with your patients at a level of touch which is beneath this stimulus threshhold so as to avoid causing the contraction-self-protective response from the organism you are attempting to observe.

The motions which you will test using the vault hold, and which Sutherland attributed to the sphenobasilar joint or synchondrosis are:

1. Flexion-extension.
2. Sidebending with convexity to the left or to the right.
3. Torsion with the great wing of the sphenoid high on the left or the right.
4. Vertical strain with the posterior sphenoid body either superior or inferior to the anterior occipital base.
5. Lateral strain with the posterior sphenoid body either left or right of the anterior basiocciput.
6. Compression or impaction of the sphenobasilar joint/synchondrosis.

Among the first five of these six sphenobasilar joint motions, the reciprocal motions are compared to determine the presence of "lesion" or motion dysfunction; i.e., the range of flexion motion is compared with the range of extension motion. Traditional cranial concept as originated by Dr. Sutherland states that when the sphenobasilar joint moves more readily into flexion and is more resistant to extension, it is called a "flexion lesion." When the sphenobasilar joint moves further into left lateral strain than into right lateral strain, it is called a "left lateral strain lesion." The lesion is named for the direction toward which the cranial base moves with the greatest facility.

When the sphenobasilar joint is compressed or impacted, examination will reveal that the joint is resistant to anterior-posterior expansion or disimpaction. There is thus no real reciprocal motion for use as a comparison. The diagnosis must be made on the basis of the therapist's experience with compressed and non-compressed patients. As your experience grows, you will gain confidence and sharpen your diagnostic acumen.

When testing for flexion or extension, the therapist should always first lay hands on, tune in and join the inherent motion of the patient. Testing for flexion or extension should only be done as the patient's body is itself moving into the flexion or extension phase, respectively. Do not attempt to initiate a flexion movement while the patient is moving into extension, or to initiate an extension movement while the patient is moving into flexion.

There is a neutral or relaxed period of time between each reciprocal motion of flexion and extension. That is, before entering the flexion phase of motion, there is a brief time of relaxed neutrality following the return from the extension phase of motion, and vice versa. It is the excursion from neutrality to the end of the range of motion which you, the therapist, will evaluate. You simply apply a little push or boost as the patient's craniosacral system moves from neutral into one or the other of the active ranges of motion. You then evaluate the response to the push or boost.

In the perfectly functioning craniosacral system, flexion and extension are the only normal sphenobasilar joint motions which are occurring when the subject is in a relaxed, supine position. However, the sphenobasilar joint/cranial base will allow for a little gently-induced, extrinsically-originated torsion, sidebending, vertical strain, lateral strain and compression-decompression. It is how much of each of these motions the craniosacral base will permit which is of interest to the therapist and which is, therefore, the subject of the testing procedures described below.

Cranial base motion patterns are positionally inducible. While you are monitoring the cranial motion, ask another person to raise or rotate one of your subject's extremities (either upper or lower). Observe what changes occur in cranial motion. A little experimentation in this manner will begin to afford the therapist an appreciation of the delicate integrity of the human body and of the significance of connective tissue tonus and tension.

Sphenobasilar/Cranial Base Flexion-Extension

Using one of the vault holds described above, exert a gentle force over the occipital squama and great wings of the sphenoid concurrently. This force is directed toward the patient's feet. When you use the first vault hold, the third and fourth fingers are not in use; the thumbs are in contact with each other and furnish proprioceptive and kinesthetic cues so that your force will be applied as equally and symmetrically as possible. After the cranium has responded to the initiating force (on the order of 5 grams), you become passive and follow the cranial motion to its restricted end point. Flexion at the sphenobasilar union is the postulated motion which is being tested. That is, the angle formed by the basiocciput and the sphenoid body becomes more acute. After reaching the end point of the flexion motion, passively follow the sphenoid wings and occipital squama back to a position of neutral balanced ease.

To test the reciprocal motion (extension) of the sphenobasilar joint/cranial base, you apply a similar, bilaterally equal force in a superior cephalad direction toward yourself. Once the motion is initiated, your force is terminated and the motion is passively followed to its restricted end point. This motion implies a lessening of the acuteness of the angle at the sphenobasilar union. Once again, the therapist passively follows the cranial bone motion to a point of neutral balanced ease. The testing may be repeated several times until you are satisfied that your impression is reliable with respect to the relative ease or restriction of the reciprocal motions. The direction *toward* which the motion is restricted is noted; e.g., restriction against the induction of flexion is called an "extension lesion" and vice versa. Always begin your testing force at the onset of the physiological flexion or extension motion, and compare the result with normal motion.

Sutherland postulated, and both the Sutherland Cranial Teaching Foundation and the Cranial Academy have traditionally taught, that the palpable, rhythmic activity perceived on the skull of the subject is the result of changes in the angle formed between the sphenoid body and the occipital base. At the junction of these two bones, the angle formed at the inferior surface of this synchondrosis is less than 180°, while the superior surface of the angle is greater than 180°. During the flexion phase of craniosacral system motion, the number of degrees of the angle formed by the inferior surface decreases. Therefore, the size of the angle formed at the superior surface must increase. The reverse is true during the extension phase of the motion; however, the angle formed by these two bones is never regarded as being a straight line. Also, during the flexion phase, the sphenobasilar joint is said to move slightly cephalad, and during the extension phase, slightly caudad (ILLUSTRATION 7-11). X-ray studies by Greenman lend some support to this idea (APPENDIX H).

SPHENOBASILAR/CRANIAL BASE SIDEBENDING

Sidebending distortions of cranial base motion, we believe, are maintained by an imbalance of tension placed upon the bones of the sphenobasilar joint by one or a combination of factors. The result is that the anterior-posterior distance between the sphenoid great wing and its paired occipital squamous bone on the same side is shorter than on the opposite side. This means that the median sagittal plane through the head is angulated slightly at the sphenobasilar joint. The flexion and extension phases of craniosacral system motion continue, but from a sidebent orientation. When this lesion pattern is discovered, it is called sidebending with convexity either left or right.

The test for sidebending lesion patterns is performed by the application of one of the vault holds described above, but with palm contact on one side to perceive convexity bulging. At the beginning of a flexion phase of the craniosacral motion, the therapist should attempt to gently approximate the occipital squamous and the ipsilateral great wing of the sphenoid. As this gentle approximation is performed, a bulging of the convexity on the opposite side is perceived with the palm of your other hand. The extent of this bulging should be mentally noted. The cranial motion is passively monitored back to neutral, then through the extension phase, and back to neutral again. As the next flexion phase begins, repeat the test on the opposite side. The amount of approximation and convexity bulging at each side of the head is compared. The lesion is named for the side at which the greater bulging convexity is perceived (ILLUSTRATION 7-12).

We repeat: the force applied by the therapist during this test is small (5-10 grams) and initiatory only. Once the sidebending has begun in response to the induced force, you become a passive monitor observing how far it will go. This is *not* a test to see how far you can push it. The sidebending force is induced during the natural origin of the flexion phase of craniosacral motion only. Essentially, you are inducing an exaggerated flexion of the sphenobasilar joint, unilaterally. Normally,

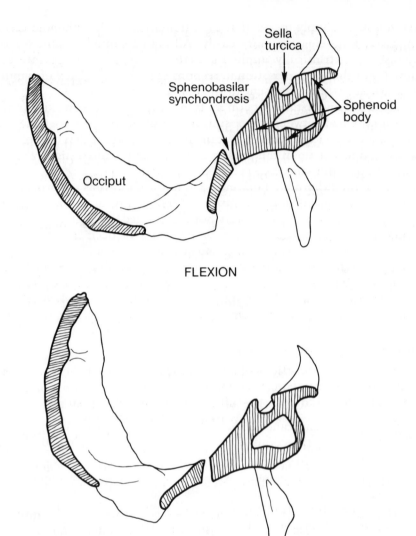

FLEXION

EXTENSION

Illustration 7-11
Flexion and Extension Phases of Craniosacral
Motion Depicted at the Cranial Base

during the flexion phase of motion the occipital squama and the great wings of the sphenoid move closer as the angle at the inferior sphenobasilar surface decreases slightly.

SPHENOBASILAR/CRANIAL BASE TORSION

This lesion is named either right or left for the side on which the great wing of the sphenoid bone moves cephalad with the most ease and excursion. A "right torsion lesion" simply means that the orientation of the sphenoid is such that the right great wing elevates more easily. All crania should exhibit some torsion in response to extrinsically applied initiatory forces. You are interested in the symmetry of the torsion motion in response to your test. Lack of symmetry means that a lesion pattern is present in the cranial base.

To better understand torsion motion, simply imagine an axis running through the patient's head between the posterior occipital protuberance (where the straight venous sinus ends) and glabella anteriorly. Then imagine that the sphenoid is tilted slightly to one side upon this axis, and the occiput is tilted slightly in the opposite direction upon the same axis (ILLUSTRATION 7-13).

The normal rhythmic flexion and extension motions are proceeding as usual, but the cranial base is operating from a torsioned orientation.

To test for torsion, the vault hold is applied. A gentle torsional motion is induced at the great wings of the sphenoid, while the occiput is stabilized relative to any torsional movement. The motion test can be initiated at the beginning of either a flexion or extension phase of craniosacral motion. If your testing force is focused more upon the wing of the sphenoid which is rising cephalad, initiation of the test should be made during the beginning of the extension phase. If you are concentrating more upon the great wing of the sphenoid moving inferiorly, then start the test at the beginning of the flexion phase. You are simply testing to determine the direction of ease toward which cranial base torsion can be induced.

CLINICAL SIGNIFICANCE AND TREATMENT OF FLEXION, SIDEBENDING AND TORSIONAL DISTORTIONS OF CRANIOSACRAL SYSTEM MOTION

The clinical significance and correction of flexion, extension, sidebending and torsional lesions of the cranial base are all discussed together for several reasons:

1. In our experience these lesions are usually secondary to some somatic dysfunction or imbalance which is extrinsic to the craniosacral system. Frequently, flexion, extension, sidebending and torsion dysfunctions of the cranial base are correctable by cranial treatment, but will often return unless the extracraniosacral system problem is itself identified and treated. These cranial base dysfunctions are often self-correcting when the primary dysfunction is remedied. We use the "spontaneous" corrections of abnormal flexion-extension, sidebending and torsion patterns as indicators of the therapeutic effect on the primary, extracraniosacral system problems. Strain and compression of the cranial base often have their origin within the craniosacral system.
2. Craniosacral motion pattern abnormalities are often transient. This is not true of the more severe cranial base strain and compression problems, which are discussed further on. The transient nature of many of these problems may be due to the fact that they are often secondary to temporary changes in the neuromusculoskeletal system. These changes are usually the result of traumas and everyday stresses.
3. Although the dysfunctions of flexion-extension, sidebending and torsion of the cranial base may be symptomatic, they are seldom seriously incapacitating and/or debilitating as may be the case with cranial base strains and compression problems.
4. The correction (at least, the temporary correction) of these lesions can usually

NORMAL

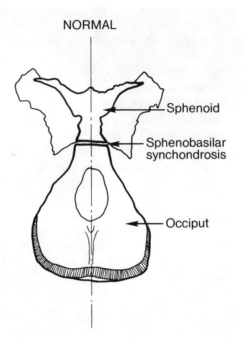

Sphenoid

Sphenobasilar
synchondrosis

Occiput

SIDEBENDING WITH
CONVEXITY RIGHT

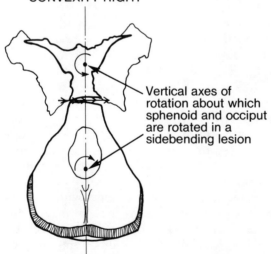

Vertical axes of
rotation about which
sphenoid and occiput
are rotated in a
sidebending lesion

SIDEBENDING WITH
CONVEXITY LEFT

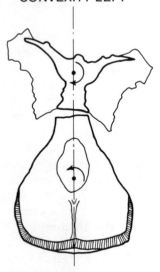

Illustration 7-12
Sidebending Lesion (Top View)

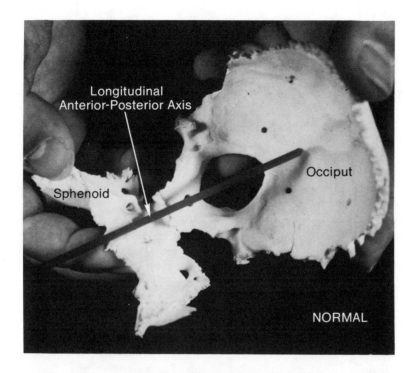

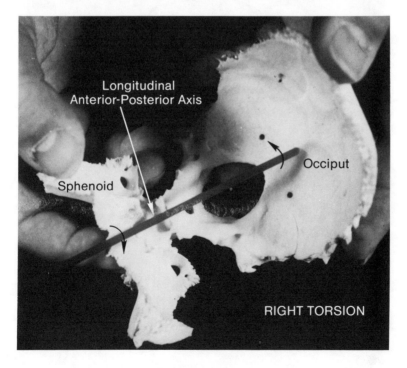

Illustration 7-13
Cranial Base Torsion

be effected by the application of indirect technique without much difficulty. The correction of cranial base strain and compression problems is frequently more difficult and may sometimes require the use of direct techniques with more individual modification in order to achieve success.

Flexion-lesion heads, in general, belong to externally rotated bodies (ILLUS-TRATION 7-14). That is, the extremities will usually be more externally rotated. The walk will often have a slight "waddling" quality, and the head will tend to be transversely wider and proportionately shorter in its anterior-posterior dimension.

The complaints of such flexed-externally rotated patients will often be related to pelvic and lumbosacral instability; annoying but seldom severe headaches; transient and numerous musculoskeletal system problems. They will frequently have endocrine dysfunction, recurrent sinusitis and nasal allergies.

This type of cranial lesion is often temporarily correctable by the use of indirect technique. That is, after it has been determined that flexion is the dysfunction, follow the motion into its extreme range of flexion, and hold against that barrier very gently. When the craniosacral system attempts to return to the neutral

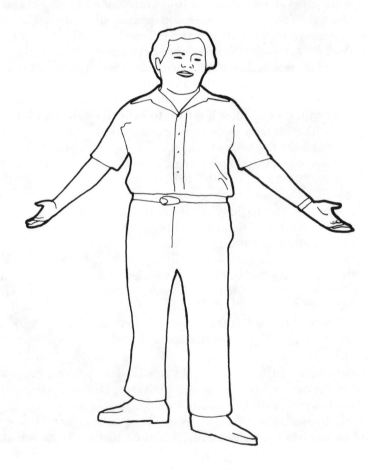

Illustration 7-14
Whole Body Habitus of Chronic Craniosacral Flexion

position, the therapist becomes immovable. Do not push against the indirect barrier: just prevent the cranium from returning to neutral. If it begins to exhibit torsion or sidebend, or proceeds into any other motion pattern, you allow that to happen. These are lesions which you have not diagnosed and which will probably correct as you prevent the return of the craniosacral system to its neutral position. You are a passive barricade. Ultimately the cranium will go further into the flexion range of motion. When this occurs, you have achieved at least a partial release of the flexion lesion pattern. As this movement into further flexion occurs, you follow, staying against the barrier but *not* pushing it. This may occur once or several times.

Finally, one of these movements of the flexion range of motion will be accompanied by a sense that the patient's head has "softened."

We cannot explain what has occurred; but once you have perceptually experienced this softening of your patient's head, you will understand what we mean. You will not likely forget the experience either. It feels as though the intracranial dura mater was contracted and suddenly relaxed, allowing all of the cranial vault bones a little more freedom of movement. We speak of this softening as the "release."

Once the release has occured, you should follow the motion back to neutral, then into the extension phase. Three or four craniosacral system cycles should be passively monitored. The flexion-extension phases of motion can then be re-evaluated to determine whether or not the correction has been made.

Usually, it seems as though the imbalance between the ranges of the flexion and extension phases of motion is about 50% corrected when a full therapeutic effect has been achieved. When you perceive this amount of improvement, it is enough.

Occasionally, the indirect barrier does not move for a considerable period of time, even though you do not allow a return to neutral by the craniosacral system. When this occurs, the therapy can often be expedited by enlisting the patient's cooperation. Simply have the patient inhale deeply and hold their breath as long as possible before exhaling. If this doesn't work, have the patient exhale forcefully and hold their breath out as long as possible. The correction, or release, usually occurs as the patient feels that they *must* resume normal breathing. Yet another method of breathing assistance by the patient is "step" inhalation and/or exhalation (deep inhalation or exhalation in a series of steps.) However, we have found that it is rarely necessary to enlist patient breathing assistance.

If none of these techniques work you are probably dealing with a severe neuromusculoskeletal somatic dysfunction which will have to be corrected before even a temporary correction of the flexion lesion pattern of the craniosacral system can be achieved.

Extension-lesion heads are usually longer in their anterior-posterior dimension and shorter transversely. The body extremities are often somewhat internally rotated (ILLUSTRATION 7-15).

When headache is a problem for the extension head patient, the pain is usually more severe and incapacitating than in flexion heads. Many migraine patients have extension heads coupled with temporal bone dysfunctions.

Our experience tells us that extension head people have fewer endocrine problems. They complain less about neuromusculoskeletal system discomfort, although they may have it. These people probably have a tendency to work it out themselves by the use of exercise.

The correction of the extension lesion is also accomplished by the use of in-

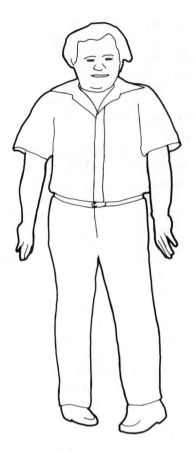

Illustration 7-15
Whole Body Habitus of
Chronic Craniosacral Extension

direct technique. You use the same approach as you did for the flexion lesion correction, except that you follow the motion to its extreme range of extension and resist the return to neutral. The craniosacral system will attempt a return to neutral against your resistance. With each cycle of craniosacral motion the system will go a little further into extension. You take up the slack each time this occurs and wait as patiently as possible. As you develop confidence in the self-corrective process with which every person is endowed, the "waiting with patience" will become easier. Actually, as your perceptual skills develop you will find this period of waiting for the release to be fascinating and instructive.

Ultimately, the release occurs and the correction has been made. You may of course enlist the patient's breathing assistance if you grow tired of waiting. As in the technique for flexion lesion, you evaluate the flexion-extension ranges of motion after you feel that the correction has been made. A 50% reduction of the range of motion discrepancy indicates that a good therapeutic effect has been achieved.

We shall consider the clinical pictures of cranial base sidebending and torsion lesion patterns together. We do this because we believe the motion dysfunction diagnosis should be made strictly on the basis of physical evaluation. The clinical syndrome should not be used to suggest the cranial base motion distortion.

Patients with sidebending and/or torsion lesion patterns of the cranial base (the same patient may have both) frequently suffer from recurrent neuromusculoskeletal system pain syndromes, headache, endocrine disorders, visual perception and motor disturbances, sinusitis, nasal and upper respiratory allergies, temporomandibular joint problems, dental malocclusion, etc. These problems are annoying but seldom are they incapacitating.

Corrections for sidebending and torsion lesions of the cranial base are made using the same indirect techniques described above. Follow the motion in its direction of greatest ease; prevent its return to neutral; wait through several cycles, taking up the slack against the barrier at the end of the range of motion after each cycle. Finally, the release will occur. Again, enlist the patient's breathing assistance as you deem necessary or as you grow tired of waiting. However, we repeat, waiting for the release is a most instructive time for the therapist.

Re-evaluation must be done following the release and correction. A 50% improvement in asymmetry of motion indicates that a correction of the cranial base dysfunction has been achieved.

Always be suspicious and search for dysfunctions elsewhere which are primary to the flexion-extension, sidebending and torsion problems of the cranial base. These primary problems are frequently, but not always, extrinsic to the craniosacral system. The sacrum usually mimes the occipital distortion in this type of cranial base dysfunction. The sacrum may also reflect pelvic or lower back problems which are primary. A piriformis muscle contracture or hypertonus can affect the sacrum and result in a sidebending or torsion lesion pattern of the cranial base. The cranial base problem will continue to recur until the abnormal influences upon the sacrum have been corrected. There are innumerable examples of cranial base dysfunctions reflecting distant somatic and visceral dysfunctions. On the other hand, cranial base dysfunction, for various reasons, may produce its effect upon the sacrum, and in this manner result in recurrent lower back or pelvic problems. All patients have their own dysfunction blueprint. The underlying problem must be discovered. This may require a great deal of tenacity on the part of the therapist.

SPHENOBASILAR/CRANIAL BASE LATERAL STRAIN

The "lateral strain lesion" patterns of the cranial base are usually more severe and incapacitating than flexion-extension, sidebending and torsional lesion patterns. They are also more likely to be primary craniosacral system dysfunctions than problems which are secondary to extracraniosacral system dysfunctions. Lateral strain patterns are frequently the result of trauma. It may be the trauma of the birthing process, or it may be a previous head injury.

Lateral strain usually presents a forehead which bulges forward on the side toward which the sphenoid body has been displaced. This is also the side for which the strain is named. For example, a left lateral strain means that the sphenoid body is displaced to the left in relationship to the basiocciput. Also, the forehead on the left side should be more prominent anteriorly. The head will have a parallelogram configuration when viewed from above (ILLUSTRATION 7-16).

In order to motion test for lateral strain, apply one of the vault holds. Induce a gentle, anteriorly directed force at the beginning of either a flexion or an extension

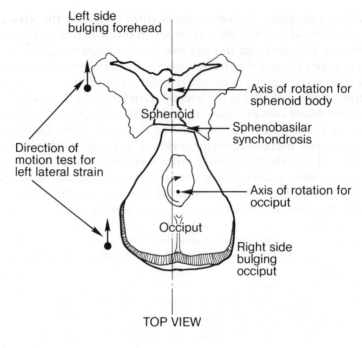

Illustration 7-16
Left Lateral Strain

phase of craniosacral system motion. This force direction is unphysiologic so that it matters little which phase of motion is used; however, it is better not to interrupt a motion phase which is already in progress. Also, for purposes of comparison, it is better to test both sides in the same manner. Test for right and then left lateral strain at the beginning of either a flexion or an extension phase.

The testing force is on the order of 5 grams. It is applied in an anterior direction at the ipsilateral occipital squamous and great wing of the sphenoid.

Traditional cranial osteopathic groups teach that the sphenoid and occiput are abnormally positioned around vertical axes, both being rotated in the same direction to produce lateral strain lesion. It is assumed this lesion pattern is maintained at the sphenobasilar joint.

If the sphenobasilar joint were indeed a symphysis, this model might be tenable. However, this is not the case. Rather, we contend that lateral strain patterns of the cranial base are probably the result of sutural dysfunction and/or abnormal dural membranous tensions. These abnormalities result in distortion at the sphenobasilar joint. This joint is actually a somewhat malleable cartilagenous bridge between the sphenoid and the occiput. The characteristic tendency of this cartilagenous bridge is more probably towards lesion correction. Thus, it is actually one of the inherent self-corrective forces of the craniosacral system.

The Sutherland model can be used to detect lateral strain dysfunction problems of the cranial base. As described above, the gentle lateral strain motion is first induced on one side, then on the other side of the patient's head. The freedom, restriction and length of excursion between the two sides is compared. The lesion is named for the side which moves furthest anteriorly with the greatest ease. For example, a left lateral strain of the cranial base is one which allows for the easiest and greatest motion anteriorly on the left side (ILLUSTRATION 7-16).

Some degree of lateral strain response to motion testing is normal. It should be bilaterally symmetrical in both ease and range of motion.

Another method of testing for lateral strain lesion of the cranial base is simply to move the sphenoid and/or frontal bone laterally, first to one side and then to the other. The occiput is held stationary during this procedure. This technique is, we believe, easier and more direct; however, it has one pitfall. If you allow the sphenoid/frontal complex to diverge from a straight transverse test line, you are actually testing sidebending, probably combined with lateral strain motion. With experience this pitfall can be overcome. Ultimately, you can learn to test the two motions, lateral strain and sidebending, almost concurrently. This test also makes use of the vault hold.

Using this second technique, the lateral strain lesion is named either left or right for the direction into which it moves further with the greatest ease (ILLUSTRATION 7-17).

The correction of lateral strain lesion of the sphenobasilar joint/cranial base is done by lesion exaggeration, as described for flexion-extension, sidebending and torsion. The indirect barrier is followed in the direction of ease until the release is perceived. Breathing assistance (inhalation, exhalation and/or step breathing) may also be required. Correction of this lesion pattern will usually take longer than correction of those patterns described previously. It requires a more extensive adjustment of the motion characteristics of the total cranial base. It usually requires

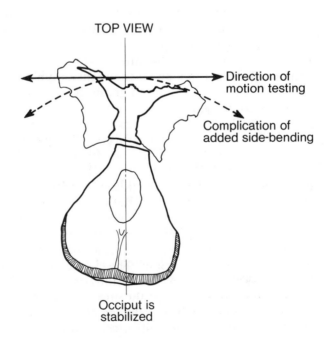

TOP VIEW

Direction of
motion testing

Complication of
added side-bending

Occiput is
stabilized

Illustration 7-17
Motion Testing for Left Lateral Strain

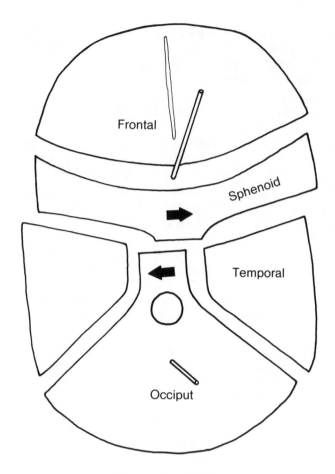

Illustration 7-18
Cranial Base Sutures in Right Lateral Strain

a mobilization of some or all of the cranial base sutures and, perhaps, several of the sutures of the cranial vault. As you maintain lesion exaggeration position, all of the necessary corrections begin to occur either one at a time or simultaneously. Be patient, take your time and let it happen. Occasionally, after the correction induced by indirect technique has been exploited to its fullest extent, it may become necessary to apply direct but *gentle* force against the lesion barrier. That is, the force is applied in the direction of restriction until a further release is obtained. This direct technique should be used only after the indirect techniques and breathing assistance have been fully utilized.

Clinically, those patients with lateral strain patterns of the sphenobasilar joint/cranial base present more severe problems.

The 3rd, 4th, and part of the 5th and 6th cranial nerves pass between the leaves of the tentorium cerebelli. Lateral strain of the cranial base imposes abnormal tension upon the tentorium cerebelli. This tension often interferes with motor function of the eye. We have corrected many cases of strabismus in children by cranial treatment aimed at the alleviation of abnormal tensions within the tentorium cerebelli. These patients, some of whom were already scheduled for surgery, were able to avoid the invasive surgical technique. Also, the motor nerves to the eye pass through the superior orbital fissure, which is formed by the greater and lesser wings and the body of the sphenoid in conjunction with the frontal bone. The tensions imposed by lateral strain lesion patterns of the cranial base can easily be visualized to interfere with the free passage of these nerves through that bony orifice.

Severe head pain is very common with lateral strain lesion of the cranial base. The first patient on which I (Upledger) used cranial osteopathy was a case of unrelenting headache of fourteen years' duration. The severity was such that the patient had been medically discharged from the U.S. Navy twelve years prior to our encounter, after having spent two years in a naval hospital. He had received disability pay since his discharge. The headaches had begun after a blow to the head inflicted by a shell casing during shipboard gunnery practice.

The patient had been referred by a neurosurgeon for a therapeutic trial by acupuncture. Cranial examination revealed a severe lateral strain pattern of the cranial base. This problem was corrected during the first treatment. Neither the lesion nor the headache returned during a seven-month follow-up period.

Since that first patient there have been many similar cases; most have resulted from trauma to the head. The direction of force of the trauma was usually oblique. In such cases, the head usually appears as a parallelogram when viewed from above (ILLUSTRATION 7-18). Personality changes frequently accompany the head pain. We have a tendency to say that the personality changes are of an emotional or psychiatric origin. Often the head pain is attributed to a psychiatric cause. We have found that both head pain and personality disorder spontaneously correct when the lateral strain lesion pattern of the cranial base is successfully corrected.

Occasionally, we have found personality disorder which improves upon correction of cranial base lateral strain and which has not been accompanied by head pain. This situation is less frequent but should be considered when personality change follows either mild or severe head trauma by as much as several months. After all, the examination for cranial motion distortion is quite innocuous when properly performed. Lesions, when found and corrected, can only work for the patient's good, whether or not they seem related to the chief complaint.

Very often, lateral strain lesion patterns of the cranial base are imposed at birth during the delivery procedure. Our studies and research experience indicate that in children the most common result of the birth-inflicted lateral strain lesion is a learning disability, usually in the area of reading (APPENDIX I). Correction of the lateral strain has resulted in dramatic improvement in reading skills in several cases. We continue to collect data in this area and plan to publish the results by 1985. Of necessity, this type of study requires longitudinal observation of several children. The mechanism for the reading problems may be that lateral strain of the cranial base creates pressure upon the great superficial petrosal nerve as it passes through the foramen lacerum. This foramen is a fibrocartilagenous opening between the sphenoid great wing and the petrous part of the temporal bone. This nerve (the great superficial petrosal) has been shown to possess the capability of influencing occipital lobe blood flow in primates by 50% of total volume delivered (OWMAN and EDVINSSON 1977). If it is compressed in the human, it seems reasonable that visual association skills could be affected. Our preliminary clinical results support this concept.

In conjunction with other craniosacral system lesions, lateral strain seems a key dysfunction in spastic cerebral palsy cases. To date, by releasing the lateral strain lesion of the cranial base along with the other lesion patterns of the temporal, parietal and frontal bones, we have successfully alleviated the spasticity in seven cases of cerebral palsy. Motor function has improved enough in three of those cases to permit almost normal function of previously hemiplegic limbs.

Remember that the flexion and extension phases of craniosacral motion continue even when a cranial base presents a lateral strain lesion pattern. The amplitude of the flexion-extension motion may be somewhat reduced, but its rhythmic movement is present.

SPHENOBASILAR/CRANIAL BASE VERTICAL STRAIN

The vertical strain lesion patterns of the cranial base are comparable in clinical significance and severity to the lateral strain problems. They are much more frequently incapacitating and debilitating than are the lesions of flexion-extension, sidebending and torsion. Vertical strain is also more likely to originate etiologically within the craniosacral system. It is common for this strain pattern to result from trauma.

The appearance of the forehead of the subject suggests vertical strain lesion, either superior or inferior. An anteriorly bulging forehead suggests superior vertical strain. Conversely, a forehead which slopes posteriorly from the anterior brow line to the coronal region usually indicates inferior vertical strain lesion.

The terms superior vertical strain and inferior vertical strain refer to the position of the body of the sphenoid (at the sphenobasilar union) in relationship to the base of the occiput where it contributes to that union (ILLUSTRATIONS 7-19-A, 7-19-B and 7-19-C).

If the sphenobasilar joint were a symphysis capable of maintaining an interosseous shear, it is conceivable that vertical strain lesions might etiologically originate from the joint itself. The sphenobasilar union is, however, a cartilagenous bar which joins these two prominent bones of the cranial base; it is not a symphysis. As stated earlier, it is a somewhat flexible synchondrosis. It will respond to tensions placed upon it by membranes attaching to sphenoid and occiput and to relevant

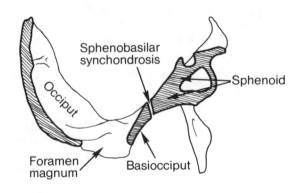

Illustration 7-19-A
Sagittal Section through Human Skull
Normal Anatomical Position

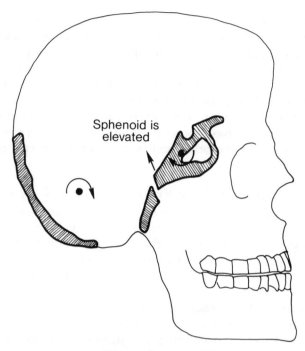

Illustration 7-19-B
Superior Vertical Strain

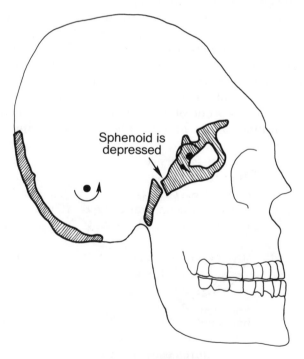

Illustration 7-19-C
Inferior Vertical Strain

sutural problems by manifesting a secondary strain pattern in its anatomy. It will seldom, if ever, evidence an aberration in its anatomy due to primary dysfunction located within the sphenobasilar union itself. Therefore, the cause for the strain pattern must be the subject of a search through the membrane system and through the cranial sutures.

Diagnostic motion testing for superior and inferior vertical strain patterns utilizes any one of the vault holds described above. The therapist should conceptualize axes passing through the occiput and sphenoid transversely. The external contact points are eccentric to the postulated axes of rotation of the two bones. Therefore, a rotation about these transverse axes can be induced by *gentle* manual force.

All normal craniosacral systems will tolerate some externally induced superior and inferior vertical strain. Lesion presence is determined by the ease and range of motion in these two directions.

There are two methods of inducing vertical strain motions in the cranial base. One is to stabilize the occiput and apply force only to the sphenoid wings. The other is to move both the sphenoid and the occiput concurrently.

In testing for superior vertical strain, when force is applied only to the great wings of the sphenoid the eccentric contact points induce an anterior "nose-dive" motion. A cephalad motion is induced at the great wings of the sphenoid when testing for inferior vertical strain.

When force is applied to both occiput and sphenoid in the course of motion testing for superior vertical strain, the occipital squama are encouraged to move superiorly while the sphenoid wings are moved inferiorly. The motions are reversed when testing for inferior vertical strain.

The approach to the correction of vertical strain lesion is similar to the approach used in the correction of lateral strain lesions since the two problems are comparable in physiological and clinical severity.

Indirect technique by the use of lesion exaggeration to the *indirect* barrier should be utilized first. If you find that the sphenoid moves easier in the inferior "nose-dive" direction which indicates superior vertical strain, you should hold, but *not push,* against the barrier at the end of the motion in the direction of ease. Take up the slack as you wait through as many cycles as are required to obtain the release or correction. The reverse of this technique is applicable for inferior vertical strain patterns. If you cannot obtain satisfactory release by this method, patient breathing assistance may be enlisted. If the correction is still not achieved, you may then resort to the continuous application of direct correction technique. Gently, but persistently, hold the cranial base against the direct restriction barrier until a release and correction occur. You should then re-evaluate for a 50% improvement in motion symmetry.

After mobilizing the strain lesion of the cranial base, conduct a search for the etiologic factors which underlie the problem.

Flexion and extension rhythmic movements of the craniosacral system, although often inhibited or restricted by vertical strain lesions, are nevertheless present. Commonly, the first clue to the presence of a vertical strain lesion is a labored quality to the normal flexion-extension motion of the craniosacral system.

Clinically, vertical strain patterns produce results similar to those induced by lateral strain patterns. Symptoms may seem bizarre until one recognizes that craniosacral system dysfunction is the common source for apparently unrelated symptoms.

The vertical strain pattern of the cranial base correlates to, and may be the cause or effect of, undue tension upon both the falx cerebri and the tentorium cerebelli. The falx (cerebri) is attached to the frontal bone, both on the cranial base and at the forehead. A bulging forehead, as found in superior vertical strain, will obviously stress the falx cerebri (ILLUSTRATION 7-20). The tension thus created is necessarily transmitted to the tentorium cerebelli and the sagittal and straight venous sinuses. Dysfunction of the sutures of the cranial base also occurs when vertical strain is present. Especially affected are the sphenofrontal and sphenopetrosal sutures.

This sutural dysfunction may then interfere with the function of nerves and blood vessels which pass through the various foramena which are formed along the paths of these sutures. Included among the affected foramena is the foramen lacerum, which passes the great superficial petrosal nerve. This nerve has a strong influence upon the blood supply to the occipital lobes of the brain. Also affected by vertical strain is the superior orbital fissure, which affords passage to the visual motor nerves. This anatomy may account for the frequent occurrence of visual problems which accompany the vertical strain lesion patterns of the cranial base.

It must also be kept in mind that the anterior attachments of the tentorium cerebelli are to the clinoid processes of the sphenoid bone. The diaphragma sellae is strongly influenced by this double-layered membrane. The orifice of this dia-

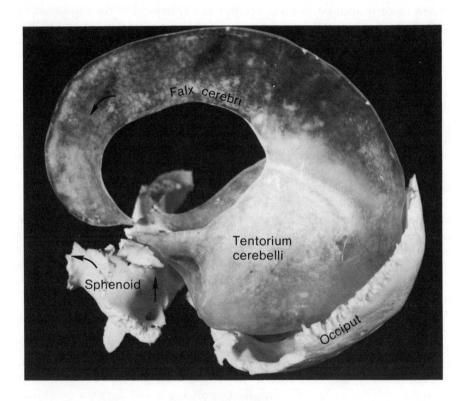

Illustration 7-20
Membrane Model Demonstrating Tension on the
Falx Cerebri with Superior Vertical Strain

phragma allows passage of the hypophyseal infundibulum, which suspends the pituitary gland from the hypothalamus. The diaphragma sellae also encloses the intercavernous and circular sinuses. It is common for correction of vertical strain patterns of the cranial base to result in "serendipitous" and concurrent benefits to the patient through the improvement of endocrine function.

With severe vertical strain patterns of the cranial base, severe head pain, sinusitis, allergies and personality disorders are the rule rather than the exception. Often the personality disorder is one which manifests violent outbursts of temper and antisocial acts. (It has been a fantasy of one of the authors to examine prison inmates for vertical strain lesions; however, to date, time has not permitted this investigation.) (ILLUSTRATIONS 7-21-A, 7-21-B and 7-21-C).

CRANIAL BASE COMPRESSION

Compared to those cranial base dysfunctions described earlier in this chapter, compression is a special problem. In both its clinical significance and the extent of its physiological effects, it is significantly more severe. The clinical symptoms which it can produce are extremely varied and may seem bizarre. One of the most consistently occurring clinical manifestations of cranial base compression is depression of mood. It is often diagnosed as an endogenous depressive neurotic condition. It may also be an underlying etiologic agent for conditions as unrelated as sciatica, childhood "autism" and allergies. We have observed the physiological and anatomical effects of cranial base compression from the bottoms of the feet to the top of the head.

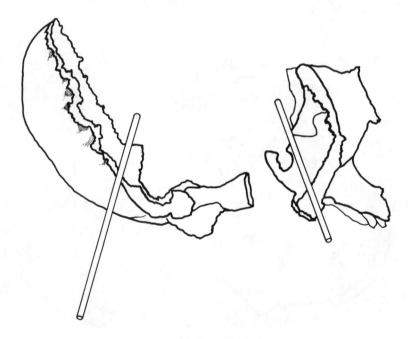

Illustration 7-21-A
The Axes of Cranial Base Motion Distortion —
Transverse Axes for Flexion, Extension and
Vertical Strain

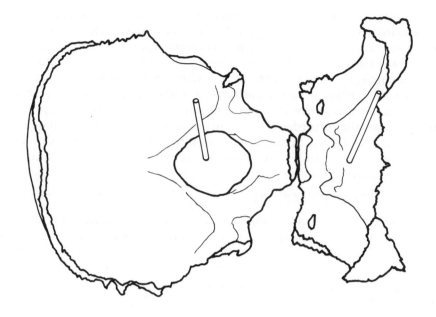

Illustration 7-21-B
The Axes of Cranial Base Motion Distortion—
Vertical Axes for Sidebending and Lateral Strain

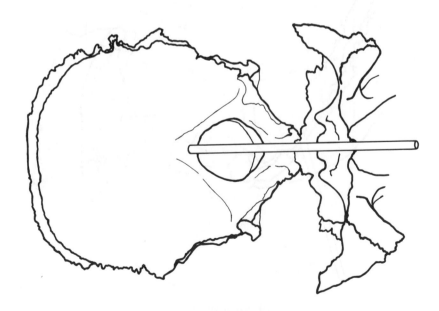

Illustration 7-21-C
The Axes of Cranial Base Motion Distortion —
Longitudinal Axis for Torsion

Our point is simply that the thorough physician should always look for cranial base compression, no matter what the patient's complaint nor how unlikely it may seem that the clinical symptom or syndrome could be etiologically related to cranial base compression.

Traditionally, the Cranial Academy and the Sutherland Cranial Teaching Foundation teach that compression refers to anterior-posterior impaction at the sphenobasilar joint between the sphenoid body and the occipital base. We would expand this concept to include any compression of the cranial base components in any direction, whether due to osseous impaction, sutural dysfunction or membranous restriction (ILLUSTRATIONS 7-22-A, 7-22-B and 7-22-C).

In our investigations of craniosacral system function in severely disabled children (cerebral palsied, autistic, seizure-disordered, learning disabled and the like), we came to the conclusion that careful physical examination of the craniosacral system can differentiate osseous from membranous restrictions of the cranial base. In fact, we carried out a double blind study involving 63 children with Dr.

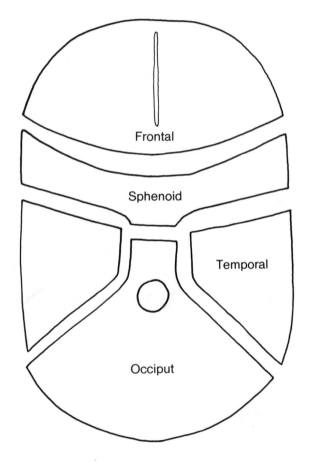

Illustration 7-22-A
Cranial Base Bones —
Normal Relationship

Bernard Rimland, Director of the Institute for Child Behavior Research in San Diego, California. Dr. Rimland, a prominent authority in the field of child psychology, developed a rating scale which diagnoses childhood autism on the basis of the historical analysis of various developmental landmarks. The child who rates above +20 on this scale is considered to be suffering from Early Infantile Autism.

After three years of work with children in the Genessee Intermediate School District Center for Autism (1978 through 1980), we postulated that the more classically autistic children in this Center for Autism suffered from a membranous (dura mater) compression of the cranial base. This tightening of the dural floor covering of the cranial cavity resulted in an elastic type of cranial base compression which was present in all directions around the compass. The restriction is elastic in quality as compared to the firm, rigid quality of osseous restriction.

To test this postulate, we examined under blind conditions 63 children who had previously been rated by Dr. Rimland. Only 5 of the 63 children had been diagnosed as autistic by Dr. Rimland using his +20 score as the cutoff point. These children

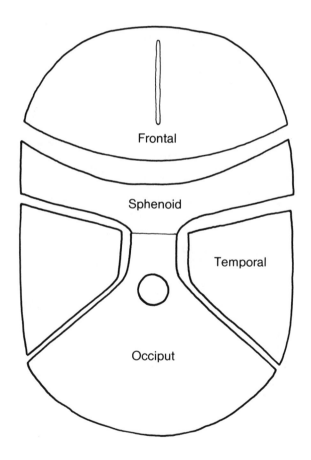

Illustration 7-22-B
Anterior-Posterior Compression
of the Sphenoid and Occiput

were rated on a scale of 1 to 10 in terms of membranous and osseous restriction. A normal mobility was rated as 1, while the most severe restrictions were rated as 10.

A positive correlation was registered between higher scores on the Rimland rating scale and our own rating of severity of membranous restriction to motion. This correlation was significant at a 0.01 level of confidence. This is a preliminary study, but suggests that further investigation would be worthwhile.

From the above information it is apparent that cranial base compression can result from several different etiologic agents. It can result from a traumatic blow to the head, which literally and mechanically impacts the bones and/or sutures of the cranial base one into the other. It can result from birth trauma in the birth canal or from forceps which have compressed the cranial base to the extent that the internal hydraulic force produced by the cerebrospinal fluid cannot effect a post-partum self-correction. It can result from an inflammatory process which has involved the dural membrane and reduced that membrane's ability to accommodate osseous growth of the cranial base. It can result from the membranous transmission of tension from a post-traumatic antero-flexed coccyx, or from lumbosacral impaction. It can result

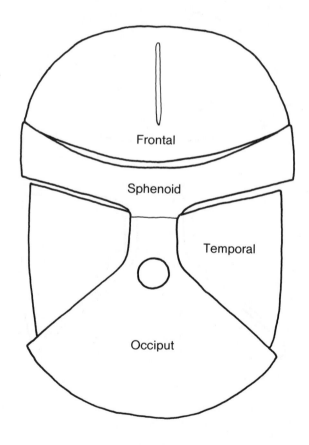

Illustration 7-22-C
Lateral Compression of the Cranial Base
(Note the Occipitomastoid Suture Compression)

from compression of the occipital condyles between the articular facets of the atlas. It also seems somehow to result from emotional trauma, although we cannot explain how this might occur.

EVALUATION OF ANTERIOR-POSTERIOR COMPRESSION OF THE CRANIAL BASE

This procedure is performed upon the supine patient using one of the vault holds. The first step is to compress the patient's head gently in an anterior-posterior direction. This is done to exaggerate and thus quickly treat transient or insignificant cranial base dysfunctions. The compressive force is induced gently and held until a lateral broadening and a release of the patient's head is perceived. Often, during this phase of the procedure, the cranial base may go into other lesion patterns such as torsion, lateral strain, etc. The therapist should passively follow these motions of the cranial base while continuing the *gentle* compressive force to the end point of release with its palpable lateral spread of the cranial vault. These other lesion patterns are actually present and are self-correcting in response to your compressive force.

The question is always asked, "How much compressive force is used?" Each cranial base is different and therefore requires a different amount of compressive force. Start with a very gentle touch and just "think" compression. This thought will telegraph a slight amount of compressive force to your hands. If nothing happens in the patient's cranial base after about 30 seconds, *very gradually* increase your force until something does happen. That something may be a flexion, a torsion, a strain pattern or any other motion. Once the motion begins, that is the amount of force you use until the release occurs.

Occasionally the release will occur without any other lesion pattern presenting itself first. This would seem to be the "perfect" cranial base, if there is such a thing. If you find yourself applying a significant compressive force (½ to 1 pound) and nothing has happened, you have increased your force too rapidly and not allowed for the patient's head to respond. Go back and start over, increasing your force more slowly, concentrating very carefully so that you do not miss the subtle changes which tell you when the force is correct. Remember that you are establishing a closed feedback or cybernetic loop by your initial contact. You must be alert to receive and process, instant by instant, the information which the patient is giving back to you.

After you have completed the compression or lesion exaggeration phase of the treatment and have obtained the release at the end of this phase, you are ready to decompress the patient's cranial base.

The deep side of the skin is ultimately, although indirectly, attached to that bone of the skull which it overlies. Using the vault hold, cradle the occiput posteriorly for purposes of monitoring its activity. You should apply enough pressure on the skin over the great wings of the sphenoid so that, by this gentle pressure, friction is created between the patient's skin and the skin of your fingers or thumbs, depending upon which vault hold is used. A *gentle* anterior decompressive force is then applied. For the supine patient, this force will be aimed directly toward the ceiling overhead.

When the amount of lifting decompressive force is adequate, the occiput will seem to settle posteriorly. Additional lifting of the great sphenoid wings is then introduced, causing the occiput to further lighten and later to settle again. More anterior decompression is applied and the process repeated until the occiput feels as though it is free and balanced to the therapist who is monitoring it posteriorly. In problem cases, this freedom between the occiput and the sphenoid may not be totally achievable during one treatment, but may require several treatments.

As you perform the decompressive phase of the treatment, you may again become aware that various cranial base restriction or lesion patterns are appearing. As you suspend the occiput like a puppet from a series of strings, these lesion patterns will often self-correct. Those lesion patterns which do not self-correct during the decompression phase may be treated specifically as described in the earlier sections of this chapter. After correction has been achieved, decompression of the cranial base is repeated for further evaluation and treatment.

The traction effect during decompression is twofold. First, the transversely orientated cranial base sutures are mobilized as the weight of the occiput, the weight of the brain and the internal hydraulic forces all inherently work together in favor of correction. Second, the attachments of the tentorium cerebelli to the clinoid processes of the sphenoid bone serve to therapeutically stretch this membrane structure between its anterior and posterior attachments to the straight venous sinus and the occiput. This tentorial traction has a relaxing effect upon the tentorial fibers and a beneficial milking effect upon the venous sinus system as it relates to the tentorium cerebelli.

You may have guessed by now that we use the compression-decompression technique described above with our favorite vault hold as a "shotgun" technique to both diagnose and treat most lesion patterns of the cranial base. Specific lesions of the cranial base are easily detected and corrected in a minimal amount of time using this approach. Occasionally, a cranial base lesion will require independent and specific corrective technique in addition to the decompression; but this is the exception rather than the rule. When these resistant lesions are identified, you may rest assured they are significant and that you have cut through the "chaff" to the "wheat."

When the occiput does not drop posteriorly or toward the floor after "lightening," you are dealing with a compression lesion of the cranial base. Experience is the only means of learning to evaluate the normal time and degree of lightening versus dropping or releasing of the occiput. If the occiput rigidly follows the anterior motion of the sphenoid as you raise it anteriorly, you probably have an osseous impaction. When the occiput seems suspended from an elastic system and the sphenoid does decompress, but offers an elastic or rebound resistance to your decompression, you are dealing with a membranous problem.

When you have applied this technique to many, many cranial bases, you will know what each feels like. The same is true in palpating for enlarged livers, precordial heaves, or in auscultating lungs and hearts. You must develop an experiential reservoir of information in your cerebral data bank in order to evaluate the degree of normalcy or abnormalcy of what you have discovered for a given patient. This is the art of practice wherein no numbers can be read from the computer to obtain normal or abnormal values. You must evaluate on the basis of what you have perceived in other patients and make judgments for which you are responsible. Fortunately, errors in judgment when performing decompression techniques have no serious ramifications. The system is very forgiving.

EVALUATION FOR LATERAL CRANIAL BASE COMPRESSION

It was during our work with autism that the concept, test and treatment technique for lateral cranial base compression were developed. In an attempt to mobilize the many severely internally rotated temporal bones, we developed what we have half-jokingly called the "ear pull" technique. It is a simple and direct technique. We have found, with practice, that it is effective in almost all types of temporal bone dysfunction, especially those involving the petrous temporal bone parts and their sutures.

The external pinna of each ear is ultimately attached by collagen fiber to the osseous ear canal of the temporal bones. When you apply *gentle* traction upon the external pinna in the direction of the longitudinal attitude of the petrous part, this traction decompresses the cranial base laterally (ILLUSTRATION 7-23). It releases the temporosphenoidal suture, the occipitomastoid suture, the occipitotemporal suture and the medial junction between the temporal petrous parts and the sphenobasilar region.

With the patient supine, the external ears (pinnae) are gently grasped (in the manner of a healing professional rather than that of an irate school ma'rm).

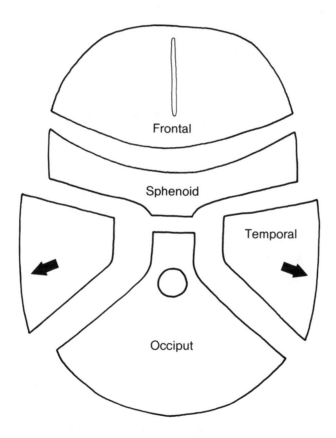

Illustration 7-23
The Effect of the "Ear Pull" Technique upon the
Sutures of the Cranial Base

Posterior lateral traction is *gently* applied in the direction which would be an extension of the osseous ear canal. The traction is applied bilaterally, as uniformally as possible. Any twisting, turning or shearing motions that come into play are not interfered with; rather, they are passively followed. Gradually, the temporal bones as anchors of the external ears will begin to move laterally. Continue your traction until a sense of softening or release is perceived on *both* sides. If, after a reasonable time, this bilateral release has not been achieved, you may need to try again at another sitting. Ultimately the release will occur.

A small force or traction over a prolonged period of time is extremely powerful, yet it does not invoke the tissue resistance and guarding by the patient which will occur if your force is too great and you are impatient. You can move a 100-foot yacht in the water with one finger if you are willing to apply your force over a prolonged period of time. The same is true in treating dysfunctions of the craniosacral system and, for that matter, in dealing with all of the connective tissue of the body. Gentle, non-threatening force which does not stimulate tissue defense reaction is the rule for maximum success.

THE CLINICAL SIGNIFICANCE OF THE MECHANICAL PROPERTIES OF CONNECTIVE TISSUES

The science of biomechanics is concerned with the mechanical properties of biological tissues. Much of our research effort at the Michigan State University College of Osteopathic Medicine's Department of Biomechanics is directed at the study of the mechanical properties of connective tissue. Robert W. Little, Ph.D., our chairman, has developed models which illustrate many of the clinically significant characteristics of connective tissues with which the therapist becomes involved when dealing with the craniosacral system, the neuromusculoskeletal system and all of the body fascia.

The research by Dr. Little and our department to date would indicate that the characteristics of connective tissue which explain the perceptions discussed above are best illustrated by the use of the spring and dashpot model which is so familiar to physicists and engineers.

The spring is essentially a linear elastic element. The force which exists in this element is dependent solely upon the state of deformation. Increasing deformation relates directly to the imposition of greater force. A constant factor which relates to the stiffness of the spring dictates the amount of deformation which will result from a given load. Stiffness means resistance to deformation. Strength refers to the maximum load the spring will carry before it breaks. Strength and stiffness should not be confused. When deforming a spring, the rate of application of load does not matter, only the amount of the load. The spring will return to its original dimensions when the load upon it is terminated.

The dashpot represents viscosity. Therefore, the rate of application of the imposed load is the important factor, for it determines the resultant deformity (ILLUSTRATION 7-24-A).

Soft connective tissues such as muscle, ligament, tendon, fascia, etc., behave as a combination of these two elements, the spring and the dashpot, as though they were in series. Bone, under load, behaves as though the spring and the dashpot were in parallel (ILLUSTRATION 7-24-B).

The research by Dr. Little and our department to date would indicate that the

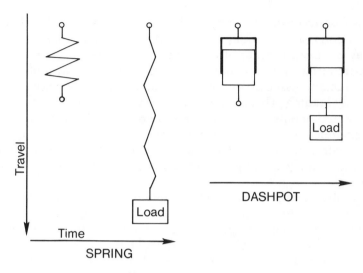

Illustration 7-24-A
Spring and Dashpot

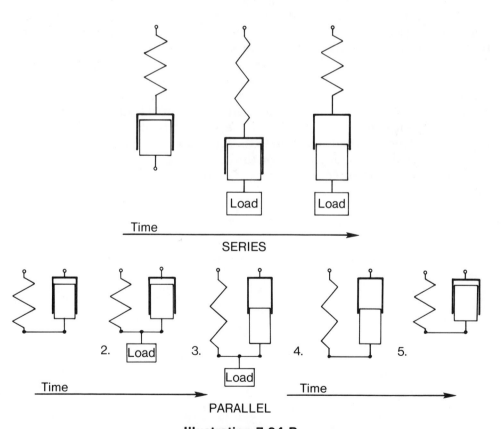

Illustration 7-24-B
Effect of Loading on the Spring-Dashpot System
in Series and Parallel

spring load is first accommodated by the stretch of the spring. Then, more slowly, the dashpot begins to move, taking the load off the spring as time passes. The tissue, therefore, has memory for the pre-loaded state as long as the spring continues to feel the load. When the dashpot has totally accommodated the load, and the spring is no longer on stretch, the tissue no longer remembers what it was prior to the deformation imposed by loading. This model illustrates very nicely the type of corrections made in the craniosacral system as we described the techniques above. From this model, it is apparent that all dashpots must accommodate all loads imposed in order for permanent corrective change to occur. This movement of the dashpot requires time. When the spring is no longer under load, the release is palpably perceived by the physician.

In the parallel model, the dashpot (viscous element) requires time to respond to the load. But when the load is imposed over time, the dashpot responds by deforming. This circumstance begins to place a load upon the spring. The transferrence of this load from dashpot to spring continues through time until the load is finally and completely transferred to spring. Later, if the load is removed, the return to the normal, undeformed state is carried out by the spring with resistance to this return initially being imposed by the dashpot. As the spring continues to load the dashpot, the undeformed state is finally reached and the load no longer exists.

In the series arrangement, there is permanent deformation when the load is removed after sufficient time has passed. In the parallel arrangement, the material returns to its original state after some time has passed.

The lesson to be learned from these models is that when dealing therapeutically with connective tissues, consider both the spring and the dashpot characteristics of the tissues. Collagen usually exists as a wavy, relaxed configuration. It does not assume a load until the elastin has been stretched by initial loading. The ground substance collagen contributes greatly to the viscous or dashpot response of the connective tissues. Careful attention to the feedback from the patient's response to your loading will successfully guide you through therapeutic techniques. The results you obtain will more often be permanent, and the accuracy of prognosis will be improved.

Chapter 8
The Spinal Dura Mater and Sacrococcygeal Complex

The dura mater, which connects the occiput with the sacrococcygeal complex, travels through the longitudinal vertebral canal where it is also known as the dural tube. Within this canal the dural membrane forms a loose sheath for the spinal cord. The endosteal layer of the intracranial dura mater is represented below the foramen magnum by the vertebral periosteum which lines this canal. The spinal dural membrane is considered to be an extension of the inner or meningeal layer of the intracranial dura mater.

Within the vertebral canal, the spinal dura mater usually has firm osseous attachments only at the entire circumference of the foramen magnum, to the posterior bodies of the 2nd and 3rd cervical vertebrae, and within the sacral canal at the level of the 2nd sacral segment at its anterior portion. It is attached to the posterior longitudinal ligament by fibrous slips. These attachments to the longitudinal ligaments are variable, and usually more pronounced caudally.

The subdural space ends within the sacral canal at the approximate level of the 2nd sacral segment. Here the spinal dura mater closely invests the filum terminale, passes out of the sacral canal via the sacral hiatus and blends with the periosteum of the coccyx. The caudal part of the dural tubular sheath, below the 2nd lumbar segment where the conus medullaris is formed, is occupied by the cauda equina.

As the spinal nerves exit the vertebral canal through the intervertebral foramena, they are covered by prolongations of the dural sheath which terminate by blending into the paravertebral fascia. These tubular prolongations of dura are more nearly transverse at the upper levels of the vertebral canal. As one descends caudad, the prolongations become more longitudinal in their orientation. This arrangement results in a greater transmission of tension into the dural tube from the lower (caudad) regions than from the upper regions. The upper transverse dural sleeve orientation allows for more freedom of longitudinal spinal dural tube motion, even when these sleeves are under tension (ILLUSTRATION 8-1).

The subdural space within the tubular dura mater is much larger than required. Most of this excess space is filled by the subarachnoid space, which allows for some independent motion between the spinal cord and the dural membrane.

The epidural space between the dural sheath and the periosteum of the vertebral canal also presents a rather large interval. This space contains venous plexuses,

131

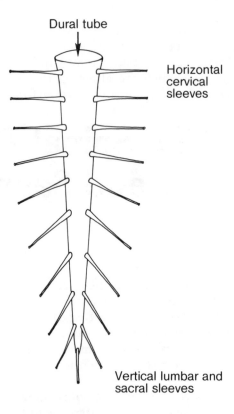

Dural tube

Horizontal
cervical
sleeves

Vertical lumbar and
sacral sleeves

Illustration 8-1
Directional Orientation of Dural Sleeves

which are analogous to the cranial dural sinuses, and loose areolar tissue.

Under normal, restful conditions, the functional anatomy of the dural connections between the occiput and the sacrococcygeal complex are such that movements of the occiput are duplicated at the sacrococcygeal end; conversely, movements of the sacrococcygeal complex are duplicated at the occiput. This occurs because of the relative freedom of motion for longitudinal gliding, which is characteristic of the dura mater within the vertebral canal.

By the same dural continuity, restrictions to motion which are imposed upon either the occiput or the sacrococcygeal complex usually are manifested as symptoms at both ends of the spinal dura mater. It is often by this mechanism that head and lower back pain occur concurrently. It is also by virtue of the attachments of the spinal dural membrane to the posterior bodies of the 2nd and 3rd cervical vertebrae that there is often a significant clinical relationship between upper cervical, head and lower back pain. The cause of this problem can begin at any one of the three regions of osseous attachment of the dural membrane. With time, it will frequently spread as symptomatic pain and dysfunction to all three regions of the body. In addition, any spinal or paravertebral somatic dysfunction of significant severity can restrict spinal dural tube mobility and thus manifest as secondary dysfunction at any or all of these three regions of osseous dural attachment.

Given the functional conditions described above, it is easy to understand the importance and usefulness of techniques which evaluate the freedom of motion of the spinal dura mater. The mobility of this dural membrane can be used to search for somatic dysfunctions which are affecting the occiput, the upper cervicals, the sacrum, the coccyx and all of the intervertebral foramena. Dural sheath mobility can also be used to locate dural adhesions which are responsible for various pain syndromes. Frequently, such dural adhesions seem to dissipate with the continued application of techniques directed at the modification of the intradural hydraulic forces, and other techniques aimed at the enhancement of the gliding motion of the dural membrane within the vertebral canal. These latter techniques utilize the leverage forces which can be developed and imposed upon the osseous attachments of the spinal dural membrane. Hence, the legs, lower back and head are often used when attempting to mobilize the spinal dura mater.

EVALUATION OF SPINAL DURAL TUBE MOBILITY

The mobility of the spinal dural tube is best evaluated by simultaneously testing the motion at the occiput and the sacrum. This can best be accomplished by one person; however, when learning and gaining experience, it is beneficial to have two therapists working together on a single patient.

When working alone, have the patient lie comfortably supine on a foam pad about 2-4 inches thick, or on an air mattress. You should sit comfortably to the patient's side so that one of your hands can cradle the patient's sacrum while the other hand cradles the occiput. The purpose of the tabletop foam padding or air mattress is to allow your hand and arm to pass under the patient's gluteal and sacral areas with minimal effect upon the patient's resting position on the tabletop.

It is important when evaluating dural tube mobility within the vertebral canal that external factors caused by the examination do not result in a tissue response of guarding or hypertonus. That is, the examination conditions and procedures must not result in an alteration of osseous motion of the occiput or the sacrococcygeal complex. Artificial alterations in motion can only too easily be induced; and incorrect information leads to incorrect diagnostic impressions and, ultimately, to ineffective treatment. We therefore cannot emphasize strongly enough the importance of patient comfort and connective tissue relaxation during the examination procedures. You must evaluate the patient's physiological motion as it is, not as it responds to your intervention.

Once you have comfortably and correctly placed one hand under the patient's sacrum and the other hand under the occiput, you can evaluate rocking flexion-extension motions of these two bones. The occiput and sacrum seem to move in synchrony and parallel in response to the rhythm of the craniosacral system. The axes of the rotational movement of the occiput and sacrum are transverse (ILLUSTRATION 8-2). The dural tube and probably the anterior and posterior longitudinal ligaments act as connectors between these two osseous anchors.

Remember that flexion and extension are rhythmically alternating movements of the craniosacral system. During the flexion phase the anterior dural tube and anterior longitudinal ligaments are tensed in a cephalad direction. This results in the rotational movement of the sacrum, as illustrated, in which the sacral apex moves anteriorly. During the extension phase of motion the posterior dural tube and the posterior longitudinal ligaments are tensed cephalad while the anterior connectors

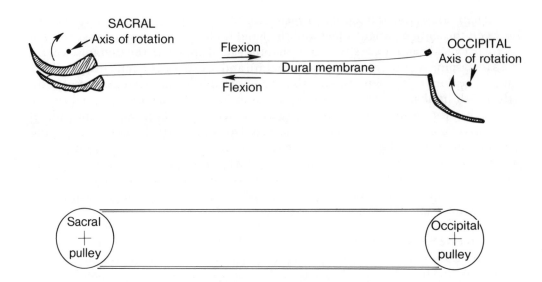

Illustration 8-2
Mechanism of Occipital-Sacral Synchrony

are relaxed. This results in an anterior movement of the sacral base as it rotates about the postulated axis in the illustration.

As you tune in to the movements of the occiput and the sacrum at the same time, there are several questions which must be answered:

1. Are the sacrum and occiput moving freely and in synchrony with each other?
2. Is one of these two bones lagging, or moving in time, slightly behind the other?
3. If there is a time lag, does the movement of the lagging bone seem to be coming from a restraint or drag imposed upon it from outside the dural membrane? Is it coming from your hand or from an extrinsically attached muscle or ligament?
4. Does the lag seem to be coming from somewhere between your hands?
5. If you sense a dural tube drag, can you locate the position of drag? Is that area tender to palpation? Is it within the dural tube, or on one of its spinal nerve sleeves?

As you answer these questions after experience with more patients, you will develop skill in localizing the causes of restriction to the free mobility of these two bones, which represent the osseous attachments of the extremes of the spinal dural tube.

As a learning experience it is beneficial to slightly inhibit the motion of either the occiput or the sacrum with one of your hands, and then to note the effect of this artificial restriction upon the motion perceived by the other hand.

When two therapists are working together to evaluate the mobility of the spinal division of the craniosacral system, one examiner uses the occiput while the other uses the sacrum. For the therapist at the head end of the patient, it is often beneficial to use a vault hold (CHAPTER 7) so that the effect of the sacrococcygeal complex can be perceived not only upon the occiput, but upon the whole cranial vault. This is an excellent learning experience.

The therapist at the sacrococcygeal end of the patient should place the arm between the supine patient's legs and the hand under the coccyx and sacrum. The sacrococcygeal complex is situated so that the sacral apex is in the therapist's palm; the sacral spine is between the therapist's third and fourth fingers, and lies parallel to them. The therapist's finger tips may be at the level of the transverse processes of the 4th or 5th lumbar vertebrae, depending upon individual hand and sacral size. It seems that the more weight which the sacrococcygeal complex therapist places upon his or her elbow, the better—so, *lean on it.* Do not try to feel with the hand which is under the sacrum. Try to meld your hand with the sacrum and allow your hand to move with it. When this has been achieved, observe what your hand is doing, that is, what the sacrum is doing. This application of the hand to the sacrococcygeal complex is identical to that which is used when there is only one therapist (ILLUSTRATION 8-3).

After both therapists have tuned in to the patient in this manner, they should communicate what is happening at the two ends of the spinal dural tube. The same questions should be answered by both therapists. One of the therapists should then impose artificial restrictions to gain perceptual experience about what a sacrum feels like when an occiput is restricted, and vice versa. The therapists can also impose deep paravertebral pressure upon the patient to perceive the effect of paraspinal somatic dysfunctions upon the function of the craniosacral system.

CAUSES AND TREATMENT OF RESTRICTIONS TO SPINAL DURAL TUBE MOBILITY

Causes of dural tube motion restriction which originate within the intracranial membrane system have been discussed previously. Suffice it here to say that each

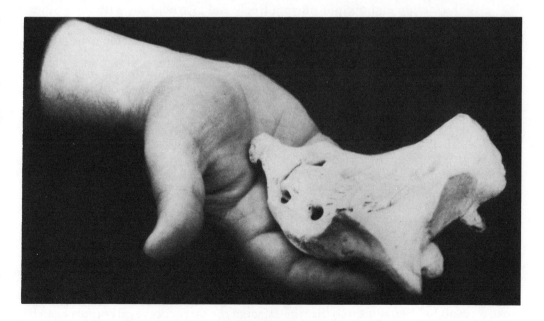

Illustration 8-3
Hand Position for Palpation of the Sacrum

intracranial membrane restriction pattern has its dural tube effect.

Extrinsic factors which affect occipital motion include all of the muscles, ligaments and fasciae connected to this pivotal bone of the skull. In most patients the suboccipital musculature is more than one inch thick. These muscles may be considered individually (CHAPTER 13). For our present purposes, however, they will be considered in aggregate. When occipital mobility is impaired by factors extrinsic to the dural membrane, the effect is felt throughout the craniosacral system. It is therefore extremely important to understand that abnormal connective tissue tensions which are directed at the occiput must be dealt with effectively before an accurate evaluation of craniosacral system motion can be performed.

The technique for release of the cranial base (CHAPTER 5) is our usual method for releasing general tension placed upon the occiput by its connective tissue attachments. This technique also releases the atlanto-occipital joints, which are also a frequent source of occipital restriction. Compression of the occipital condyles is a cause of severe craniosacral system dysfunction and requires effective treatment before one can expect the craniosacral system to function normally.

As stated above, the spinal dural membrane is attached within the vertebral canal to the posterior surfaces of the 2nd and 3rd cervical vertebrae. Somatic dysfunction of these vertebrae, which is either primary or secondary to somatic dysfunction elsewhere, will always result in craniosacral system motion impairment. These somatic dysfunctions must be corrected.

We prefer to use position and hold techniques to release upper cervical somatic dysfunctions which are influencing craniosacral system mobility. Any therapist with the sensitivity required to perceive craniosacral system motion can begin to use position and hold techniques. In this technique, position the patient either sitting or lying supine (ILLUSTRATIONS 8-4-A and 8-4-B). The head is guided with one hand while the other hand holds the neck and monitors local tissue tension. The muscles of the neck are brought into maximum relaxation or softening by positioning the head. In the beginning, you will have to resort to a great deal of positional trial and error. In order to achieve maximum relaxation of the cervical musculature, gentle and precise positioning is necessary. After you gain experience, it will seem as though the patient's head guides itself to the proper positions (APPENDIX E).

As some of the muscles relax, the optimal position changes. This is a dynamic, not a static treatment technique. Our research with connective tissue has shown that such tissue literally posseses memory (CHAPTER 7). As you discover positions in which tissue has been strained or stressed, the strain or stress pattern will dissipate from those tissues. Often, as correction occurs, you will feel heat emanating from the area of involvement; also, you may notice a rather rapid, pulsating activity. The position should be held until both heat emanation and pulsation cease. If the position is changed prior to the end of these corrective phenomena, full therapeutic effect will not be achieved.

There are many other methods of correcting somatic dysfunctions (MITCHELL 1979); in expert hands, most of these methods are acceptable. The method which we have described is noninjurious. When properly applied, this method is extremely effective. Be patient with the patient: that is the key. Use whichever technique you are most comfortable with and which achieves the proper therapeutic effect.

We have yet to encounter a paravertebral somatic dysfunction of more than transient nature which does not express itself as a drag upon the spinal dural tube.

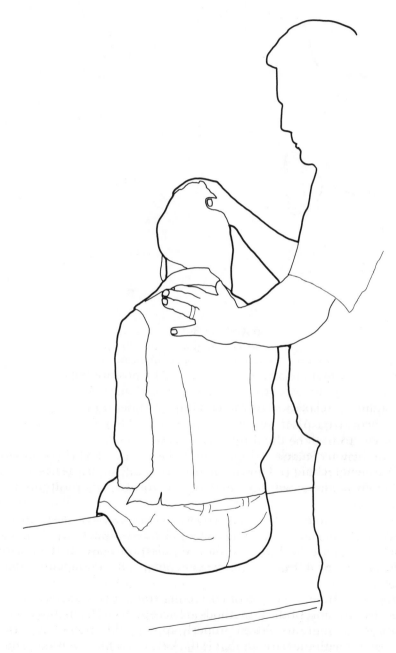

Illustration 8-4-A
Position and Hold Technique for the Neck —
Patient Seated

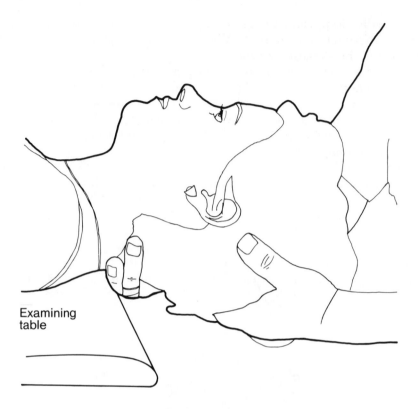

Illustration 8-4-B
Position and Hold Technique for the Neck —
Patient Supine

Evaluation of spinal dural tube mobility, as described above, can be effectively used to locate significant paraspinal somatic dysfunctions. When found, they must be corrected in order to free the dural tube from its motion restriction.

Once again, any technique at which you are expert and which is effective is acceptable. The correction of the somatic dysfunction will immediately remove the dural tube restriction; therefore, dural mobility can be used as an indicator of your therapeutic success.

There are three simple methods, all of which are safe and effective, for mobilizing the spinal dural tube and correcting contributing paraspinal problems.

The first is to exercise the dural tube motion from both ends. Gently, but firmly encourage the synchrony of the motion of the occiput and sacrum, and gently, but persistently encourage an increase in the amplitude of motion through 30-50 cycles of flexion-extension. Frequently, you can overcome the dural membrane restriction in this way; as you do, the paraspinal somatic dysfunction will self-correct.

The second method of correcting significant paraspinal lesions which influence craniosacral system function is the application of CV-4 technique through several still points (CHAPTER 4). As the patient progresses through a series of still points or interruptions in craniosacral rhythm, they will often experience pain at the locus of the somatic dysfunction as they approach each still point. During the still point, the pain will usually disappear. As long as the pain can be induced by CV-4 application, the somatic dysfunction is present. When the pain can no longer be induced, you have corrected the somatic dysfunction.

The third method of mobilizing paraspinal somatic dysfunction is simply the "direction of energy." This technique is based upon the fact that all living human beings are batteries, generators and capacitors in the literal, electrical sense. Your skin is the insulator which holds in your electricity and which protects you from environmental electrical phenomena which could interfere with your electrical health and functioning.

When you place your skin into intimate contact with the skin of another human being, some of the resistance of these two insulator skins seems to be lost. Ultimately, the two capacitors (you and your patient), by virtue of the increasing conductivity of the skin, become one. Although this may sound rather romantic, it can also be used therapeutically.

When a paravertebral somatic dysfunction is discovered, you need only place one finger over each of the transverse processes of the involved vertebra, and the other hand *very gently* upon the top of the patient's head so that the parietals and their sutures are mostly covered by this hand (ILLUSTRATIONS 8-5-A and 8-5-B).

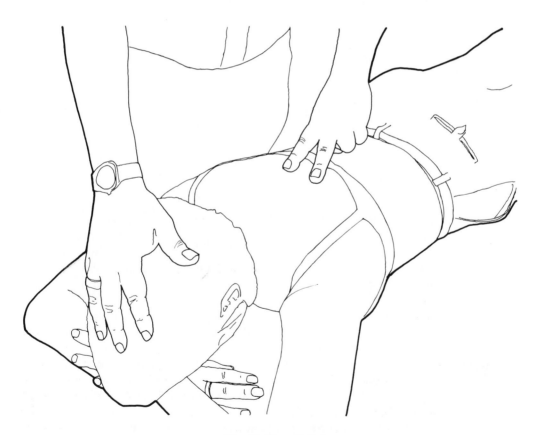

Illustration 8-5-A
Correction of Somatic Dysfunction by
Direction of Energy — Patient Prone

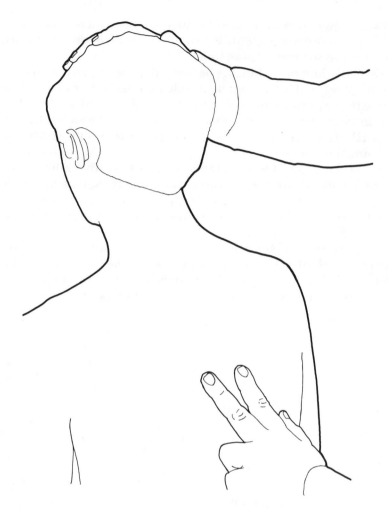

Illustration 8-5-B
Correction of Somatic Dysfunction by
Direction of Energy — Patient Seated

After about 30-60 seconds, you will perceive a gentle motion beginning; it is as though the involved vertebra is autonomously beginning to move. When this occurs, gently follow the motion while maintaining your contact over the transverse processes. Usually the next occurences will be heat and pulsating at the locus of the somatic dysfunction. Continue your technique until the motion, heat and pulsation are all no longer perceptible. The somatic dysfunction has corrected at this time.

Occasionally, a somatic dysfunction involves a structural problem which is too severe for this technique to totally correct. In such cases, a simple joint articulation after the direction of energy may be required to complete the correction. The somatic dysfunctions which seem to be corrected best by the direction of energy technique are those which are maintained by soft tissue contracture rather than by osseous malalignment.

Another cause of severe craniosacral system dysfunction is compression of the lumbosacral junction (L5-S1). This problem is often the underlying cause of recurrent cranial base compression, which results in head pain, intellectual dysfunction and psychoneurotic depression. The cranial base must, of course, be decompressed, as described in Chapter 7, during the same treatment session. Also frequently involved is compression of the occipital condyles, which must also be treated concurrently. The third part of the triad of compression is often at the lumbosacral junction. This simply means that the lumbar vertebral articular facets have become wedged into the articular facets of the sacrum. Probably as a protective mechanism, the connective tissues splint to prevent further injury and in so doing also contribute to the continuation of the problem. We would guess that this condition usually results from a fall upon the sacrococcygeal complex although it may also result from soft tissue hypertonus, which is or was adaptive to other problems of the neuromusculoskeletal system. We have also found this problem with some regularity in autistic children. Here we believe that it occurs because of constant cephalad dural traction upon the sacrum.

The only test we know of to diagnose this condition involves a direct attempt at decompression of the sacrum from the lower lumbar vertebrae (ILLUSTRATIONS 8-6-A and 8-6-B). Place one hand under the sacrum of the supine patient. It is sometimes helpful if the patient's knees are bent. Bring your other hand in from the patient's side so that the spines of the lumbar vertebrae are between your fingers, which are oriented transversely with the fifth finger in the space between the spines of the 5th lumbar

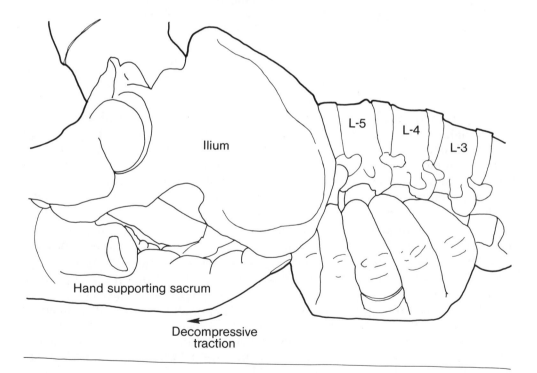

Hand supporting sacrum

Decompressive
traction

Illustration 8-6-A
Lumbosacral Decompression — Hand Placement for
Diagnosis and Treatment

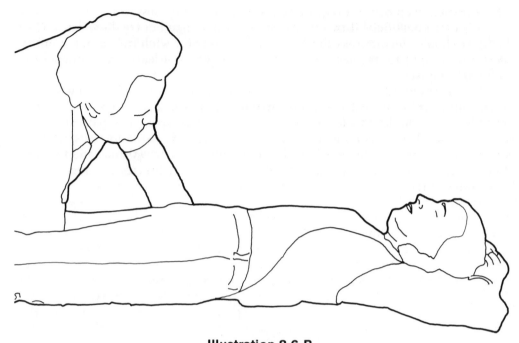

Illustration 8-6-B
Lumbosacral Decompression — Position for
Examination and Treatment

and the 1st sacral vertebrae. The fourth finger is between the spines of the 4th and 5th lumbar vertebrae. The rest of your fingers simply support the patient's lumbar spine.

Now stabilize the lumbar vertebrae with one of your hands. With the hand on the sacrum, apply a caudad traction upon the sacrum. This traction begins with a very small force and is gradually increased. The 5th lumbar vertebra and 1st sacral segment should separate easily. If your force becomes too great, you will feel the tissues begin to contract against you. This tissue response indicates that you should reduce the traction. If no separation of the lumbosacral junction occurs, you have a localized osseous compression of that junction. For treatment, hold the force of your traction beneath the level of tissue response until decompression occurs. This may take several minutes. If there is some separation but still some restriction, apply the same treatment until release occurs. The restriction very often seems to correct in a ratchet-fashion, alternating from side-to-side like a drawer that is being pulled out when stuck.

When the lumbosacral junction decompresses upon traction but seems to spring back as though it were being held together by elastic, the compression is due to increased tension upon the dural tube from above. Frequently this tension can be traced through the dural tube to the falx and tentorium cerebelli, and then through the falx cerebri to glabella. The tentorium causes compression of the cranial base, sphenoid to occiput, and the falx cerebri causes posterior retraction of the frontal bone. All of these problems must be corrected during a single treatment session. Repetitions of correction are usually required; it seems as though the dural membranes possess memory and require repeated reeducation sessions.

It is often beneficial if two therapists can work together on these cases. One therapist should decompress the lumbosacral junction while the other simultaneously decompresses the head. This can provide a valuable learning experience for the two therapists.

Another method of treatment which we have found very useful, and which we utilize following localized decompression of the lumbosacral junction, is to flex the pelvis by using the legs as levers (ILLUSTRATIONS 8-7-A and 8-7-B). The patient's body weight immobilizes the lumbar vertebrae and decompressive force is applied. Anterior pressure may be added to the suprapubic area to enhance the fulcrum effect of the lumbar vertebrae. This technique probably reeducates the tissues which have been maintaining the lumbosacral compression and all of its secondary effects.

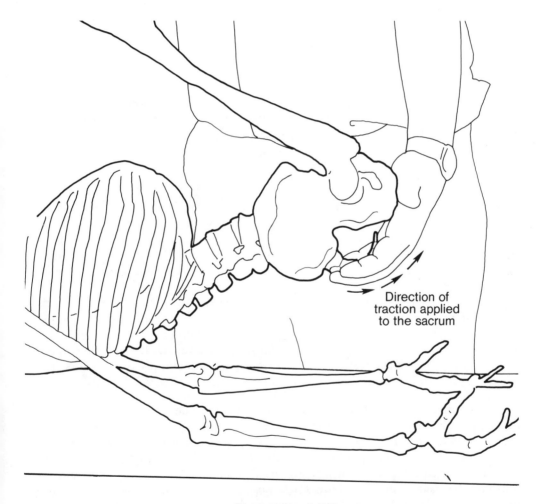

Direction of
traction applied
to the sacrum

Illustration 8-7-A
Use of Legs as Levers in Lumbosacral
Decompression — Hand Position Relative to Bony
Structures

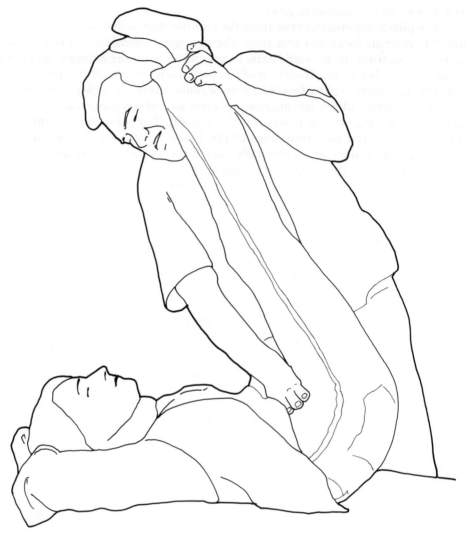

Illustration 8-7-B
Use of Legs as Levers in Lumbosacral
Decompression — Added Suprapubic Force

Use a slow application of this technique allowing the tissues to accommodate as you proceed. If the pelvis tends to sidebend or rotate as you flex, allow this to happen. As the tissue relaxation permits more and more flexion, continue to take up the slack. The patient's legs should be kept straight; the knees should not be bent. If the technique is painful, you are proceeding too fast; back off a little and continue. We seldom use this technique initially. Rather, we use it after decompression has been performed locally at the lumbosacral junction. It is often beneficial to have a second therapist balance the cranium as this technique is performed.

Extradural factors which impact the sacrum's ability to accommodate the movement of the craniosacral system include all muscles and ligaments which attach to it as well as the sacroiliac joints.

The piriformis muscles arise from the anterior sacrum between the 1st, 2nd, 3rd and 4th anterior foramena and from the grooves leading from these foramena. Origin is also from the greater sciatic foramen and from the anterior surface of the sacrotuberous ligaments. Insertion of the piriformis muscle after it passes laterally through the greater sciatic foramen is via a tendon into the superior border of the greater trochanter of the femur, just posterior to and sometimes blended with the tendon of the obturator internus and the gemelli. The piriformis is innervated by branches of the 2nd and sometimes of the 1st sacral and 5th lumbar nerves. The muscle acts to abduct and externally rotate the femur. It may also have some extension effect on the thigh (ILLUSTRATION 8-8).

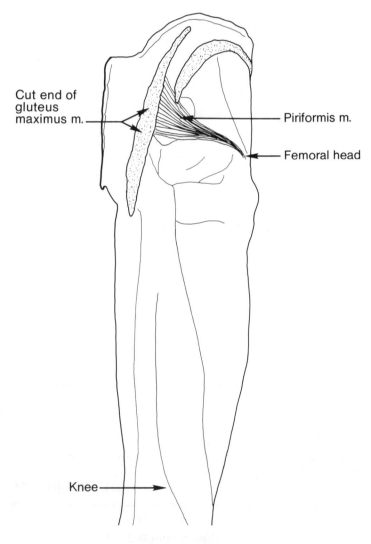

Illustration 8-8
Piriformis Muscle

Contracture of this muscle is common in patients suffering from lower back pain and sciatica. It will always serve to drag upon the sacrum, and therefore the mobility of the craniosacral system is at least partially compromised when the piriformis is abnormally hypertonic. This deleterious effect upon the craniosacral system may explain the general malaise and personality change which frequently accompanies piriformis muscle problems. The piriformis muscle, when unilaterally hypertonic, has a tendency to pull the sacrum to one side. This situation of sacral position will be duplicated at the occiput.

There are many techniques for correction of piriformis muscle hypertonus. One of the most effective in our experience makes use of the principle of reciprocal innervation. The patient must perform an exercise which tightens the opposite piriformis for 3 to 5 minutes, at least three times daily and whenever the affected muscle is painful (ILLUSTRATION 8-9).

The exercise is performed by having the patient lie on the floor parallel to and with the good (non-painful) side next to the wall. Under your direction, the patient must be taught to palpate the tight piriformis. Then, while lying on the floor, the good leg is flexed at the hip with the knee comfortably flexed, until the tissue change is palpable in the contracted piriformis. While maintaining this degree of thigh

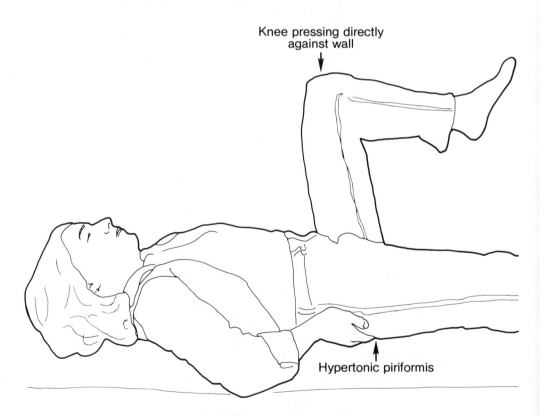

Knee pressing directly
against wall

Hypertonic piriformis

Illustration 8-9
Self-Help Exercise Used to Relax
Hypertonic Piriformis Muscle

flexion, and monitoring the tight piriformis with a finger, the patient presses the knee of the non-involved side against the wall in a lateral direction. The force against the wall is increased and continued until the tight piriformis can be felt to relax. The exercise is completed when this relaxation is perceived. Repetition of this exercise three times daily will cause the chronically contractured piriformis muscle to respond favorably over a period of days to weeks. As this occurs, the craniosacral system will function more efficiently.

The iliacus muscles are the flat, triangular muscles which fill the iliac fossae. They arise from the superior two-thirds of the fossae, from the inner lips of the iliac crests, from the anterior sacroiliac and iliolumbar ligaments and from the dorsum of the sacral base. The fibers converge as the muscle runs inferiorly and inserts into the lateral side of the psoas major, the lesser trochanter, the capsule of the hip joint and the body of the femur. The iliacus muscle is innervated by branches of the femoral nerves, which usually originate from the 2nd and 3rd lumbar nerve roots. The muscle acts to flex the thigh and tilt the pelvis forward.

When in a state of abnormal contracture, the iliacus maintains the sacrum in a position which corresponds to the extension phase of the craniosacral system motion (ILLUSTRATON 8-10). Unilateral contracture will then contribute to sacral torsion, which is mimed by the occiput. Bilateral contracture contributes to

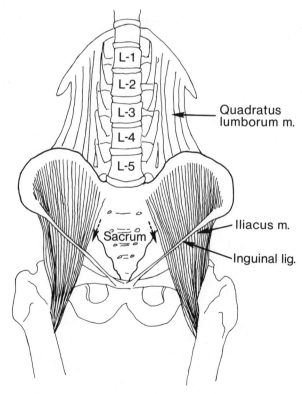

Illustration 8-10
Iliacus Muscle (Arrows Indicate How This Muscle
Can Interfere with Free Sacral Mobility)

extension lesioning, which is reflected in the occiput and therefore in the whole cranial base. Techniques to relax the iliacus are numerous. It is our experience that mobilization of the upper lumbar vertebrae by the direction of energy techniques described previously are very effective. Reciprocal innervation techniques which flex the thigh against resistance will also cause relaxation of the contralateral iliacus muscle.

The gluteus maximus muscles are the broad muscles which account for much of the muscle bulk of the buttocks. They are roughly rectangular in shape. They arise from the posterior gluteal lines, the tendons of the sacrospinous muscle masses, the dorsum of the sacrum throughout its entire length, the dorsum of the coccyx and the sacrotuberous ligaments. They insert into the gluteal tuberosities of the femur and the iliotibial bands of the fascia lata. The innervation of the gluteus maximus is from the inferior gluteal nerve which receives contributions from the 5th lumbar and the 1st and 2nd sacral nerve roots.

The gluteus maximus is a very powerful extensor, adductor and lateral rotator of the thigh. When the thigh is stable, it acts to extend the trunk. Hypertonus of this muscle unilaterally tends to immobilize the sacrum and rotate it slightly away from the muscle. Bilateral hypertonus immobilizes the sacrum, which causes a drag upon the craniosacral system.

The gluteus maximus can be relaxed by utilization of the principle of reciprocal innervation or by means of deep pressure upon the motor point (ILLUSTRATION 8-11). Deep pressure can be performed by a thumb, a knuckle or even an elbow. Pressure should be applied at the locus of maximum tenderness and continued until the muscle is perceived to have relaxed.

The multifidus muscles consist of a number of fasciculi which fill up the grooves on both sides of the spinous processes of the vertebrae from axis to sacrum. The fasciculi arise laterally on the vertebrae, ascend two to four segments and insert into the appropriate spinous processes above (ILLUSTRATION 8-12).

The multifidus is innervated by appropriate branches of the spinal nerves. It sidebends the spine when acting unilaterally and it extends the spine when acting bilaterally. Multifidus hypertonus contributes to sacral immobility, acting against craniosacral system flexion when bilaterally hypertonic. When unilaterally hypertonic, it promotes sacral sidebending or torsion, which is reflected in the occiput and cranial base as abnormal motion patterning.

Hypertonus of the multifidus is effectively treated by the position and hold technique described earlier in this chapter for decompression of the lumbosacral junction. The straight legs of the supine patient are flexed toward the chest. As you wait for the tissues to release, you will achieve multifidus relaxation.

The complex ligaments of the pelvis all influence sacral motion when they are in a state of unbalanced tension. These tensions are treated by balancing posture, mobilizing the pelvis and releasing the pelvic diaphragm (CHAPTER 5). The major ligaments which must be kept in mind are the sacrococcygeal, sacrogluteal, sacroiliac, sacrosciatic, sacrospinous and the sacrotuberous. It must also be remembered that many of these ligamentous structures serve as muscle attachments (as do the fasciae) and therefore transmit tensions, which originate in the appropriate muscles, to the sacrum.

Two very common injuries which adversely influence craniosacral system function and are often the underlying cause of headache and autonomic dysfunc-

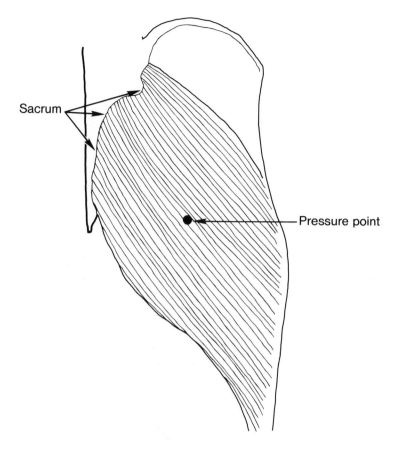

Sacrum

Pressure point

Illustration 8-11
Gluteus Maximus Muscle

tion are impaction of the sacrum between the ilia, and anterior flexion of the coccyx.

Impaction of the sacrum between the ilia occurs from a fall upon the ischial tuberosities where the downward motion of these tuberosities is suddenly halted by a hard surface, and the momentum of the sacrum and the structures above the sacrum drive it caudad between the ilia. Seldom does this occur with perfect symmetry, so there is usually a sidebending component in the lesion pattern (ILLUSTRATION 8-13).

The best treatment for this condition is to place the index finger inside the rectum and grasp the sacrum between the index finger and thumb. Stabilize the ilia with the other hand and move the sacrum cephalad until it "floats free," or mobilizes. The patient is best placed in the lateral recumbent position with the knees comfortably flexed toward the chest. Patient assistance may be utilized by having the patient exert medial force upon both anterior superior iliac spines so that the posterior regions of the ilia spread laterally and aid in releasing the impacted sacrum.

Anterior flexion of the coccyx due to injury is another very common cause of cephalgia and pelvic autonomic dysfunction. Anteroflexion of the coccyx causes increased tension to be transmitted through the posterior part of the dural tube to

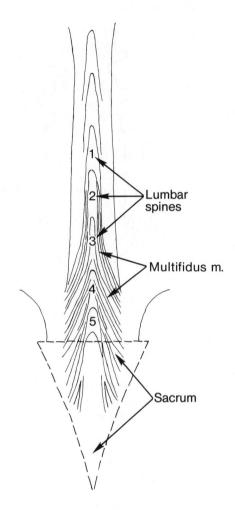

Illustration 8-12
The Multifidus Muscles

the foramen magnum. It can then be transmitted via the falx cerebelli to the straight sinus, to the falx cerebri, and may, on occasion via the flax cerebri, show itself as a frontal headache. More often, the tension disseminates after it reaches the occiput and results in occipital headache.

The treatment for anteroflexion of the coccyx is to place the patient in a lateral recumbent position. Insert the index finger in the rectum. Gently grasp the coccyx between the thumb and index finger, and *gently but firmly* mobilize it.

Frequently, both in cases of sacral impaction between the ilia and anteroflexion of the coccyx, the headache can immediately be induced and removed by lesion exaggeration and reduction. This circumstance suggests a cause and effect relationship between sacrococcygeal complex somatic dysfunction and head pain. Similar cause and effect relationships can often be demonstrated between sacrococcygeal complex problems and low back, pelvic and/or visceral pain.

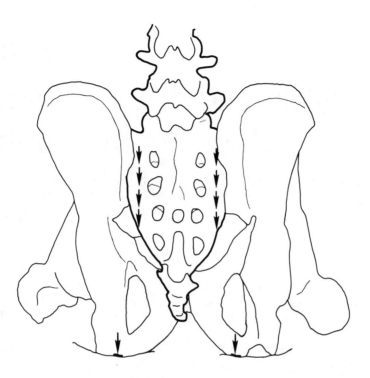

Illustration 8-13
Sacrum and Ilia (Arrows Indicate Direction of
Compacting Force)

Chapter 9
Diagnosis and Treatment of Osseous and Sutural Dysfunctions of the Cranial Vault

The cranial base, which is the floor of the cranium, has been considered in Chapter 7. In this chapter we will consider the cranial vault, which is its sides and roof. Embryologically, the base is derived from cartilage, and the sides and roof from membrane.

The parietal bones are the only bones of the sides and roof of the vault which do not also contribute to the cranial base. It is obvious, therefore, that our division is somewhat artificial. The remainder of the sides and roof of the cranial vault are made up of the frontal bone, the great wings of the sphenoid, the temporal squama and mastoid portions, and the occipital squama.

The sutures which we will consider here are the coronal, sagittal, lambdoidal, occipitomastoid, temporoparietal, sphenosquamal, sphenofrontal and the sphenoparietal. Other sutures related to the cranial vault have either been discussed previously in relation to the cranial base or will be discussed later in Chapter 12, which deals with the mouth, face and the temporomandibular joints.

The physical nature of the suture determines the type of motion in which it participates, and which it will allow. Traditionally, Western anatomy has taught that skull sutures are junctural fibrosae or synarthroses (PRICHARD 1956, JACOB and FRANCONE 1974, WARWICK and WILLIAMS 1978). They have been regarded as immovable joints. The suture is that form of articulation in which contiguous bone margins are united by connective tissue. Our research clearly demonstrates that sutures do allow small amounts of movement between their component bones (RETZLAFF 1978, APPENDIX G, APPENDIX J). Sutures not only contain connective tissue, but also rich vascular networks, nerve plexuses and receptors. In our laboratory we have traced a single dendrite from the sagittal suture of the monkey through the dural membrane, into the brain substance and then into the wall of the third ventricle of the brain.[1]

Cranial sutures (ILLUSTRATION 9-1) are classified as follows:

1. *Sutura dentata:* toothlike projections, as in the sagittal suture.
2. *Sutura serrata:* the bone edges are serrated, as are the teeth of a saw. An example is the metopic suture.

---

[1]This work is presently in progress by Retzlaff, et. al.

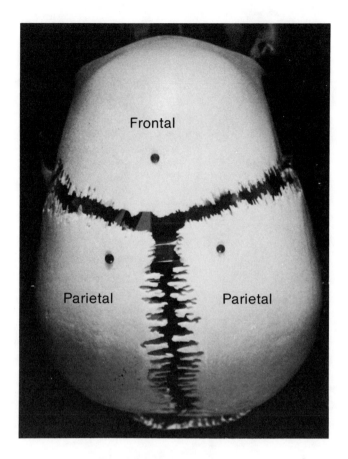

Illustration 9-1
Types of Sutures on Exploded Skull

3. *Sutura lumbosa:* in addition to the interlocking, there is a beveling so that the bones overlap one another, as in the coronal suture.
4. *Sutura squamosa:* formed by the overlapping of contiguous bones with very broad, beveled margins. An example is the temporoparietal suture.
5. *Sutura plana:* simple apposition of contiguous rough surfaces, as in the intermaxillary suture.
6. *Schindylesis:* a thin plate of one bone is received into a cleft formed by other bone(s). Examples of the schindylesis can be seen between the vomer and the ethmoid, and between the vomer and the maxillae-palatines as they form the hard palate.
7. The *synchondrosis* is not strictly a suture. It is illustrated by the cartilage bridge formed between the occiput and the sphenoid.

Our own impressions suggest that in the sutures which present interdigitation, the longer the digital projections, the greater the motion in that region of the suture (ILLUSTRATION 9-2-A).

The squamosal suture components are beveled and grooved. This morphology indicates the direction of motion which these sutures perform (ILLUSTRATION 9-2-B).

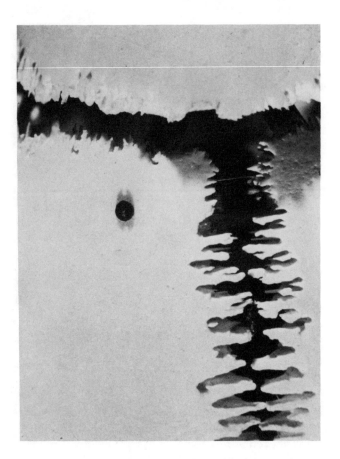

Illustration 9-2-A
Varying Lengths of Digits at Sagittal Suture

Dr. Sutherland and his followers postulate specific movement around specific axes for each of the cranial vault bones. When you consider the cranium as a mechanical model, it does indeed become obvious that movement of one bone induces movement in other, related bones until the whole cranium is seen to move in response to the initial driving force (MAGOUN 1966). Our contention is that the driving force is the changing fluid pressure: the cranial bones move to accommodate these subtle changes in cerebrospinal fluid pressure.

When one suture or bone of the cranial vault becomes restricted in its motion for any reason, it causes a distortion in the motion of the whole cranial vault as adjustment is made for this localized motion restriction. The CV-4 technique is an example of iatrogenically induced restriction of occipital bone motion. The result is a small but significant increase in the motion of all other sutures and bones of the craniosacral system. If the CV-4 technique were to be continued long beyond its therapeutic usefulness, it could become a severe restricting lesion to the cranio-sacral system, as in occipital somatic dysfunction.

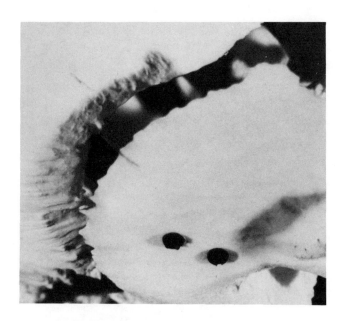

Illustration 9-2-B
Beveled and Grooved Temporoparietal Suture

ACCOMMODATIVE MOVEMENTS OF THE CRANIAL VAULT BONES

In order to gain a view of the accommodative movements of the bones of the cranial vault, we shall consider these bones individually. Although we present postulated axes of motion for each bone of the vault, you should keep in mind that the best way to discover the typical movements of the cranial bones is not to learn them academically but to *experience* these movements perceptually.

The movements vary from one patient to another. The norms vary for each vault bone. The movement is dependent upon many factors, not the least of which is head shape. We are most interested in the quality of the motion, whether the perceived movement is smooth, whether the bone is moving against resistance, whether the range of motion is abnormally limited, etc. If a vault bone seems to be moving freely but in a motion pattern which deviates from the model which we shall propose here, you should catalog this fact in your mind but do not necessarily attempt to "normalize" its motion pattern, or even consider it as abnormal for that patient.

In order to understand the movement of the cranial bones it is essential that you experience the motions of many crania. You may not be able to verbally describe what you feel, but you will perceptually understand the movements and, ultimately, their meanings and related symptoms.

SPHENOID

As the sphenoid moves into the flexion phase of the craniosacral motion cycle, its posterior aspect moves cephalad, and its anterior parts take an anterior-inferiorly directed "nose-dive." The transverse axis of rotation is approximately halfway between the anterior and posterior borders of the body, when cut through the midsagittal plane. It is horizontally level with the bottom of the sella turcica (ILLUSTRATION 9-3).

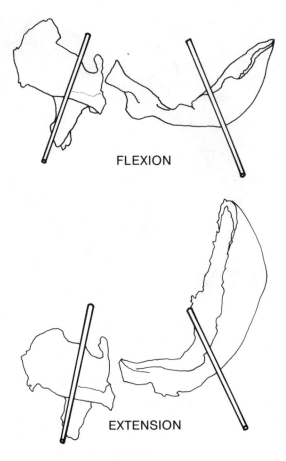

FLEXION

EXTENSION

Illustration 9-3
Sphenoid and Occiput (Note Transverse Axes)

As the sphenoid bone rotates about this axis during cyclic flexion and extension of the craniosacral system, the great wings have a significant effect upon the vault bones with which they articulate, namely, the frontal, temporals and parietals (ILLUSTRATION 9-4). Additionally, it must be kept in mind that the sphenoid in the cranial base works in conjunction with the occiput, the ethmoid, the vomer and the petrous temporals (ILLUSTRATION 9-5). When you consider the effects of the sphenoid upon the other bones of the floor, sides and roof of the cranial vault, you must also keep in mind the secondary concurrent effects of all of these bones upon other bones with which they articulate.

The eccentrically placed great sphenoid wings rotate anteriorly at their superior borders during flexion. The sphenoid, via the sphenofrontal suture, therefore induces the inferior part of the frontal to move anteriorly. Since the axis of rotation of the frontal is above the bone margin affected by the sphenoid wing, the frontal rotates in the opposite direction. At the same time the ethmoid, influenced by the sphenoid body, is helping to carry the transverse axis of the frontal bone anteriorly and may thereby act against the effect of the sphenoid wings upon the

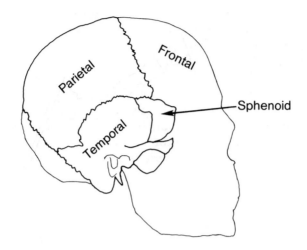

Illustration 9-4
Vault Articulations of the Sphenoid

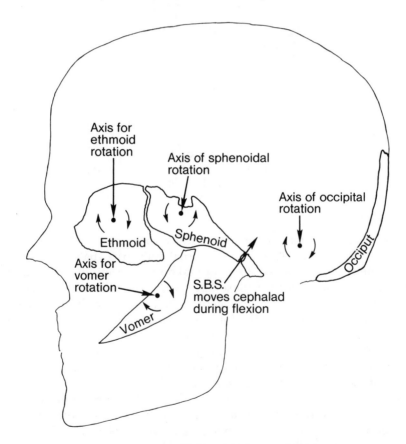

Illustration 9-5
Interrelated Movement of the Cranial Base
Bones During Flexion

frontal. Our impression of frontal motion during flexion is that of a posterior rotation about a transverse translatory axis which is moving in an anterior and inferior direction.

The posterior margin of the sphenoid wing also has sutural contact with the anterior margin of the temporal squamous. This posterior margin of the sphenoid wing is very close to the axis of rotation of the sphenoid body. The effect, therefore, is probably more to inhibit than to activate temporal motion. The temporal bone, strongly influenced by the occiput, in turn exerts a governing effect upon the sphenoid. The angle of the occipitomastoid suture, with its change in bevel, allows for a wobbling motion between these two bone margins (ILLUSTRATION 9-6).

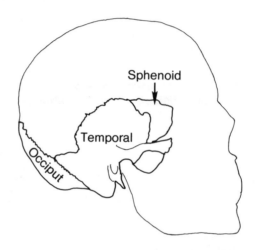

Illustration 9-6
Relationships Among the Sphenoid, Temporal
and Occiput

TEMPORAL BONES

The temporal squama rotate eccentrically about bilateral axes which are externally located approximately at the external auditory canals, and internally pass through the petrous portions of the temporal bones to their medial junctions at the sphenobasilar regions. Because these axes run diagonally and anteriorly as they travel from the periphery toward the center, they cause a wobbling rotation of the temporal squama. During the flexion phase of craniosacral system motion, the transverse distance between the superior margins of the temporal squama increases as they move anteriorly. This broadening of the transverse distance between the superior margins of the paired temporal squama, together with the anterior movement of these superior margins, is referred to as external rotation of the temporal bones. The movements are reversed during the extension phase of craniosacral system motion: the transverse distance between the superior margins of the temporal bones decreases as these margins move posteriorly. This movement is called internal rotation of the temporal bones. All paired bones of the body externally rotate during craniosacral system flexion, and internally rotate during extension (ILLUSTRATION 9-7).

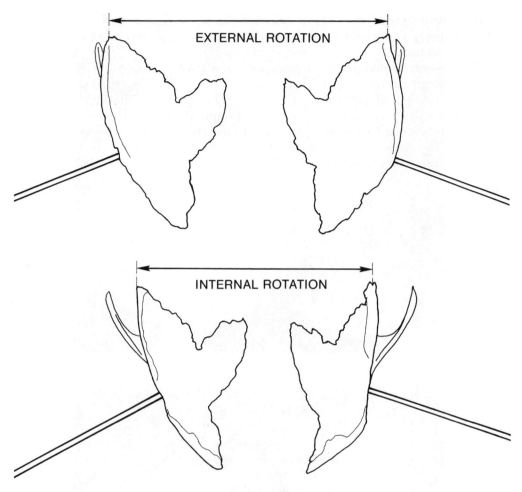

Illustration 9-7
Temporal Motion (Note Axes and Difference
in Distance Between Squama)

OCCIPUT

During the flexion phase of craniosacral system motion, the anterior occipital base (basiocciput) moves cephalad; the squamal part moves inferiorly and anteriorly in an arc about a transverse axis located above the foramen magnum, approximately level with the superior nuchal line.

As the occiput moves into flexion in response to changing fluid pressure, it drives the temporal into external rotation. The greatest force is at the point of the bevel change of the occipitomastoid suture (ILLUSTRATION 9-8).

PARIETAL BONES

The parietals and temporal squama are relatively free to glide up and down upon each other as long as they don't shear. This means that when the temporal superior margins move anteriorly into external rotation, the parietals also move for-

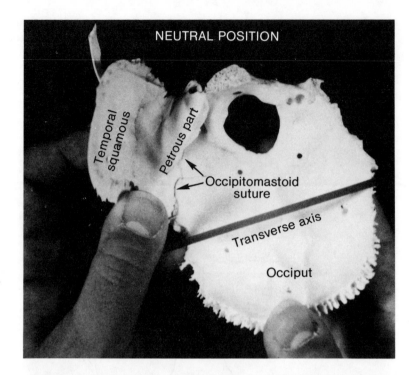

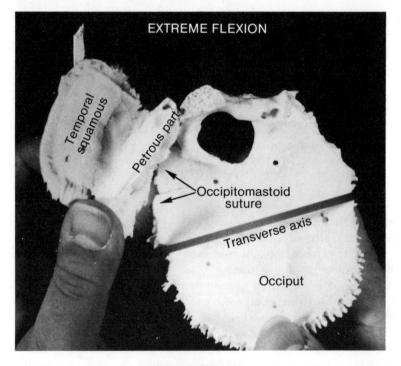

Illustration 9-8
Relationship Between Occiput and Temporal
(Note Axis)

ward as they spread laterally. This anterior motion is allowed by the interdigitations between the occiput and the parietals at the lambdoidal sutures. The parietal spread during external rotation is allowed by the digits of the sagittal suture.

THERAPEUTIC TECHNIQUES FOR THE CRANIAL VAULT

PARIETAL LIFT

The parietal bones are mobilized by a technique called the parietal lift. To perform this technique you should be seated above the patient's head. Your fingertips are placed gently in contact with the lateral aspects of the parietal bones, bilaterally. The fingerpads of the fifth fingers are in contact with asterion, anterior to the lambdoid sutures and just above the temporoparietal sutures. The other three fingers of each hand are placed about one centimeter apart and must be above the temporoparietal sutures (ILLUSTRATION 9-9). Your thumbs are now crossed upon each other above the patient's head. They do not touch the scalp. Then, after finger placement is rechecked, *gentle* pressure is exerted to compress the lateral aspects of the parietal bones medially (ILLUSTRATION 9-10). If the temporal bones are pressured, the technique will not work and may, in fact, precipitate a worsening of the clinical symptoms. The amount of pressure exerted on the parietal bones is on the order of 5 grams. The thumbs, in contact with each other, are used to steady the hands. This gentle pressure on *only the parietal bones* is held constant for several minutes (usually 3-5 minutes will suffice). As the temporoparietal sutures disengage, it will feel as

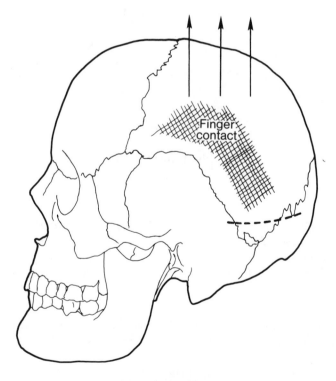

Illustration 9-9
Finger Placement for Parietal Lift

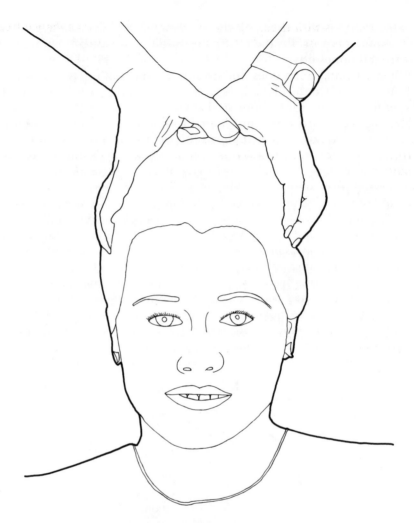

Illustration 9-10
Hand Position for Parietal Lift

though the parietal bones are moving superiorly and spreading very slightly—allow this to happen. *Do not suddenly release your pressure on the parietal bones.* Do it gradually; otherwise, you may cause the symptoms to worsen. Usually, when this release is felt, the patient will remark that pressure within the head has been relieved (APPENDIX D).

FRONTAL LIFT

The frontal seems to rotate posteriorly while its axis moves anteriorly; it also seems to broaden transversely during the flexion phase of craniosacral system motion, as though the metopic suture was still patent.

As we stated at the beginning of the chapter, the best way to learn the movements of the vault bones of the cranium is to discover them with your hands. Variation in normal motion of frontal bones from head to head is great. Each patient carries the motions with them; all the examiner should do is enhance freedom of motion as much as possible, then study the motions that are present to learn what it is that frontal bones do.

When a frontal bone does not seem to be moving freely, the technique for mobilization is the frontal lift (ILLUSTRATION 9-11). With the patient supine, place your hands gently over the frontal bone so that your third or fourth fingers are grasping the ridges of the frontal bone, just lateral to the orbits of the eyes. An anteriorly directed lifting traction is then applied until the frontal bone is felt to release and float free. If specific sutural restriction becomes apparent during this technique, the procedure may be interrupted in order to mobilize the suture. These techniques for sutural mobilization are discussed below.

Frequently, the frontal seems to be immobilized or restricted by the falx cerebri. This type of restriction will show itself as an elastic resistance to your lifting traction. When this occurs, simply use a direction of energy technique through the falx cerebri until release is perceived (ILLUSTRATION 9-12). The energy is best directed by placing one finger at the base of the occiput pointing at the anterior falx cerebri. Two fingers of the other hand should be laid parallel to, and on either side of the anterior falx cerebri attachment to the frontal bone. You will first perceive heat, then pulsating, then some movement as the falx releases. When all of these activities are ended, you may stop the direction of energy technique. Re-apply the frontal lift technique to evaluate your results.

Specific corrections for sphenoid and occiput have been described in Chapter 7

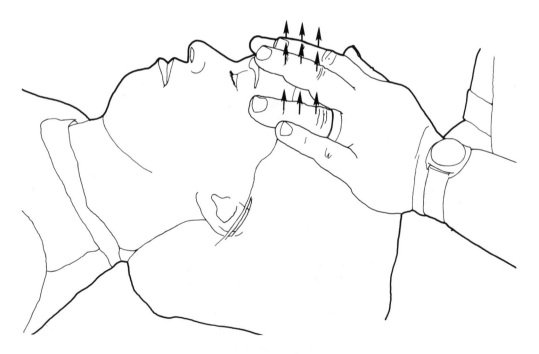

Illustration 9-11
Hand Position and Direction of Traction
for Frontal Lift

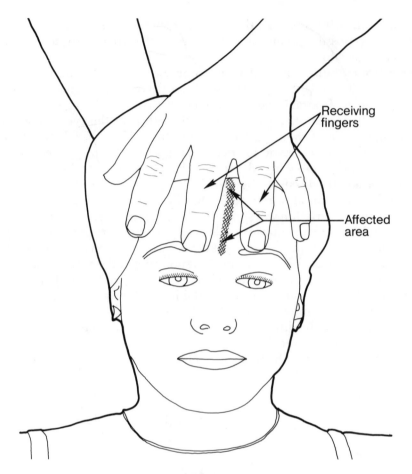

Illustration 9-12
Hand Position for Direction of Energy Technique
to Falx Cerebri

and will be further considered in Chapter 10. Specific techniques for temporal bone dysfunctions are described in detail in Chapter 11.

SPECIFIC SUTURAL RESTRICTIONS

Specific sutural restrictions (APPENDIX D) are best treated by the direction of energy technique. To perform this technique, place the pad of one of your fingers upon the restricted suture and point across the greatest diameter of the cranial vault. Gently palpate the part of the cranium toward which you are pointing with your whole hand. After a few seconds you will perceive a pulsating motion with your palpating hand. When you feel this pulsation, place one finger of your palpating hand upon the center of the pulsating area, and point directly across the cranium at the restricted suture. Then gently place two of your fingers on either side of, and approximately parallel with the restricted suture. It is as though you will receive the energy between these two fingers which you are sending from the other side through

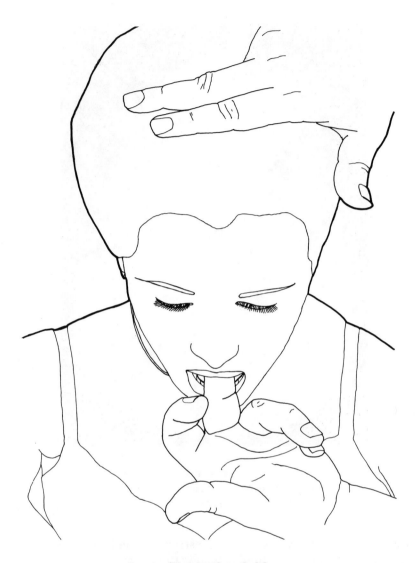

Illustration 9-13
Hand Position for Direction of Energy Technique
from Hard Palate

that finger. First, you will feel heat and pulsation at the restricted area, then the bones (one under each finger) will begin to move independently of each other as if struggling to get loose. You should encourage these independent motions very gently. Finally, when you feel the release of restriction, the correction has been made.

Sutures such as the coronal and sagittal, located on the top of the cranial vault, are best treated by directing energy from the midline of the hard palate (ILLUSTRATION 9-13). With the directing finger inside the patient's mouth, point at the restriction and receive with your other fingers placed parallel to the restricted suture on the

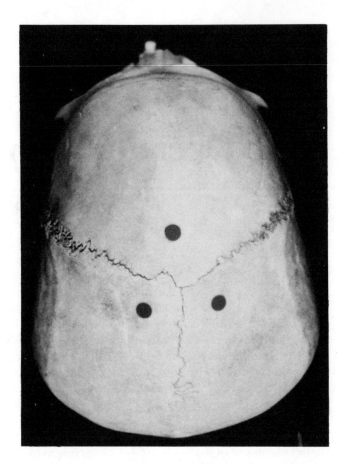

Illustration 9-14
Finger Placement for Receiving Energy
at Junction of Three Bones

external surface of the patient's head. If the restriction involves the juncture of three bones as it would at the bregma, three receiving fingers may effectively be used, one on each bone, while the energy is directed with the other hand (ILLUSTRATION 9-14).

Although we do not know the mechanism of action of this technique, it has been very effective in our hands and in those of many of our students. Try it before you reject it as being too esoteric.

Chapter 10
The Occipital Condyles

The occipital condyles occupy a critical position in the craniosacral system at the meeting point between the cranium and the spine. Somatic dysfunction of the occipital condyles is never without serious consequences. Do not overlook the possibility of occipital condylar compression as the cause of a multitude of syndromes.

Although it may be said that a chapter devoted solely to one part of one bone is not in the best holistic tradition, we hope that by focussing upon the occipital condyles you will be able to better understand their role in the body as a whole.

EMBRYOLOGICAL DEVELOPMENT OF THE OCCIPUT

In order to get a "feel" for the occipital condyles, we must take a brief look at the embryological development of the skull itself. The first signs of the membranous skull are found in the sphenobasilar region and around the auditory vesicles. Mesoderm is generated from the basilar area up and around the ectodermal brain until the brain is enclosed by the membrane. This enclosure is called the membranous cranium. The enclosure is interrupted by spaces where large nerves and blood vessels are afforded passage into and out of this membranous vault.

Before the membranous vault is completed above, the basilar area begins to develop into cartilage so that the cranial base is cartilagenous and the sides and roof of the cranial vault are membranous. By the end of the fourth week of gestation, the cranial vault enclosure is usually completed.

The cartilagenous development of the base of the occiput begins from two mesodermal growth centers located on both sides of the notocord. These centers will ultimately form the anterior margin of the foramen magnum as medial growth occurs. Lateral growth from these centers will form the hypoglossal canals. The occipital condyles are also produced from these centers. It is from the lateral regions of the occipital cartilage that its nuchal plate develops and extends around the primitive brain to form the posterior margin of the foramen magnum.

Occipital cartilage growth also spreads forward toward the forebrain where it encounters cartilage development arising from the sphenoid centers. The sphenobasilar synchondrosis is formed at the juncture of these two cartilage developments.

As the occipital cartilage grows lateralward it meets cartilage coming from the auditory capsules. The juncture of these two cartilages forms the jugular foramena, the foramena lacerus and the sutures which separate the occiput from the petrous temporal bones.

The cartilagenous ossification centers give rise to all of the bones of the occiput (except the interparietal squama), the petrous and mastoid parts of the temporal bones, the sphenoid (except for the pterygoid plates and the parts of the great wings which are most lateral), and all of the ethmoid bone. The rest of the cranium is formed from membrane.

At birth, the condylar parts of the occiput are not ossified completely; there is still cartilage present. The presence of this cartilage allows for some flexibility. If and when the condylar parts of the occiput are forced anteriorly during hyperextension of the head on the neck as a phase of the delivery process, they may become wedged into the narrowing receptacle formed by the articular surfaces of the atlas. If the self-correcting hydraulic force of the craniosacral system fails to correct this circumstance, and if craniosacral treatment is not effectively performed, the condylar compression may persist (ILLUSTRATION 10-1).

Since cartilage is somewhat malleable and bone grows in the direction of lesser resistance, this compression or jamming of the occipital condylar parts between the receiving articular surfaces of the atlas can easily result in abnormal growth and

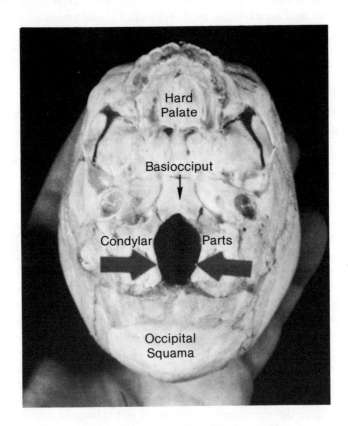

Illustration 10-1
Inferior View of Fetal Skull (Arrows Indicate
Direction of Condylar Compression)

morphological development of the occiput. This will contribute to asymmetry of the skull and its dural membranes (ILLUSTRATION 10-2). As a result, malformation of the foramen magnum, the occipital condyles, the hypoglossal canals, the foramen lacerum and the jugular foramen may occur. The clinical implications of these malformations are extremely varied and may be very serious.

Through the foramen magnum passes the caudal end of the medulla oblongata, the meninges and their blood vessels, the vertebral arteries, the accessory nerves, the anterior and posterior spinal arteries, the tectorial membranes and the alar ligaments. Abnormal pressure about the foramen magnum which results in its deformation can therefore indeed set the stage for problems resulting from pressure on any of these structures.

Compression of the condylar parts can easily result in hypoglossal canal maldevelopment. This condition gives rise to clinical symptoms relating to dysfunction of the hypoglossal nerve, e.g., motor coordination problems, atrophy or maldevelopment of the tongue. The compression of the occipital condyles between the articular surfaces of the atlas may also interfere with normal function of the suture between the occiput and the petrous temporal parts of the base of the cranium. This interference will appear as clinical syndromes relating to deformation and/or dys-

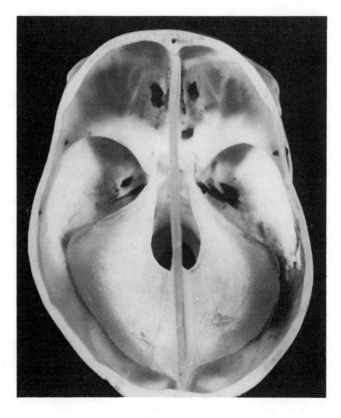

Illustration 10-2
Floor of Cranial Vault Viewed from Above
Showing Asymmetrical Dural Membrane

function of the jugular foramena, the foramena lacerum and the atlanto-occipital joints themselves. Since the occiput is not completely ossified until approximately the age of six years, early correction of abnormal forces on the occipital condyles can have an extremely beneficial effect upon the health of a child for the duration of his or her life.

Through the jugular foramena passes the jugular venous drainage of blood from the cranial vault. Therefore deformation or dysfunction of these foramena often results in symptoms relating to intracranial fluid congestion such as brain dysfunction or head pain. Also the 9th, 10th and 11th cranial nerves pass through these foramena. Dysfunction of these nerves can result in gag reflex problems, taste abnormalities of the posterior third of the tongue, problems with speech and swallowing, cardiac arrythmias, digestive and elimination problems relating to vagal control of stomach and lower bowel, and abnormal tonus of the sternocleidomastoid and trapezius muscles. The foramen lacerum is partially filled with fibrocartilage. It is also intimately related to the great superficial petrosal nerve and the auditory tube. Symptoms related to the auditory tube often result from occipital condyle compression, as do symptoms related to impairment of blood supply to the occipital lobes of the brain. This blood flow is strongly influenced by the great superficial petrosal nerve (OWMAN and EDVINSSON 1977).

DIAGNOSIS AND TREATMENT OF OCCIPITAL CONDYLAR SOMATIC DYSFUNCTION

As is so often the case with the craniosacral system, the diagnosis and treatment of occipital condylar somatic dysfunction are inseparable. The diagnosis is simply a determination of whether or not the occipital condyles are free to disengage posteriorly from between the articular surfaces of the atlas. If this freedom is not present, the treatment is to establish the desired mobility and then to spread the condylar parts laterally as much as possible after they have been disengaged from the atlas.

Diagnostic and therapeutic consideration of the occipital condyles comes as a natural follow-up to the release of connective tissue restrictions of the cranial base as described in Chapter 5. These extradural connective tissue restrictions must be released before reliable and accurate evaluation of the condition of the occipital condyles can be accomplished.

The diagnostic technique is performed with the patient supine. The occiput is gently cradled upon the palmer surfaces of your hands and fingers. Your fingertips are allowed to intrude as far as is comfortably possible along the inferior surface of the patient's occiput in an anterior direction. You then gently attempt to move the inferior surface of the occiput posteriorly around its postulated transverse axis (ILLUSTRATION 10-3). The traction or force used is minimal. If the force is too large the patient's tissues will react by tightening or contracting. The evaluation cannot be made when the connective tissues attached to the occipital base region are in a state of contraction.

If the occipital condyles are not compressed between the articular surfaces of the atlas, the occiput will seem to float freely around the axis. If the occipital condylar parts are dysfunctional between the articular surfaces of the atlas, the occiput will resist the motion you are trying to induce.

When the motion tests indicate that the condylar parts are restricted at the

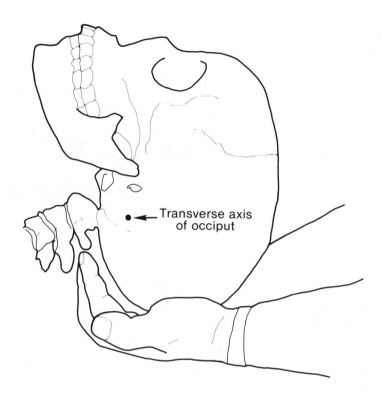

Transverse axis
of occiput

Illustration 10-3
Hand Position for Diagnosis and Treatment
of Condylar Compression

atlas, the first step of the treatment is instituted without changing the hand positions
on the occipital region. Simply continue the gentle urging of the occipital condyles
to disengage themselves posteriorly from the wedge formed by the articular surfaces
of the atlas until you gradually perceive a posterior gliding of the occipital base in
response to your traction. If traction is too forceful, nothing good will happen. After
disengagement has occurred, induce a lateral spread into the condylar parts. This
phase of the treatment technique has a tendency to help decompress the foramen
magnum. It will also help release restriction at the jugular foramena.

In order to achieve this lateral spreading of the condylar parts, slowly
approximate your elbows using your arms as levers, and your hypothenar eminences
and palms as the fulcrum. If you can imagine projections from your fingertips into
the condylar parts, you can see the projected effect of bringing your elbows closer
together. Continue this second phase of the treatment until the release is perceived.

Compression of the condylar parts is often accompanied by cranial base and
lumbosacral compression. Based upon the observations of numerous practitioners
of craniosacral therapy, this problem is causally related to "hyperkinetic" behavior
in children (APPENDIX I), to severe cephalgia in adults (MILLER 1972) and to various
respiratory distress syndromes in infants and newborns (FRYMAN 1966). We have often
wondered whether severe dysfunction of the occipital condylar parts is not
contributory to sudden infant death syndrome.

Chapter 11
Temporal Bone Dysfunction

The paired temporal bones both contribute significantly to the cranial base by their petrous portions and to the lateral walls of the cranial vault by their squama, tympanic and mastoid parts (ILLUSTRATIONS 11-1-A, 11-1-B, 11-1-C and 11-1-D). Projecting anteriorly from the inferior part of the squama are the temporal zygomatic processes, which articulate with the zygomatic bones of the face. As will be seen, these zygomatic processes are quite useful as levers in the treatment of temporal bone dysfunction.

Embryologically, the temporal bone is ossified from eight centers. The temporal bone of the newborn infant is in three parts: squama, petromastoid and tympanic ring (ILLUSTRATION 11-2).

The tympanic ring, which offers attachment to the tympanic membrane, fuses with the squama shortly before term. The petromastoid and squamal parts of the temporal bones unite during the first year of life.

The temporal bones articulate with the occiput, parietals, sphenoid, mandible and zygomatic bones.

PHYSIOLOGICAL TEMPORAL BONE MOTION

Our findings and impressions with respect to temporal bone motion largely concur with those described by Dr. Sutherland (MAGOUN 1966). He postulated that the temporal bones rotate around axes which follow a line approximately 1 centimeter inferior to the petrous ridges and which enter the cranial vault through the external ear canals (auditory meatuses). These axes are almost horizontal when the head is in the upright position. The axes angle anteriorly as they move medially following the angle of the petrous ridges of the temporal bones.

During the flexion phase of craniosacral system motion, the superior borders of the temporal squama move anteriorly. Because of the direction of the axes, they also move laterally; the transverse distance between the superior parts of the temporal squama is therefore increased. This is a part of the external rotation of the temporal bones.

As the superior squamal regions move anteriorly and broaden, the zygomatic processes move inferiorly and the mastoid tips move superiorly and posteriorly. At the same time, the transverse distance between the mastoid tips decreases. The

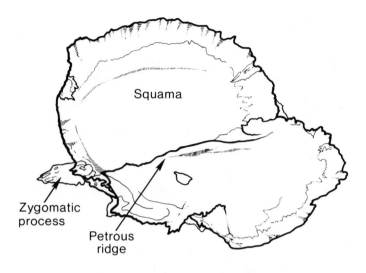

Illustration 11-1-A
Temporal Bone — Internal View

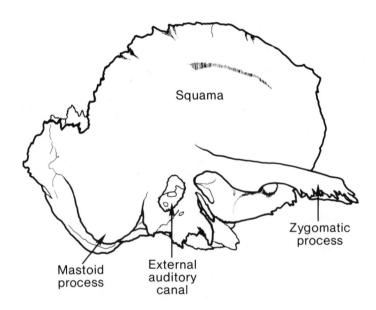

Illustration 11-1-B
Temporal Bone — External View

whole picture is therefore somewhat like that of a wheel or gear moving in a small arc on a bent axle. These wheels or gears move back and forth during flexion and extension describing very small arcs. Dr. Sutherland has described this movement as similar to that of a "wobbly wheel."

Since the petrous ridge attachment of the tentorium cerebelli is above the postulated axis of temporal bone rotation, the external rotation phase of temporal

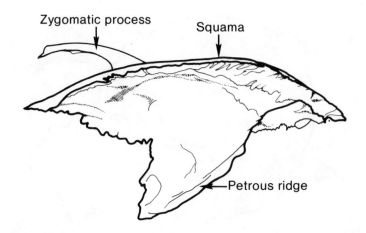

Illustration 11-1-C
Temporal Bone — Superior View

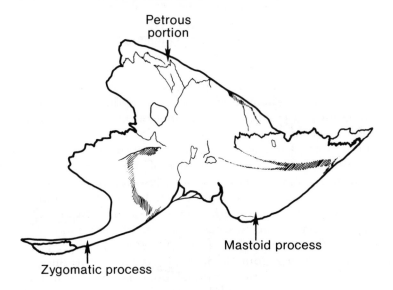

Illustration 11-1-D
Temporal Bone — Inferior View

bone motion causes the anterior borders of the tentorium cerebelli to move slightly anteriorly. The effect is to tighten this membrane. The membrane acts as a diaphragm, causing a fluctuation of cerebrospinal fluid. Granted the movement is small, but small movements in extremely sensitive areas create large effects.

The movements of internal rotation of the temporal bones are just the opposite of those described above. Temporal bone internal rotation corresponds to the extension phase of craniosacral system motion.

The squamous part of the temporal bone is part of the site of origin of the powerful temporalis muscle. This muscle inserts upon the ramus and angle of the

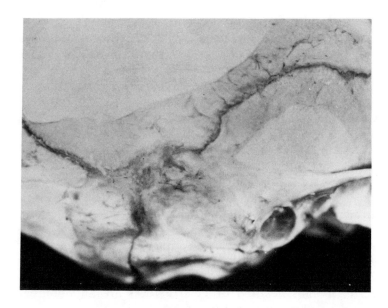

Illustration 11-2
Fetal Temporal Bone — Note Membranous Aspects

mandible and is used in the chewing process. It exerts a strong force upon the temporal squama, causing them to externally rotate during muscle contraction.

The zygomatic process of the temporal bone offers attachment for the masseter muscle, another powerful muscle used in chewing. The effect of masseter muscle contraction upon the temoral bone is external rotation via its levering action upon the zygomatic process. The superior border of the zygomatic process provides attachment for the temporal fascia which descends from above. This fascia moderates the force of external rotation exerted upon the temporal bone by the temporalis and masseter muscles during the process of mastication. The articulation of the anterior end of the zygomatic process of the temporal bone with the zygomatic bone of the face is in the nature of a serrated suture. The effect of this relationship is to transmit zygomatic process movement into the zygoma.

The mastoid process of the temporal bone is strongly influenced by the attachment of the sternocleidomastoideus muscle, which crosses the occipitomastoid suture and also attaches to the occiput. The splenius capitis, longus capitis and digastricus muscles also attach to the mastoid processes of the temporal bones. Abnormal tonus of any of these muscles tends to pull the mastoid process inferiorly, thereby internally rotating the temporal bone. The postulated axis of rotation of temporal bone motion is approximately through the external auditory meatus. The axis angles forward (anteriorly) as it extends medially; therefore this force, imposed upon the mastoid process, tends to rotate the temporal squama posteriorly. This movement is referred to as internal rotation of the temporal bones. It corresponds to extension of the cranial base, and causes the transverse dimension of the cranial vault at the superior borders of the squama to decrease.

The actions of the muscles which attach to the mastoid processes are countered by the actions of the masseter and temporalis muscles which attach to the zygomatic arch (process) of the temporal bone (ILLUSTRATION 11-3).

The temporal bone styloid processes provide attachments for the stylohyoideus and styloglossus muscles. During contraction, these muscles inhibit temporal bone motion. They act much as an anchor which drags upon the temporal bone.

The temporal bones are a very common cause of craniosacral system problems, not only because of their numerous muscle attachments but also because of the extensive sutural articulations which are present around their boundaries. We have a tendency to consider only those sutures which are available to direct palpation on the surface of the cranial vault. This is a serious error of omission. We must also keep in mind the fact that these sutures extend into the cranial base all the way to the basiocciput and the sphenobasilar synchondrosis (ILLUSTRATION 11-4).

Additionally, remember that the temporal bones offer generous attachment for the tentorium cerebelli along their petrous ridges and laterally along the internal surfaces of the mastoid parts and squama.

Because of the numerous muscle and dural membrane attachments, as well as the extensive and varied sutural articulations, the proper dynamic equilibrium of the temporal bones is in constant jeopardy. The unfavorable influences of muscles, sutures, fasciae, membranes and other structures are all potential sources of temporal bone dysfunction (ILLUSTRATION 11-5).

Clinically, the symptoms related to temporal bone dysfunction can best be appreciated by considering the list of nerves and blood vessels which pass through and are thus intimately related to these bones.

NERVES PASSING THROUGH THE TEMPORAL BONES	BLOOD VESSELS PASSING THROUGH THE TEMPORAL BONES
acoustic	internal carotid artery
chorda tympani	stylomastoid artery
facial (C.N. VII)	internal jugular vein
greater petrosal	occipital artery
sympathetic plexus of internal carotid	inferior petrosal sinus
	middle meningeal vessels
semilunar ganglion of trigeminal (C.N. V)	tympanic branch of maxillary artery
	internal auditory branch of basilar artery
tympanic branch of glossopharyngeal (C.N. IX)	internal cochlear branches to jugular
auricular branch of vagus (C.N. X)	

The most common clinical problems involving temporal bone dysfunction relate to hearing, balance, pain and vagotonia. In addition, because the motor nerves to the eye pass between the layers of the tentorium cerebelli, and the tension of these membranes is influenced by the temporal bone, we have found frequent, sudden and lasting relief of strabismus effected by temporal bone mobilization and balancing. Dyslexia always seems to correspond to temporal bone dysfunction, and reading skill is sometimes quickly improved following successful mobilization and balancing of the temporal bones. We have also found the temporal bone to be etiologically related to many cases of persistent and/or recurrent arm and shoulder pain syndromes. Bilateral medial compression of the temporal bones has been a consistent finding in the autistic children we have examined and treated. (Approximately 100 autistic children have passed through our clinic to date.) Certain aspects of autistic behavior which are discussed in Chapter 15 are improved when lateral

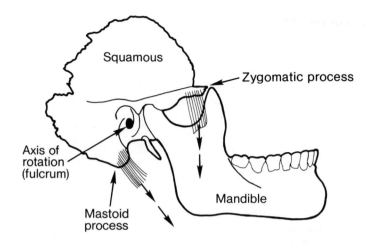

Illustration 11-3
Balance of Muscle Action on the Temporal Bone

temporal bone decompression is successfully performed.

EVALUATION AND TREATMENT OF TEMPORAL BONE FUNCTION AND DYSFUNCTION

There are three major techniques which we have found most useful when dealing with the temporal bones.

MASTOID TIP TECHNIQUE

This technique is used for motion evaluation and treatment. Interlace your fingers to support the supine patient's occiput. Place your thumbs so that they cover the mastoid processes and tips of the temporal bones. Then gently apply medial pressure bilaterally, upon the patient's mastoid tips. This pressure has the effect of *springing* the superior borders of the temporal squama laterally.

From the description of physiological motion above, you can see that you are encouraging one component of external rotation of the temporal bones by medially compressing the mastoid tips. As the other component (the rotational component) comes into play, you should simply go with it. Do not impede or inhibit the rotation about the transverse axis in any way.

Evaluate the symmetry of temporal bone motion. Asymmetry, when perceived, can often be successfully treated by rocking the temporal bones. Rocking is accomplished by applying pressure first to one mastoid tip and then the other in rhythm with the craniosacral system. This encourages external rotation first in one temporal bone, and then the other. Several cycles of this type of movement will usually free the restricted temporal. One or the other temporal bone will thereupon become still for one-half cycle and then begin moving in synchrony with its mate on the opposite side.

If this treatment technique is unsuccessful, it will often make obvious a specific sutural restriction. Sutural restrictions involving the temporal bones are quite common. They are successfully treated by the direction of energy techniques described in Chapter 9.

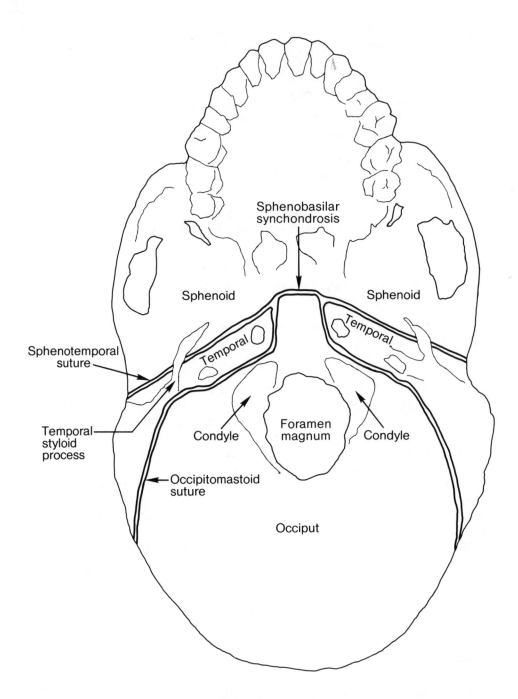

Illustration 11-4
Cranial Base — Inferior View

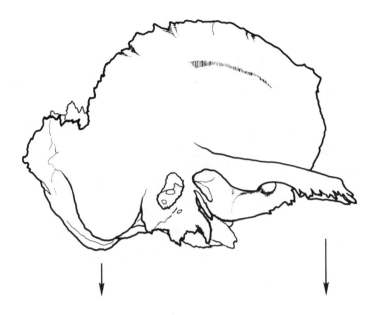

Illustration 11-5
Effects of Muscle Action (Arrows) on Temporal Bone
(Fulcrum Is in the External Ear Canal)

CIRCUMFERENTIAL MOTION TESTING AND TREATMENT TECHNIQUE

Apply this technique by inserting your middle fingertips in the supine patient's ears in such a manner that your fingers act as extensions of the axis for the rotational component of temporal bone motion (ILLUSTRATION 11-6). Then lay your fourth fingers in contact with the mastoid processes of the temporal bones, while keeping your index fingers in contact with the zygomatic processes of the temporal bones. Evaluate rotational movement around your middle finger extensions of the temporal bone axes for symmetry and ease of motion. Motion testing is always performed in synchrony with the patient's own craniosacral system rhythm. As you perceive this rotational motion, the broadening and narrowing of the temporal squama will also become apparent.

When you encounter restrictions to the motion, induce alternate movements; carry one temporal bone into external rotation and the other into internal rotation. This treatment has an excellent therapeutic effect upon the sutures related to the petrous parts of the temporal bones in the cranial base, especially those sutures between the occiput and temporal bones. When you feel the release of the restricted temporal bone, be alert to one of the bones tending to stop for one-half cycle so that the other bone will catch up, restoring synchrony of motion between the two temporal bones.

Always leave the temporal bones in neutral. Never take your hands off the patient when the bones are in either extreme internal or external rotation. Never leave the temporal bones out of synchrony. Otherwise, you may cause nausea, vomiting, vertigo or even seizure activity.

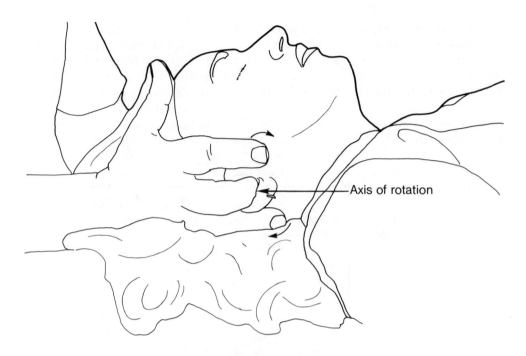

Illustration 11-6
Circumferential Motion Testing and Treatment
(Arrows Indicate the Direction of Force for
Encouragement of External Rotation)

TEMPORAL BONE DECOMPRESSION:
THE "EAR PULL" TECHNIQUE

Through our rather extensive work with autistic and other severe behaviorly disordered children, we have discovered the phenomenon of medially compressed temporal bones. This type of temporal bone dysfunction allows for some physiological temporal bone motion. It is the quality of this motion which seems abnormal. The perception is that these bones are moving as if in a highly viscous medium. Put simply, it is as though the system is "gunked up" with molasses. When only one of the temporal bones is so involved, of course, the lack of symmetry of free motion is apparent. On the other hand, when both temporal bones are medially compressed, motion symmetry is present; but the quality of motion is abnormally restricted. The temporal bones seem to drag on the whole system. Considering the extensive functional influences that the temporal bones have throughout the craniosacral system, it is not surprising that their dysfunction does indeed affect the efficiency of the whole system.

It was more or less out of frustration that we developed the "ear pull" technique for the diagnosis and treatment of temporal bone medial compression. We knew that something was impeding or dragging on temporal mobility. The thought that these bones could be medially compressed occurred. It then seemed that the direct approach to such a problem would be the most efficacious. Since that time, our experience with the ear pull technique has been very positive.

The external ear (pinna) is attached by fibers to the osseous part of the external ear canal as this canal penetrates the temporal bone. The external ear canal more or less approximates the direction of the petrous part of the temporal bone as it extends anteromedially into the cranial base. To perform the ear pull technique, simply place gentle traction posterolaterally on both external ears in the direction which would roughly be an extension of the posterolateral petrous projections of the bones (ILLUSTRATION 11-7). Once traction is begun, the directions will become self-determining. Begin the traction equally and bilaterally, allowing the direction of movement to be determined by the inherent patterns of the tissues. This directional modification will be in a state of constant dynamic change as the temporal bones decompress from the sphenobasilar region of the cranial base (floor of the cranial vault).

It is our habit to grasp the cartilage of the external ear on a transverse level with, and immediately posterior to the external auditory meatus (ear canal). Grasp both ears simultaneously with the patient lying comfortably supine. Begin the force of traction very lightly and *gradually* increase it until you feel a motion response. If the ears want to turn or slide in one direction or another, go with these movements. *Do not impede any movement.* If you should decide in advance that the ear must move along

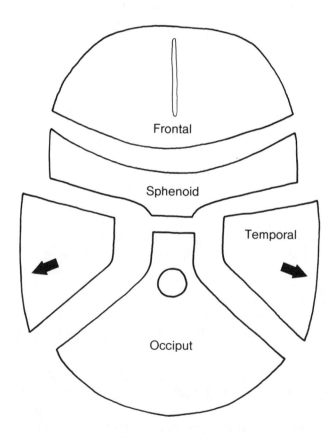

Illustration 11-7
Direction of Traction for the "Ear Pull" Technique

a certain vector, you will become a hindrance to the correction. Be flexible. Continue your posterolateral traction, but adapt to any other vector modification which seems to be present.

If the temporal bones move easily in response to your traction, no compression was present. If they do not move easily, hold, and if necessary, gently increase your traction until a release is perceived.

Since we have begun testing and treating the majority of our patients with this technique, we have found many otherwise undetected medial compressions of the temporal bones.

It can surely be argued that "if you look for it, you'll find it." But to this argument we would counter that if you don't look for it, you won't find it. The ear pull is an innocuous technique. It requires only a few minutes. When medial compression is discovered and corrected, the rewards are great. In view of these circumstances, it would seem somewhat remiss not to test and treat your patients for medial compression of the temporal bones.

THE TEMPOROPARIETAL SUTURE

Because this suture is a particularly frequent source of clinical problems, we will consider it independently.

Several mechanisms underlying sutural dysfunction are possible. One which has been almost completely overlooked is hypertonus or contracture of the temporalis muscle. This muscle is frequently and chronically contracted under conditions of emotional stress, dental malocclusion and/or temporomandibular joint dysfunction.

The anatomy of the temporalis muscle shows that during its contracted state it is capable of producing compression of the temporoparietal suture. The insertional attachments of the temporalis muscle are the ramus of the coronoid process and the anterior border of the ramus of the mandible. The muscle arises from the floor of the temporal fossa and from the temporal fascia. The temporal fossa extends superior to the temporoparietal suture. Therefore, contraction of the temporalis muscle causes the parietal bone to move in an inferior direction thereby producing a compression of the temporoparietal suture contents. The potential results of this sutural compression include ischemia and pressure on nerve receptors and plexuses located intrasuturally (APPENDIX G).

The anatomy of this suture is such that temporalis muscle contraction will produce a gliding motion of the parietal bones' sutural surface inferiorly after the superior motion of the mandible is effectively resisted by the approximation of the upper against the lower molar teeth, or by the surfaces of the mandibular ramus coming into opposition with the roof of the mandibular fossa of the temporal bone.

The bony surfaces of the temporoparietal suture are beveled and grooved in such a way that a sutural shearing force is generated by contraction of the temporalis muscle (ILLUSTRATION 11-8). This shear may longitudinally stress the collagen (Sharpey's) fibers that appear to be innervated. It may also reduce the cross-sutural physical dimensions and produce intrasutural pressure ischemia, as well as disrupt normal neurogenic reflex activity resulting from pressure stimulation of receptors. It may also interfere with normal nerve fiber conduction.

DIAGNOSIS AND TREATMENT OF DYSFUNCTION
OF THE TEMPOROPARIETAL SUTURE

The diagnosis of symptoms (head pain—cerebral dysfunction) resulting from

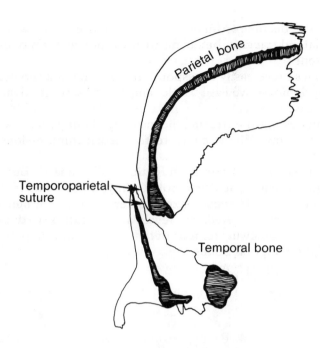

Illustration 11-8
Bevel of the Temporoparietal Suture

dysfunction of the temporoparietal suture is usually straightforward. Sutural compression, when exaggerated, will quickly increase symptom severity if the examination is done during an exacerbation. If the patient's condition is quiescent during the examination, the symptom complex can often be induced in a matter of minutes (APPENDIX G).

The technique for diagnosis of temporoparietal sutural dysfunction is performed with the patient lying comfortably supine. You should be seated cephalad so that you can comfortably grasp the patient's mandibular angle with your crooked fingers. Your elbows should rest comfortably upon the table so that the distal parts of your palms overlie the patient's temporomandibular joints, and the more proximal parts of your hands cover the temporoparietal suture.

Exert a light cephalad traction with your crooked fingers (usually the index or middle fingers) which are grasping the mandible in the notch just anterior to the angles. Apply the traction on both sides as equally as possible. As you very gradually increase the traction force, you will perceive compression at the temporomandibular joints. A swaying and balancing activity by the mandible may ensue as these joints impact. Follow any of these motions and let them achieve a balance for you. After the temporomandibular joints are compressed and balanced, the temporal squama will usually activate, moving side to side as they begin to balance. Follow and continue your traction. The shearing effect at the temporoparietal sutures will next occur. It is when this shearing occurs that the symptomatic patient will let you know. As stated above, the existing pain will worsen; the quiescent, clinical syndrome will recur.

Once you are satisfied that the diagnosis involves a compression of the temporoparietal suture, the treatment is to directly decompress the suture. The technique for decompression of the dysfunctioning temporoparietal suture is to reverse the traction on the mandible so that the temporomandibular joints decompress or disimpact first. The temporal bones then balance, and finally the temporoparietal sutures are opened and mobilized as the temporal squama glide inferiorly. This sutural mobilization can be palpated by the palms of your hands which overlie the sutural regions.

The caudally directed traction on the mandible is accomplished by gently grasping the skin over the angles and rami with just enough force so that you have a non-sliding friction between your fingers and the patient's skin. The skin is attached on its deep side indirectly to the bony surface of the mandible. Once the slack is taken up, the skin traction exerts a force upon the patient's mandible which is ultimately applied to the temporoparietal sutures. Continue traction to the point of palpable release or restoration of sutural motion.

Another very effective technique for the mobilization of the dysfunctional temporoparietal suture is the direction of energy or V-spread technique which was described in Chapter 9.

Chapter 12
The Mouth, Face and Temporomandibular Joint

The mouth, face and temporomandibular joint shall all be considered together in this chapter because they are functionally inseparable. In our experience, most clinical problems relating to this region arise from the temporals, or the maxillae and vomer. Such problems usually concern the relationship of these bones with the sphenoid, and therefore with the cranial base.

Ordinarily, the palatine, nasal and zygomatic bones will self-correct when temporal, maxillary, vomeral and sphenoidal relationships are corrected. Occasionally, a nasal, palatine or zygomatic dysfunction will require specific attention. We make this point because we believe that in the majority of cases it is a waste of time to correct secondary problems of the nasal, palatine and zygomatic bones first.

The problems associated with the temporomandibular joints are usually not effectively corrected until the temporal bones are balanced first. The techniques for these joints, described in Chapter 11, do in fact correct temporal bone imbalance at the same time that the joint dysfunction is treated.

The interrelationships of the bony structures of the mouth and face are extremely complex (ILLUSTRATION 12-1). The absence of dural membrane attachment to these structures simplifies diagnosis and treatment considerably, enabling the therapist to develop rational diagnosis and treatment along more grossly mechanical lines. Without the direct influence of the craniosacral hydraulic system, self-correcting mechanisms are weaker in this area. Direct therapeutic techniques are thus more effectively used.

Problems which primarily involve the nasal and zygomatic bones and their sutures are usually the result of direct trauma. These problems, when primary, become very apparent when you are motion-testing the rest of the mouth and face. They will usually, but not always, produce compensatory dysfunctions.

MAXILLAE, PALATINES, AND VOMER

We consider these bones as a single, complex functioning unit which anchors more or less to the sphenoid bone (ILLUSTRATIONS 12-2-A and 12-2-B). The maxillae comprise the major part of the hard palate. In the majority of cases, the palatines may be regarded as inserts or washers between the lateral pterygoid plates of the sphenoid and maxillae. When, however, specific palatine restrictions are present,

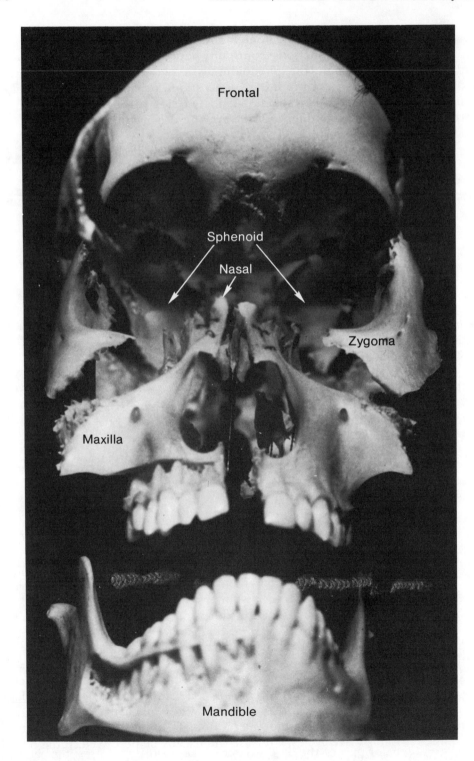

Illustration 12-1
Exploded View of the Bones of the Face

they may require specific palatine bone mobilization techniques.

The vomer provides functional continuity between the superior surface of the hard palate at the midline and the sphenoid (ILLUSTRATION 12-3). This bone is extremely flexible and often falls victim to intraosseous strain, or strain within itself, like a torsioned piece of steel. When sphenomaxillary lesion patterns are identified and corrected, the vomer component must *always* be dealt with in order to obtain a satisfactory and lasting result.

When the functional anatomy and the direct and indirect relationships of the hard palate with the sphenoid are thoroughly understood, many previously mystifying clinical syndromes become comprehensible.

The maxillae articulate with each other, and also with the nasal (ILLUSTRATION 12-4), frontal, ethmoid, zygomatic, lacrimal, inferior nasal concha, palatine and vomer bones; and inconstantly directly with the lateral pterygoid plates of the sphenoid (but always indirectly via the palatines). From this list of articulations you can see that normalizing maxillary bone function is extremely important to the mobility and normalcy of the majority of the structures of the anterior head.

The muscles which attach to the maxillae include the pterygoideus medialis, buccinator, obliquus inferior oculi and the orbicularis oculi and oris. Dysfunction of the maxillae will therefore often manifest as abnormalities of facial expression and eye movement.

Nerves which are intimately related to the maxillae include the infraorbitals, the maxillary divisions of the trigeminal nerves, the nasopalatine, the greater palatine and the anterior, middle and posterior alveolar nerves. Pain, neuralgia, sinusitis, rhinitis, toothache, and the like are symptoms which frequently are related to maxillary dysfunction.

Through the maxillae also pass the infraorbital, anterior and posterior superior alveolar and greater palatine blood vessels.

MAXILLARY BONE MOTION EVALUATION AND TREATMENT

The maxillary bones externally rotate as the cranial base flexes, and internally rotate as the cranial base extends. To evaluate maxillary function, place the palmar surfaces of the third and fourth fingers of one hand along the biting surfaces of the supine patient's upper molars. The great wings of the sphenoid should be monitored simultaneously by the thumb and index finger (or middle finger) of the other hand.

The molar biting surfaces widen in their transverse dimension as the sphenoid bone moves into flexion. The transverse dimension between molar biting surfaces narrows as the sphenoid enters the extension phase of craniosacral system movement.

One maxillary bone often moves a greater distance than the other. Loosen the restriction somewhat by indirect technique first, and then complete the correction by applying direct technique against the restriction barrier. For example, if the right maxilla will not move laterally as far as the left during the flexion phase of cranial base motion (called external rotation of the maxillae), follow both maxillae medially and resist the next cycle of external rotation. When maxillary internal rotation occurs again, follow and exaggerate this motion. Then external rotation is again resisted. After four or five cycles, a release will usually be perceived. If the release does not occur after seven or eight cycles, do not offer further resistance to external rotation of the maxillae.

Whether or not you have felt a release during your application of the indirect

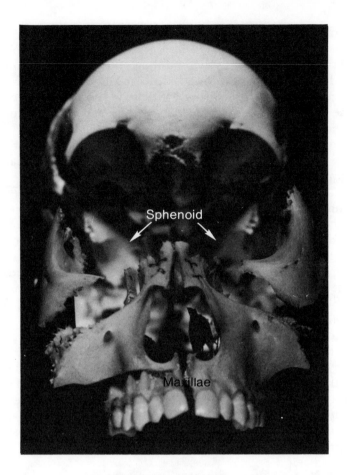

Illustration 12-2-A
Anterior View of Hard Palate

technique, you should next apply direct technique. *Gently* force the affected maxilla through the restriction barrier until it seems as though both maxillae are moving evenly. Your corrective force should be gentle, but firm and constant. Remember: a small force over a longer period of time is as effective and much less traumatic than a large force.

After making this correction, the maxillae should always be restored to synchronous movement with the sphenoid before terminating the treatment.

Other maxillary problems we have identified include sphenomaxillary torsion, shear and impaction.

SPHENOMAXILLARY TORSION

In sphenomaxillary torsion, it is as if the hard palate and the sphenoid are rotated in opposite directions about a vertical axis which passes approximately through the point of intersection of the sagittal and coronal sutures on the vault. This area is referred to as bregma.

To test for sphenomaxillary torsion, use the same hand positions described

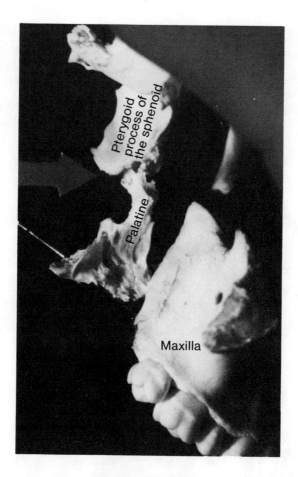

Illustration 12-2-B
Lateral View of Maxilla, Palatine and Sphenoid

above in testing for normal maxillary internal and external motion in relationship to sphenoid flexion and extension. Through your finger contact with the biting surfaces of the upper molars, the hard palate is rotated about the vertical axis (ILLUSTRATION 12-5), first in one direction, then in the opposite direction. Stabilize the sphenoid with your other hand.

Sphenomaxillary torsion is not a normal physiological motion, but all normally functioning patients which we have examined possess enough motion tolerance to allow for some torsion of the hard palate in relation to the sphenoid.

The force you apply should be very gentle, but sustained for 10 to 15 seconds to allow time for the hard palate to follow your lead. The amount of torsion should be bilaterally symmetrical. If the movement is not equal in both directions, a spheno-maxillary torsion restriction is present. This restriction is corrected by lesion exaggeration for 10 to 15 seconds or until release is perceived. This initial step is *always* followed by direct correction. Direct correction is applied gently but firmly against the abnormal restriction barrier until the barrier is felt to yield. You should then wait 3 to 5 minutes and re-evaluate.

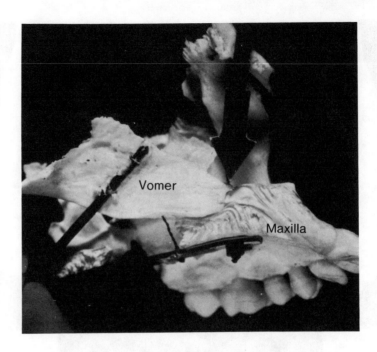

Illustration 12-3
Medial View of Vomer and Maxilla

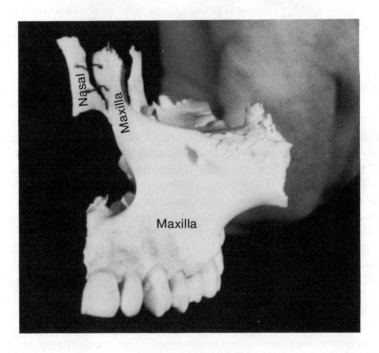

Illustration 12-4
Maxilla and Nasal Bone

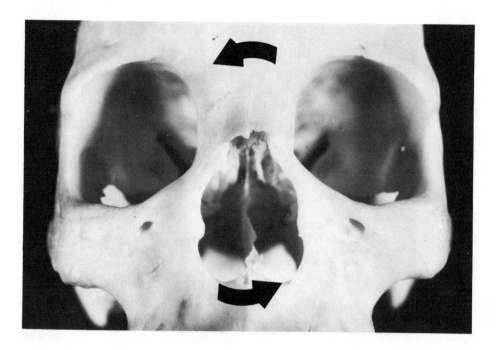

Illustration 12-5
Sphenomaxillary Torsion

Following correction of a sphenomaxillary torsion dysfunction, the palatines and vomer *must always* be evaluated and treated as described later in this chapter.

SPHENOMAXILLARY TRANSVERSE SHEAR

Another problem which we have discovered in the sphenomaxillary relationship is that of transverse shear. As the name implies, sphenomaxillary transverse shear means that the hard palate has been abnormally moved on a transverse plane to either the left or right in relation to the sphenoid. To test for this problem, you must maintain the sphenoid in a stable position in the transverse plane. Then move the hard palate laterally on a transverse plane parallel to the plane of the sphenoid. Neither the hard palate nor the sphenoid should be allowed to rotate when performing this test (ILLUSTRATION 12-6).

The sphenomaxillary shear is not a normal physiological motion. When the test is performed gently with persistent force, some transverse shear motion will occur. Place the palmar surfaces of the third and fourth fingers of one of your hands against the biting edges of the upper molars on the supine patient. Stabilize the sphenoid with the thumb and index or middle finger of your other hand. We find it useful to contact the thumb of the hand which is examining the hard palate with the dorsum of the other hand so as to provide relative motion cues. Urge the hard palate to move parallel to the sphenoid, without rotation, first to one side and then to the other. Enough time should be allowed in both directions to permit the patient's bony structure to follow the force you are applying. The motion response should be symmetrical; if it is not, a transverse shear restriction of the sphenomaxillary complex is present.

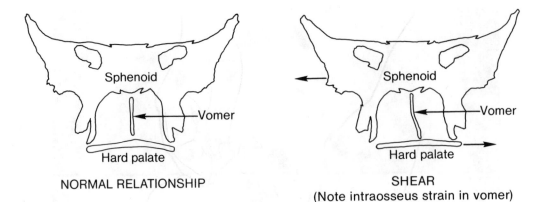

Illustration 12-6
Sphenomaxillary Shear

Sphenomaxillary shear is corrected by first using indirect technique to loosen the dysfunction. This is followed by direct technique through the restriction barrier. In summary, first exaggerate the motion in the direction toward which it most easily moves. Hold against the extreme range-of-motion barrier for 10 to 15 seconds, or until a release is perceived. Then take the hard palate in the opposite direction and hold against the restriction barrier. Continue your *gentle* force against this restriction barrier until it seems to release. Return the hard palate to neutral, follow a few cycles and then re-evaluate. After the sphenomaxillary shear is corrected you *must* evaluate the palatines and vomer. (These techniques are described later in this chapter.)

SPHENOMAXILLARY IMPACTION

Impaction of the sphenomaxillary complex is uncommon, but when present it can prove to be a most puzzling and perplexing problem until it is discovered. Sphenomaxillary impaction simply means that, due to some abnormal force, the maxilla and sphenoid are pushed together, impacting the palatine bone (or bones) between them. It also often involves the impaction of the vomer into the sphenoid. The first clue to this impaction problem is indicated when you perceive a lack of independent motion between the sphenoid and either one or both maxillae; the sphenoid and maxilla seem to move as a unit. Vomerosphenoidal impaction is discovered when testing vomer motion, which is described later in this chapter.

When your suspicion has been aroused, attempt to disimpact the affected bones by using light traction. The patient is supine with the mouth comfortably open. Grasp the anterior maxillae between your thumb, index and middle fingers. A piece of gauze is helpful to prevent slipping. Place your thumb and fingers above the alveolar ridges of the maxillae, with the thumb on the external surface and the fingers behind the ridges (ILLUSTRATION 12-7).

Use your other hand to stabilize and monitor the sphenoid bone. Place your thumb and index or middle finger over the great wing regions of the sphenoid.

With the sphenoid held still, use the thumb and fingers which are grasping the anterior maxillae to exert a gentle, steady and anteriorly-directed traction. The hard palate should glide anteriorly in a smooth and well-lubricated manner. If this does

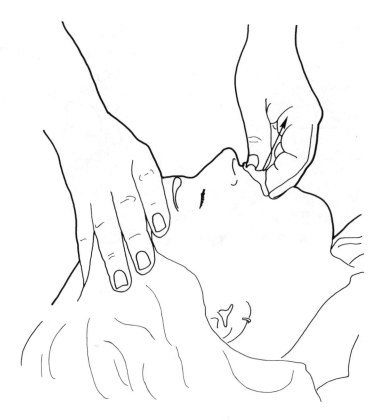

Illustration 12-7
Hand Position for Release of
Sphenomaxillary Impaction

not seem to occur, you should be able to decide whether resistance to the anterior glide is from one side, the other side, both sides or the midline. Unilateral resistance indicates ipsilateral maxillary impaction with the sphenoid. Bilateral resistance indicates bilateral sphenomaxillary impaction. Midline resistance indicates vomer impaction with the sphenoid, the maxillae or both. The treatment is to continue the anterior traction until you perceive a release and the hard palate glides freely in a balanced manner.

When the treatment is completed, the palatines and vomer should always receive individual attention to achieve free mobility and balance. These techniques are described below.

PALATINE BONE MOTION EVALUATION AND TREATMENT

The palatine bones interpose as functional connecting links between the maxillae and the lateral pterygoid plates of the sphenoid bone (ILLUSTRATION 12-8). They are therefore subject to forces from both sources, and can easily become dysfunctional secondary to either maxillary or sphenoidal problems.

The palatines articulate with the sphenoid, ethmoid, maxillae, inferior nasal concha, vomer and with each other (ILLUSTRATIONS 12-9-A and 12-9-B). The muscular attachments are from the tensor veli palatine, the musculus uvulae and the medial

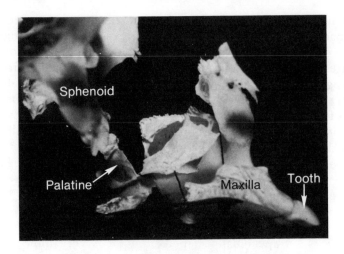

Illustration 12-8
Palatine Between Sphenoid and Maxilla

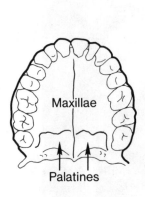

Illustration 12-9-A
Hard Palate — Inferior View

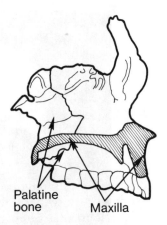

Illustration 12-9-B
Hard Palate — Sagittal Section

pterygoideus. Nerves which are intimately related to the palatine bones are the greater and lesser palatines, and sensory fibers from the palatine, nasopalatine and glossopharyngeal nerves. Blood vessels which pass through these bones include the descending palatine branch of the maxillary artery, the ascending palatine branch of the facial artery and the palatine branch of the ascending pharyngeal artery.

Frequently, correction of maxillary and sphenoidal restrictions will result in a more or less spontaneous correction of the palatines; however, they should always be evaluated individually and mobilized when necessary. We usually do this evaluation and treatment after maxillary and sphenoidal corrections have been completed, since the successful corrections of these problems often obviates the need for specific palatine corrections.

The technique for evaluation and treatment of the palatine is the same. The diagnosis is made only as the treatment is performed. Slip one finger along the medial borders of the upper molars of the patient, just past the last molar but still on the hard palate. Keep this finger about one-quarter inch medial from the molar borders. Exert gentle pressure upon the palatine bone in a cephalad direction until the bone is felt to disengage from the maxilla and to glide slightly cephalad. After the bone moves as far cephalad as it will move with ease, exert gentle pressure upon it in a lateral direction. Hold this pressure until the bone rotates externally. Repeat the procedure on the opposite side of the patient's mouth.

Resistance to motion, of course, indicates abnormal restriction. Easy and early compliance to your pressure means no restriction. To correct restriction, hold gentle pressure until there is compliance.

VOMER MOTION EVALUATION AND TREATMENT

The vomer is a trapezoidally-shaped bone. It is very thin, and is situated vertically in the sagittal plane (ILLUSTRATION 12-10). The posterior and inferior part of the nasal septum is formed by the vomer. The posterior superior border of the

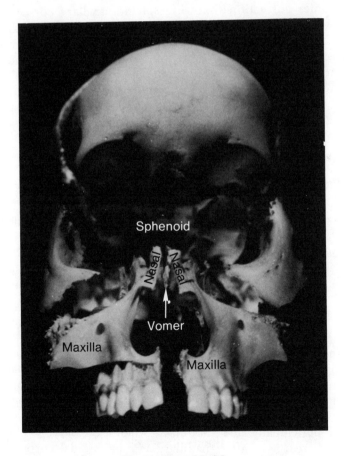

Illustration 12-10
Position of Vomer

vomer is thickened and presents a deep furrow; it receives the rostrum of the sphenoid. The alae of the vomer articulate with the medial pterygoid plates of the sphenoid and the sphenoidal processes of the palatine bones. The inferior border of the vomer articulates with the crest on the superior surface of the hard palate formed by the maxillae and the palatines. The anterior border is longer and fuses with the perpendicular plate of the ethmoid above. The posterior border is free and separates the nasal choanae (ILLUSTRATION 12-11).

The vomer moves about a transverse axis located in its mid-region, as illustrated. The anterior inferior aspect of the vomer moves superiorly as the sphenoid goes into flexion. As the posterior inferior aspect of the vomer, which is in contact with the hard palate, moves superiorly, the sphenoid is moving in extension.

Observe coordination of these motions by placing one finger on the midline of the hard palate and simultaneously monitoring sphenoid movement (ILLUSTRATION 12-12). Use direct technique to correct vomer restrictions, which interfere with coordinated motion between the vomer and the sphenoid.

VOMER TORSION

In the sections above on sphenomaxillary torsion and transverse shear, we have emphasized vomer correction following sphenomaxillary correction. To effect correction of vomer torsion, use your finger in the patient's mouth to torque the vomer about a vertical axis as the sphenoid is stabilized with the thumb and index or middle finger of your other hand. Indirect loosening is first performed for 10 to 15 seconds or until a release is perceived, then direct technique is applied against the intraosseous torsion of the vomer. The force must be sustained until the vomer

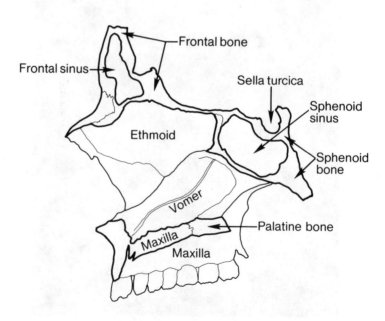

Illustration 12-11
Sagittal Section through Anterior Skull
Showing Position of Vomer

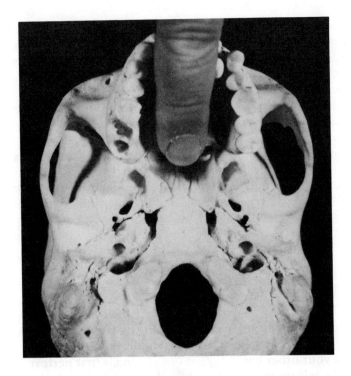

Illustration 12-12
Finger Position for Evaluation and Treatment of Vomer

follows. You will notice a release of resistance when the correction is completed.

The contact points for the finger applying the torque in the patient's mouth are the posterior midline of the hard palate with the tip of the finger, and the back of the front incisors and the posterior surface of the alveolar ridge anteriorly. We cannot overemphasize that a gentle force over a long time is the proper method of correction.

VOMER SHEAR

To correct intraosseous vomer shear resulting from sphenomaxillary transverse shear, use the same application of your hands to the patient's head as for vomer torsion. The only difference is that the forces applied are not torquing; they are lateralward in two parallel planes. Move the sphenoid and vomer in opposite directions on parallel and transverse planes. Indirectly loosen first, then follow with the direct approach to correct the intraosseous strain.

For all diagnostic tests and corrections of the hard palate in relation to the sphenoid, the sphenoid is stabilized and the testing or corrective force is applied to the hard palate. If the sphenoid is not stabilized, the testing or corrective forces will be transmitted into the cranial base through the sphenoid. Iatrogenic cranial base dysfunctions may be introduced in this way.

ZYGOMATIC BONES

The zygoma has three articulating or sutural surfaces. These surfaces are serrated so that the movements of the three bones with which the zygoma articulates influence its mobility. Functionally, the zygoma may be regarded as a triangle. Its superior articulation is with the frontal bone. Its posterior articulation is with the zygomatic process of the temporal bone, and its anterior articulation is with the zygomatic process of the maxillary bone.

During the flexion phase of craniosacral system motion, the zygoma externally rotates about a diagonal axis which passes through points slightly below the glabella and the angle of the mandible. During external rotation the transverse dimension between the superior aspects of the two zygomata increases slightly (ILLUSTRATION 12-13).

Functionally, the zygomatic bones act as connectors between the bones with which they articulate. They contribute significantly to the inferior and lateral aspects of the orbits of the eyes.

Zygomatic dysfunction can either be a reflection of frontal, temporal or maxil-

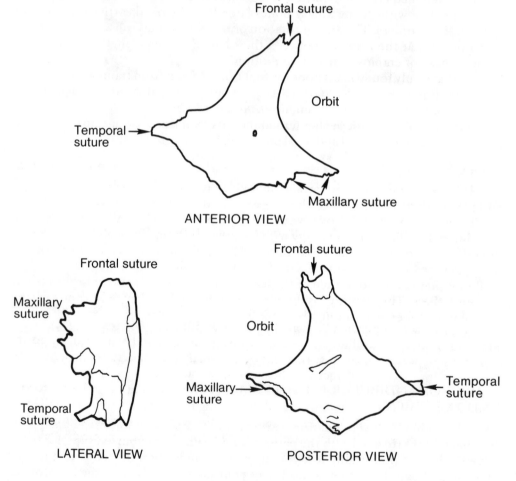

Illustration 12-13
Zygoma

lary bone dysfunction, or it can be the result of trauma. It is seldom dysfunctional for any other reason. A dysfunctional zygoma from trauma can produce secondary clinical problems to the dysfunctions of the bones with which it articulates.

Correction of zygomatic dysfunction first involves the mobilization of its sutures, and then the mobilization of the bone itself. Sutural mobilization can be accomplished by either direct disimpaction by grasping the two bones involved (since they are so readily accessible), or by the application of direction of energy technique with appropriately placed V-spread.

The zygomatic bones are usually directly mobilized by placing the index finger inside the mouth but external to the maxilla and grasping the zygoma between index finger and thumb. Indirect, and then direct technique are applied to mobilize the bone about the axis described above.

THE NASAL BONES

The nasal bones are roughly rectangular in shape. They articulate with each other on their medial sides and with the frontal bone above (just below the glabella). They articulate with the maxillary bones laterally. The nasal cartilage meets with their inferior borders. The axis of rotation of the nasal bones runs in a longitudinal direction so that the distance between their lateral borders lengthens during the flexion phase of craniosacral system motion.

We have only found nasal bone dysfunction to result from trauma. Diagnosis of sutural dysfunction is made on the basis of tenderness to palpation and lack of nasal bone motion in response to craniosacral system activity. The nature of the dysfunction is of course dependent upon the nature of the trauma. Impaction of the sutures between the frontal and nasal bones can be corrected by direct traction upon the nasal bones, using the skin of the nose as the vehicle, while the frontal is stabilized (ILLUSTRATION 12-14).

In order to mobilize the intranasal bone sutures or the nasomaxillary sutures, you can attempt to encourage the external rotation phase of nasal bone motion using two finger pads, as you would use magnets, to draw the lateral aspects anteriorly. The direction of energy with V-spread technique can also be extremely effective in mobilizing the nasal bones. We frequently use three fingertips to disimpact the frontonasal suture. One fingertip is applied at glabella on the midline, while another is applied to each of the nasal bones; this arrangement forms a tripod of your fingers. The "energy" is directed from the midline just below the external occipital protuberance (inion).

Acupuncture is another excellent method of mobilizing the sutures of the nasal bones. Intradermal placement of very fine (high gauge) needles overlying the affected suture will usually result in sutural mobilization in a matter of 30 seconds.

TEMPOROMANDIBULAR JOINT EVALUATION AND TREATMENT

The technique for evaluation and treatment of the temporomandibular joint (APPENDIX G) is performed with the patient lying supine. Seat yourself superior to the patient's head. Comfortably rest your arms and hands upon the table next to, and extending above the patient's head. Lay your hands gently over the sides of the patient's head so that the ears and temporal regions are covered by the base of the palms. The temporomandibular joints will almost be covered by the base of the

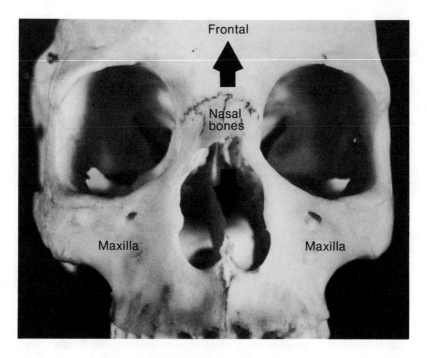

Illustration 12-14
Direction of Force for Release of
Frontonasal Impaction

fingers. We like to hook our middle fingertips under the angle of the mandible so that they fit into the notch. A gentle cephalad or superiorly directed traction is then exerted on both sides of the mandible as equally as possible. The force is gently and slowly increased until you perceive action or change at the temporomandibular joints as those joints are impacted by the traction. Usually, the mandible will then tend to swing back-and-forth or from side-to-side. Follow this motion without offering any resistance. At the same time, continue your superiorly directed traction. Lateral or anterior-posterior motions of the mandible reflect the inherent balancing process induced by your traction. Once this balancing process is completed, the lateral or anterior-posterior motions will stop.

If you continue traction in a cephalad direction, you will feel activity in the temporal bones. We do not believe you can have temporomandibular joint dysfunction without temporal bone dysfunction. The mandible will exert a force in the mandibular fossae of the temporal bones (ILLUSTRATION 12-15). This cephalad-directed force causes the temporal bones to move cephalad and begins to disengage the temporoparietal sutures, as described previously in Chapter 11.

Since the level of these sutures is angled superiorly and externally, and since it is at an acute angle, the temporal squama are forced to move laterally by the cephalad traction. This phenomenon can easily be felt at the palms of your hands. It causes a shear at the suture as the lateral borders of the parietal bones also attempt to move cephalad. The parietals are restricted in their cephalad movement by the falx cerebri and are forced into external rotation by your traction (ILLUSTRATION 12-16).

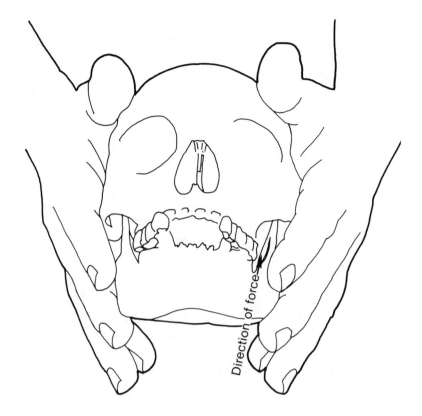

Illustration 12-15
Hand Placement for First Phase of
Temporomandibular Joint Technique

During this time the temporal bones, through their petrous ridges, are stretching the tentorium cerebelli, which is now acting as a diaphragm. This changes the fluid pressure inside the cranial vault. You will feel a considerable amount of fluid motion, membranous change and balancing in the course of this procedure. The temporal bone will move and balance in many directions. Let this happen; simply continue your cephalad traction. Finally, all the activity will stop and you will perceive a balance. The point of balance is the end of this part of the technique.

The next step is to apply caudally directed traction to the mandible. Apply enough pressure with your hands against the mandibular rami to exert this caudad force. Because the skin is attached indirectly on its deep side to the bone of the mandible, by simply taking the slack out of the skin and then continuing to apply traction, the force will thereby be transferred to the mandible. Do not try to actually grasp the mandible.

During your caudally directed traction, the temporomandibular joints will disengage and balance. Then the temporal bones will move inferiorly in response to mandibular traction. This will again activate the dural membranous diaphragm and cause a movement of cerebrospinal fluid inside the cranial vault. The temporoparietal sutures will disengage and shear in the opposite direction, and the parietals

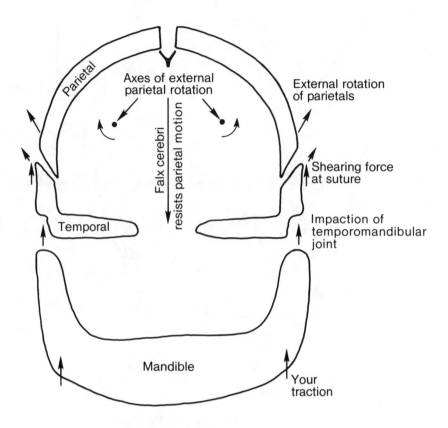

Illustration 12-16
Cephalad Traction Phase of
Temporomandibular Joint Technique

will move from external to internal rotation. Continue the caudally directed traction until all this activity has quieted down and a balance has been achieved.

When completed, you have not only effectively treated the temporomandibular joints, but you have also corrected the temporal bone involvement, mobilized the temporoparietal sutures, partially mobilized the parietal bones, caused fluid exchange in the cranial vault and balanced the dural membranes. This is truly an excellent "holistic technique" for the craniosacral system and all that it affects.

Chapter 13
Extrinsic Neuromusculoskeletal System Dysfunctions Which Influence The Craniosacral System

Many structures which are extrinsic to the craniosacral system may cause restrictive effects within that system. This chapter is therefore designed to deepen your awareness of the influence which muscles, ligaments, fasciae, scars and articular somatic dysfunctions may have on the workings of the craniosacral system. This awareness will lead to a more complete understanding of your patients and their problems. While the description of specific treatment techniques for each problem is beyond the scope of this book, such methods as position and hold, local release and somatoemotional recall and release which are described elsewhere in the text may be used to treat many of the dysfunctions discussed here. It is assumed that the reader will also apply other treatment modalities with which he or she is most familiar.

You will notice a great deal of repetition in this chapter. It is intentional. Each muscle and its action is described in connection with each of the bones discussed. Because most of the muscles attach to at least two different bones, most of the muscles are described at least twice. We have all been frustrated, angered and perhaps deterred by having to flip back and forth from page to page to clarify details in difficult areas of a reference text. We have therefore chosen to sacrifice some of the fluency of the narrative so as to provide a more useful reference guide.

MUSCLES

Abnormal tonus or imbalance of paired muscles which attach directly to the osseous boundaries of the craniosacral system exerts a powerful influence upon the delicate movements of the craniosacral system. Such imbalance impairs the mobility of the bones involved in this system, namely, the bones of the skull, vertebral column, sacrum and coccyx.

The effect of muscle hypertonus which does *not* directly relate to one of the bones of the craniosacral system is much less, owing to the dampening effect and the flexibility of the body in general.

The muscles which frequently cause impairment of the limited but free mobility of the craniosacral system are described and grouped below according to the bones to which they attach.

OCCIPUT

The occiput seems to be the bone most commonly responsible for craniosacral system dysfunction due to abnormal muscle tonus. This is probably because the occiput is the anchor for many muscles which respond with hypertonicity to the tensions of daily living. The effects of occipital immobility upon the dural membrane system are immense. Occipital immobility is often caused by muscle hypertonus. The occiput offers firm attachment for the posterior borders of the tentorium cerebelli, the posterior aspect of the falx cerebri and the posterior and inferior aspects of the falx cerebelli. Through these unique dural membrane attachments, the occiput must therefore exert a strong influence upon the straight venous sinus, the transverse venous sinuses, the confluence of sinuses, the posterior sagittal sinus and the occipital sinus. Occipital bone dysfunction can thereby interfere with venous sinus function. Fluid congestion in the venous sinus system influences the cerebrospinal fluid reabsorption system (arachnoid villae), which is located largely in the sagittal sinus.

Within the straight sinus, and also influenced by occipital bone function, is a small body which resembles an arachnoid granulation (GRAY'S ANATOMY, 39th British Edition, pp. 693-94). This body projects into the floor of the straight sinus near its junction with the great cerebral vein. It contains a sinusoidal plexus of blood vessels which acts as a ball-valve control mechanism when engorged with blood. Under these circumstances, it asserts significant control upon the outflow of the great cerebral vein which, in turn, affects the absorption of cerebrospinal fluid into the venous system.

The extremely firm attachment of the dural membrane to the foramen magnum is another factor which must be considered. Occipital bone dysfunction due to muscle hypertonus must affect the accommodative function and mobility of the spinal dural tube. Note also that the dura mater is firmly attached to the posterior aspects of the second and third cervical vertebral bodies within the vertebral canal. The occiput and the upper cervical vertebrae may thus be regarded as a single functional unit. These bones also share many extradural muscle attachments.

Muscles which attach to the external surface of the occiput and therefore influence its function are discussed below.

Longus Capitis

This muscle arises from the anterior tubercles of the transverse processes of C3, 4, 5 and 6 and inserts upon the inferior surface of the basilar part of the occipital bone.

Rectus Capitis Anterior

This muscle arises from the anterior surface of the lateral mass of the atlas and inserts upon the inferior surface of the basilar part of the occiput, immediately posterior to the insertion of the longus capitis and anterior to the foramen magnum.

Both of these muscles act to forward bend or flex the head on the spine since their insertions are located anterior to the occipital condyles. The innervation of these muscles is from branches of the 1st, 2nd and 3rd cervical nerves.

Hypertonus of the longus capitis and the rectus capitis anterior acts upon the occiput to inhibit the physiological flexion motion of the occipital base (ILLUSTRA-TION 13-1). Bilateral hypertonus of these muscles would tend to produce an extension lesion pattern of the cranial base, while unilateral involvement contributes to a torsion lesion pattern of the cranial base.

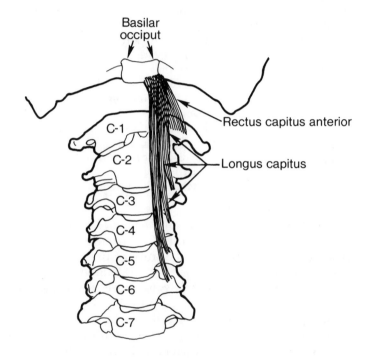

Illustration 13-1
Anterior Aspect of Cervical Spine and Occipital Base

Rectus Capitis Lateralis

This short, flat muscle arises from the superior surface of the transverse process of the atlas and inserts into the inferior surface of the jugular process of the occiput. It laterally sidebends the head. It is innervated by a branch from the loop formed by the 1st and 2nd cervical nerves.

Unilateral hypertonus of the rectus capitis lateralis contributes to a torsion lesion pattern of the cranial base. The proximity of this muscle to the jugular foramen is also of great importance. When these foramena become partially obstructed by tissue contracture, the result is increased venous back-pressure within the semi-closed cranial vault, contributing to intracranial congestion and cephalgia (APPENDIX D) and many other conditions. The glossopharyngeal (C.N. IX), vagus (C.N. X) and spinal accessory (C.N. XI) nerves also pass through the jugular foramena. Increased muscle tonus in this area can therefore produce dysfunction of these cranial nerves, which in turn may result in other problems set forth below.

IXth CRANIAL NERVE	Xth CRANIAL NERVE	XIth CRANIAL NERVE
Loss of gag reflex	Aphonia or dysphonia	Sternocleidomastoid
Slight dysphagia	Dysphagia	muscle dysfunction
Loss of taste to posterior	Regurgitation of fluid	Trapezius muscle
third of tongue	through the nose	dysfunction
Uvular deviation	Pharyngeal and laryngeal	Hypertonus of cervical
Loss of sensation to	spasms	musculature (which
pharynx and posterior	Esophageal spasms	further compounds the
tongue	Cardiospasm	problem at the jugular
Loss of motor control of	Pylorospasm	foramen)
posterior pharyngeal	Paralysis of soft palate	
wall	Pain, paresthesias or	
Increased salivation	anesthesia of pharynx,	
	larynx or external	
	auditory meatus	
	Cough	
	Respiratory disorders	
	Salivary disorders	
	Cardiac arrhythmias	
	Gastric dysfunction	
	Intestinal dysfunction	

Rectus Capitis Posterior Major

This muscle arises from the spinous process of the axis and inserts into the lateral part of the inferior nuchal line of the occiput and immediately inferior to this line. This muscle forms the medial border of the suboccipital triangle, bilaterally. The muscle is innervated by branches of the suboccipital nerve, which is derived from the 1st cervical nerve and inconsistently from the 2nd cervical nerve. The muscle extends the head and rotates it to the same side. Since the attachment of these muscles to the occiput is posterior to the occipital condyles, bilateral hypertonus of these muscles contributes to extension of the head on the neck and to flexion lesion patterns of the cranial base. Unilateral hypertonus contributes to torsion lesion patterns.

Rectus Capitis Posterior

This muscle arises from the tubercle on the posterior arch of the atlas and widens as it inserts into the medial part of the inferior nuchal line. It is innervated by branches of the suboccipital nerve.

Obliquus Capitis Superior

This muscle arises from the superior surfaces of the transverse processes of the atlas and inserts into the occiput posterior to the inferior nuchal line and lateral to the rectus capitis posterior. It is innervated by branches of the suboccipital nerve and serves to extend and sidebend the head. Therefore, hypertonus of the muscle contributes to flexion and torsion lesions of the cranial base through its influence upon the occiput.

Obliquus Capitis Inferior

This muscle does not attach to the occiput directly, but does form the inferior border of the suboccipital triangle. Therefore, it greatly influences the occiput via its origin upon the spinous process of the axis and its bilateral insertion upon the transverse processes of the atlas. It too is innervated by branches of the suboccipital nerve. It serves to rotate the atlas on the axis, and turns the head ipsilaterally. Hypertonus of this muscle will affect occiput function through its influence upon the mobility of the axis and atlas, and upon the condition of the tissues of the suboccipital triangle. One must also keep in mind the dural attachments between the occiput and the axis.

The suboccipital triangles are bounded laterally by the obliquus capitis superior, inferiorly by the obliquus capitis inferior and medially by the rectus capitis posterior major (ILLUSTRATION 13-2). All of these muscles are innervated by branches of

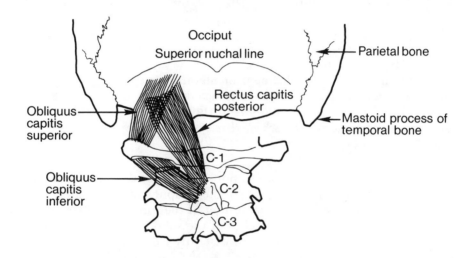

Illustration 13-2
Posterior View of Upper Cervical Spine and Occiput

The suboccipital triangles are bounded laterally by the obliquus capitis the suboccipital nerve. The innervation fibers contribute to the contents of the triangle. Muscular hypertonus of the walls of the suboccipital triangle can produce irritation of the suboccipital nerve which will, in turn, produce further hypertonus of the walls of the triangle, etc. This is a self-perpetuating problem which will ultimately cause dysfunction of the cranial base via the occiput, and dysfunction of the dural tube through its attachments to the posterior bodies of the upper cervical vertebrae.

The posterior atlanto-occipital membrane and the posterior arch of the atlas form the floor of the suboccipital triangle. The posterior atlanto-occipital membrane is broad and thin; it connects to the posterior margin of the foramen magnum and the posterior arch of the atlas. The membrane covers the groove in the atlas, which permits passage of the vertebral artery and suboccipital nerve. Anteriorly, it adheres tightly to the dura mater. Stress on this membrane due to abnormal neuromusculoskeletal function may interfere with proper function of the vertebral artery and suboccipital nerve.

The superficial cover of the suboccipital triangle is formed by the semispinalis capitis muscle and a layer of dense fibro-fatty tissue which lies just beneath this muscle.

Semispinalis Capitis

This muscle arises from C1 through C6 (inconsistently from C7), and from the articular surfaces of C4, 5 and 6. The muscle inserts by means of its tendon to the occiput between the inferior and superior nuchal lines. It is innervated by branches of the dorsal division of the cervical nerves. This muscle is a powerful rotator of the head toward the opposite side and can contribute significantly to cranial base dysfunction by immobilizing the occiput in a flexion lesion pattern if bilaterally restricted, and by contributing to a torsion lesion pattern if unilaterally hypertonic.

Trapezius

This superficial, triangular muscle arises from the external occipital protuberance and bilaterally from the medial third of the superior nuchal lines of the occiput. It also originates from the ligamentum nuchae, the spinous processes of C7 and all thoracic vertebrae. The muscle inserts into the posterior borders of the lateral third of the clavicles, the medial margins of the acromion processes and the posterior borders of the spines of the scapulae (ILLUSTRATION 13-3).

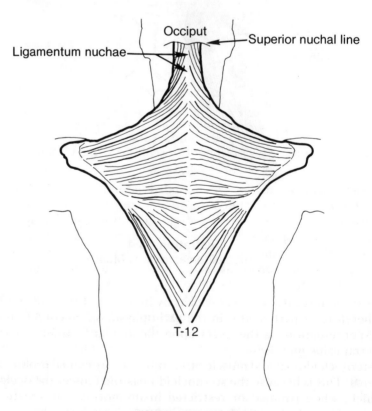

Illustration 13-3
Trapezius Muscle

Dysfunction of the trapezius immobilizes the occiput in a flexion lesion pattern. The trapezius must often be restored to a normotonic condition before the cranial base can be functionally corrected. Innervation of the trapezius muscle is by the spinal accessory nerve (C.N. XI), which passes through the jugular foramen. Trapezius hypertonus can cause dysfunction at the jugular foramena, which irritates the spinal accessory nerve (C.N. XI) and causes further trapezius hypertonus, another self-perpetuating neuromusculoskeletal problem.

Sternocleidomastoideus

This muscle arises from the sternum and clavicle (ILLUSTRATION 13-4). It inserts into the lateral surface of the temporal mastoid process and the lateral half of the superior nuchal line of the occiput. The muscle is innervated by a branch of the

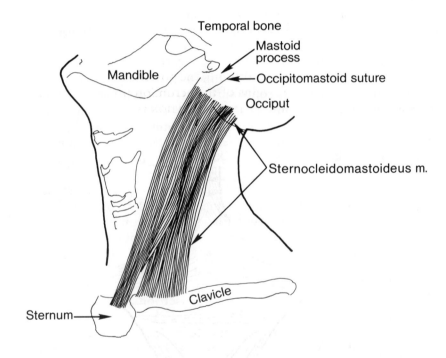

Illustration 13-4
Sternocleidomastoideus Muscle

spinal accessory nerve (C.N. XI) as well as by branches of the 2nd and 3rd cervical nerves. Therefore, it participates in the pathophysiological condition of dysfunctional self-perpetuation via the effect upon the jugular foramen described earlier under the trapezius muscle.

The sternocleidomastoid muscle offers more severe cranial problems than does the trapezius. This is because the sternocleidomastoid crosses the occipitomastoid suture which, when jammed or restricted in its motion, can create severe and incapacitating symptoms. It also can cause temporal bone dysfunction which, through its influence on the tentorium cerebelli, may cause severe problems.

Constrictor Pharyngeus Superior

This muscle arises from the pterygoid plate of the sphenoid, the pterygomandibular raphe, the alveolar process of the mandible and the side of the tongue. It inserts into the occiput by an aponeurosis to the pharyngeal spine on the basilar part. The muscle is innervated by branches of the pharyngeal plexus. It assists in deglutition.

The clinical significance of this muscle is difficult to appraise, but from a mechanical point of view its structure would indicate that hypertonus may contribute to sphenobasilar flexion and compression lesion.

Occipitalis

This muscle arises from the lateral two-thirds of the superior nuchal line and inserts into the galea aponeurotica. It is innervated by branches of the posterior auricular branch of the facial nerve. Although a weak muscle, we are sure that chronic hypertonus of this muscle can contribute to occipital bone dysfunction.

TEMPORAL BONES

The temporal bone is composed of the squamous, petrous and mastoid parts. The squama and mastoid parts contribute to the lateral aspects of the cranial vault; the petrous portions contribute to the floor or base of the cranial vault.

Numerous muscular attachments to the temporal bones render them quite vulnerable to motion dysfunction. Generous attachments of dura mater to the temporal bones make them extremely significant in terms of general craniosacral function. The numerous and varied sutural articulations must all be working correctly to insure proper temporal bone function. Further, the relationship of the temporal to the auditory apparatus, the mechanisms of equilibrium, and the numerous blood vessels and nerves with which it is connected make it extremely significant clinically. There is always more to learn about temporal bone function; when you observe closely, each contact will teach you something new.

Sternocleidomastoideus

This muscle has firm and significant insertion across the occipitomastoid suture from the occiput to the lateral aspect of the mastoid process of the temporal bone. The muscle arises from the sternum and the clavicle. It is innervated by the spinal accessory nerve (C.N. XI) and by branches of the 2nd and 3rd cervical nerves.

Hypertonus or contracture of the sternocleidomastoid is common and results in severe dysfunction of the temporal bone. Since its attachment is posterior to the normal axis of rotation of that bone, sternocleidomastoid contraction causes a posterior rotation of the temporal bone with a reduction of the transverse dimension of the superior aspects of the temporal squama, i.e., internal rotation.

Clinically, rotational dysfunction of the temporal bones may be etiologically related to any visual motor problem. This occurs because the IIIrd, IVth, Vth and VIth cranial nerves pass between the leaves of the tentorium cerebelli. Rotational dysfunction of the temporal bone places increased tension into the anterior cerebellar tent at the petrous ridges. The tentorial attachment is moved posteriorly from the clinoid processes of the sphenoid. Correction of this anatomico-physiologic dysfunction of the temporal bone often rapidly and dramatically corrects strabismus and nystagmus.

The temporal bone contribution to the jugular foramen must also be kept in mind. Dysfunction of the temporal bone produces abnormal tension in the adnexal tissues of the jugular foramen and therefore interferes with function of the IXth, Xth and XIth cranial nerves. It also results in impairment of venous outflow through these foramena, and a secondary increase in venous back pressure within the cranial vault and thus into the cerebrospinal fluid. The latter effect is created by a reduction of resorption of cerebrospinal fluid into the venous system via the arachnoid villae. This sequence of events often results in vascular and fluid congestion-type headaches accompanied by gastrointestinal distress or visual disturbances. Release of the temporal bone dysfunction is essential for a good clinical result.

The occipitomastoid suture dysfunction, which may be caused by chronic hypertonicity of the sternocleidomastoid, is often related clinically to dyslexia in learning disabled children. It may also cause head pain, nausea and personality changes.

Temporalis

This muscle arises from the whole of the temporal fossa, which includes the temporal squama as well as the lateral parts of the parietal squama, the great wings of the sphenoid and the postero-lateral parts of the frontal bone. The muscle crosses the temporoparietal suture, the sphenosquamous and the coronal suture. It is inserted into the medial surface of the apex and the anterior border of the mandibular rami. The muscle is innervated by branches of the anterior and posterior deep temporal nerve, which passes between the heads of the lateral pterygoid muscle after arising from the mandibular trunk of the trigeminal nerve (C.N. V).

The temporalis muscle is the largest muscle of mastication (ILLUSTRATION 13-5). Its anterior fibers close the mouth; its posterior fibers draw the mandible posteriorly. The gross and microarchitectural design of the temporoparietal sutures indicates that when the teeth are tightly approximated, contraction of the temporalis will

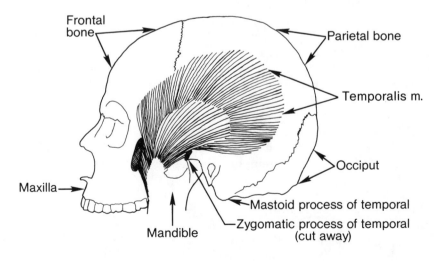

Illustration 13-5
Temporalis Muscle

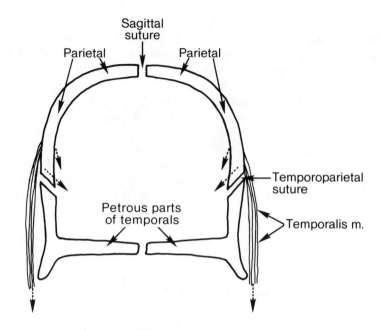

Illustration 13-6
Effect of Temporalis Muscle Contraction on the
Temporoparietal Suture

draw the parietal bone downward (ILLUSTRATION 13-6). The temporoparietal suture is classified as a squamous type suture which permits the two surfaces to slide upon each other. Accordingly, the intrasutural nerve fibers and vasculature will be compressed or stressed when the temporalis contracts. If the condition persists, the suture then becomes ischemic and painful due to the local effect on the sympathetic perivascular plexus (APPENDIX G). The sensory nerve endings in the suture are also compressed. This condition contributes to localized and distant referred pain.

Ongoing temporalis contracture, such as that which results from dental malocclusion or chronic anger, tension or fear, will ultimately result in chronic temporoparietal sutural dysfunction as well as parietal bone dysfunction. The latter will contribute to dysfunction of the sagittal sinus and impaired resorption of the cerebrospinal fluid in that region.

Clinical experience indicates that sagittal sinus and parietal bone dysfunction will result in episodes of mild to moderate cerebral ischemia. These effects are reversible when the dysfunctions of the temporoparietal and sagittal sutures are corrected and the parietal and temporal bones are mobilized.

Digastricus

This muscle consists of an anterior and a posterior belly which arise respectively from the inferior border of the mandible near the symphysis, and from the mastoid notch of the temporal bone. The two bellies of this muscle join inferior to the body of the mandible and end in a tendon which perforates the stylohyoideus muscle and then passes through a fibrous loop which attaches to the hyoid bone (ILLUSTRATION 13-7).

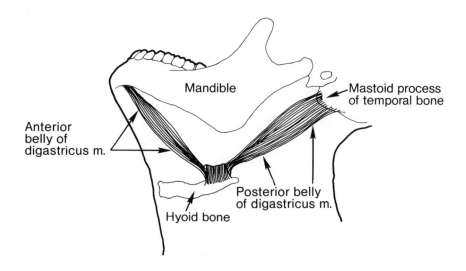

Illustration 13-7
Digastricus Muscle

This muscle raises the hyoid bone and assists in opening the jaw when the hyoid is stabilized from below. It is innervated in its anterior belly by branches of the mandibular trunk of the trigeminal nerve (C.N. V) and in its posterior belly by branches of the facial nerve (C.N. VII). A frequent variation is that the posterior belly of the digastricus may arise partially or entirely from the styloid process of the sphenoid bone rather than from the temporal.

The digastricus often is involved in anxiety and hysteria. It contracts and interferes in a subtle manner with temporal bone motion. It creates a tendency toward internal rotation of the temporal. It produces an elastic restriction which is easily overlooked by the clinician. Digastricus dysfunction in the posterior belly will also result in hyoid tightness. This may be the only clue a less experienced clinician will perceive. Anterior digastricus hypertonus causes a tenderness to palpation along its course on the inferior region of the mandible.

Digastric hypertonus should always be suspected in cases of hoarseness or loss of voice, and in pain around the hyoid bone. Occasionally, temporal bone dysfunction will be the apparent cause of digastricus contracture. Correction of temporal bone dysfunction will correct and release the digastricus muscle.

Longissimus Capitis

This muscle arises from the transverse process of the 1st through the 5th thoracic vertebrae and from the articular processes of the 4th through the 7th cervical vertebrae. It inserts into the posterior margin of the mastoid process of the temporal bone deep to the splenius capitis. The muscle is innervated by branches of the middle and lower cervical nerves. It serves to extend the head and to sidebend and rotate the head ipsilaterally. When in an abnormal state of contraction, it can result in temporal bone dysfunction by causing posterior internal rotation of the bone and immobilizing it in that position.

Splenius Capitis

This muscle arises from the lower half of the ligamentum nuchae and from the spinous processes of the 7th cervical through the 4th thoracic vertebrae. It inserts into the mastoid process of the temporal bone and into the occiput; it therefore crosses the occipitomastoid suture. The muscle also is innervated by branches of the middle and lower cervical nerves. It serves to extend the head and neck and to sidebend laterally and rotate ipsilaterally.

Because this muscle attaches to both the temporal and the occipital bones and crosses the suture, it plays a significant role in dysfunctions of the craniosacral system.

Contracture or hypertonus of the splenius capitis muscle causes the temporal bone to go into posterior rotation of the squamous portion and internal rotation of the petrous portion. It induces flexion of the occipital contribution to the cranial base and thereby contributes to a "flexion head" with internally rotated temporal bones. It also contributes to immobility of the occipitomastoid suture which contributes to learning disabilities such as dyslexia, head pain, gastrointestinal symptoms, personality changes and many other problems. Innervation is from the middle and lower cervical dorsal roots.

Masseter

Some fibers of this muscle arise from the inferior surfaces of the zygomatic processes of the temporal bones. The attachment of the muscle crosses the suture and therefore it also arises from the inferior surface of the zygomatic bone. The masseter inserts into the mandible and closes the jaw. The innervation of the masseter muscle is from the mandibular division of the trigeminal nerve.

Hypertonus of the masseter muscle will contribute to an anterior rotation of the temporal bone (synonymous with external rotation) as the bone moves about its diagonal axis (ILLUSTRATION 13-8).

Clinically, problems of emotional stress and tension which result in chronic

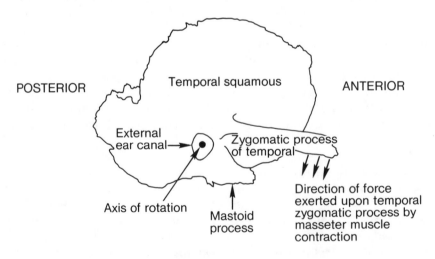

Illustration 13-8
Effect of Masseter Contraction on Temporal

clenching of the jaw and dental malocclusion significantly contribute to a chronic external rotation of the temporal bone. When cranial examination reveals this condition, always look at the tonus of the muscles of mastication.

Stylohyoideus

This muscle arises from the posterior and lateral surfaces of the styloid process of the temporal bone. It inserts into the body of the hyoid bone at its junction with the greater cornua. The muscle is innervated by branches of the facial nerve (C.N. VII). It acts to draw the hyoid superiorly and posteriorly.

Contracture of this muscle is usually a result, rather than a cause, of craniosacral system dysfunction. It contributes to the chronically tight feeling in the hyoid region which is a frequent complaint of anxious and hysterical patients. This symptom can often be alleviated by mobilization of the cranial bones.

Styloglossus

This muscle arises from the anterior and lateral surfaces of the styloid and from the stylomandibular ligament. It passes between the internal and external carotid arteries, then divides into the longitudinal part which inserts into the side of the tongue, and the oblique part which joins the hyoglossus muscle. The styloglossus muscle is innervated by the hypoglossal nerve (C.N. XII). It draws the tongue up and backwards in the mouth.

Contracture of this muscle is usually a result, rather than a cause, of craniosacral system dysfunction.

Auriculus Posterior

This muscle arises from the mastoid portion of the temporal bone and inserts into the lower portion of the cranial surface of the external ear. It is innervated by the posterior auricular branch of the facial nerve (C.N. VII). The muscle draws the external ear posteriorly and aids the occipitofrontalis in moving the scalp. Abnormal tonus of this muscle sometimes may result from dysfunction of the temporal bone and may be considered a suggestive sign of craniosacral system problems.

SPHENOID

The sphenoid is considered the mechanical "keystone" of the rhythmic accommodative motion of the skull. Muscles which, by their abnormal tonus, may inhibit or interfere with normal sphenoid function or motion are of considerable clinical significance. The major osseous articulations of the sphenoid are with the vomer, ethmoid, frontal, occipital, parietals, temporals, zygomatics, palatines and maxillary tuberosities.

It takes no great imagination to recognize that the sphenoid, if inhibited in its mobility, will place significant drag on the motion of the whole craniosacral system. The muscles which attach to the sphenoid are discussed below.

Pterygoideus Medialis

This muscle arises from the medial surface of the lateral pterygoid plate of the sphenoid, the pyramidal process of the palatine bone and the tuberosity of the maxilla. It inserts by tendonous attachments into the inferior and posterior parts of the medial surface of the ramus and angle of the mandible. The muscle is innervated

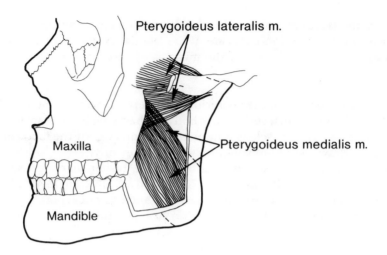

Illustration 13-9
Pterygoideus Muscles

by the medial pterygoid nerve from the mandibular division of the trigeminal nerve. Its position medial to the mandible is similar to the masseter on the outside. It is divided and offers passage to the lateral pterygoid muscle (ILLUSTRATION 13-9).

The medial pterygoid muscle is powerful; it acts with the masseter to close the jaw. Chronic problems, such as dental malocclusion, tension, anger and anxiety, which cause hypertonus of the medial pterygoid muscle, result in significant dysfunction of the craniosacral system. It is difficult to predict the symptoms which may result from chronic medial pterygoid hypertonus because the physiological effect of the muscular dysfunction is upon the "keystone" of the craniosacral system. There will always, however, be dysfunction which involves the relationship between the sphenoid, maxillary and palatine bones. The temporomandibular joint is also a frequent focus of difficulty when the medial pterygoid muscles are in a state of hypertonus.

Pterygoideus Lateralis

This muscle arises from the inferior part of the lateral great wing of the sphenoid, the infratemporal crest and the lateral pterygoid plate. It inserts into the anterior part of the condyle of the mandible and the articular disc of the temporomandibular joint. The muscle is innervated by the lateral pterygoid nerve from the mandibular branch of the trigeminal nerve (C.N. V). It opens the jaw, protrudes the mandible and moves the mandible from side to side.

Our clinical experience indicates that contracture or hypertonus of the lateral pterygoid muscles is frequently involved in dysfunction of the temporomandibular joints. Owing to the powerful nature of the muscle and its generous attachments to the sphenoid, this muscle is often etiologically related to craniosacral system dysfunction. It contributes to reduced mobility of the sphenoid, usually holding it in the extension position.

Lateral pterygoid hypertonus is often overshadowed by other lesion patterns and is difficult to discover until many layers of adaptive lesion patterns have been removed. It is a frequent cause of recurrent craniosacral and temporomandibular joint problems.

Temporalis

This muscle has firm attachment to the external surface of the great wing of the sphenoid as this bony surface contributes to the temporal fossa. These anterior temporalis fibers run almost vertically, deep to the zygomatic arch, and attach to the anterior coronoid process of the mandible. By this mechanism, temporomandibular joint problems and temporalis muscle contractures cause dysfunction of the sphenoid. This abnormal tension imposed by the temporalis upon the sphenoid wing, if unilateral, can contribute to torsion and sidebending dysfunction of the cranial base. If the increased tension imposed by the temporalis is bilateral, it may immobilize the sphenoid in a vertical strain position which, because of its immobility, may be mistaken for a sphenobasilar compression.

You must also keep in mind the attachments of the temporalis muscle to the frontal and parietal bones. These multiple attachments of the temporalis muscle to the various bones of the cranial vault make it a prime suspect when searching for the principal cause of osseous immobility.

Tensor Veli Palatini

This muscle arises from the sphenoid fossa at the base of the medial pterygoid plate, the spine of the sphenoid and the lateral wall of the cartilage of the auditory tube. It then descends vertically between the medial pterygoid plate and the medial pterygoideus muscle. It ends in a tendon which passes around the pterygoid hamulus, from which it is separated by a small bursa. The tendon then inserts into the palatine aponeurosis and the horizontal part of the palatine bone. The innervation to the tensor veli palatine is usually from the accessory nerve (C.N. XI) via the pharyngeal plexus. The muscle classically tenses the palate during the process of deglutition.

The muscle is significant in clinical craniosacral work because sphenoid bone dysfunction can cause change in its tonus. This change in tonus may increase tension on the auditory tube and become the hidden etiology for difficult-to-define symptomatology of the auditory system. It may also be the cause of recurrent middle ear problems related to impaired fluid drainage via the auditory tube.

Constrictor Pharyngeus Superior

This muscle arises from the inferior posterior surface of the medial pterygoid plate and its humulus, from the pterygomandibular raphe, the alveolar process of the mandible and, by a few fibers, from the side of the tongue. It inserts into the median raphe and an aponeurosis which leads to the pharyngeal spine of the occipital base. The muscle is innervated by branches from the pharyngeal plexus. It participates in the act of deglutition. It is partially by this muscle that the cranial base may cause difficulty with swallowing.

PARIETAL BONES

The parietal bones form much of the sides and roof of the cranial vault. The point of maximum convexity on the external surface of each parietal bone indicates the origin of ossification of the bone. If this point is abnormally prominent, it indicates that there was or is resistance to peripheral expansion of the bone, probably due to increased dural membrane tension. The parietals are extremely important in craniosacral system function. They strongly influence the function of the sagittal sinus and, therefore, the cerebral venous circulation and the reabsorption of cerebrospinal fluid into the venous system.

The nature of the suture between the temporal squama and the parietals allows for a gliding motion between these two bones (ILLUSTRATION 13-10). The intrasutural contents include blood vessels, nerves and connective tissue fibers. An extreme shearing of the suture resulting from external stress can therefore produce intrasutural ischemia, neurogenic stimuli due to pressure, and connective tissue strain, all of which may become symptomatic (APPENDIX A).

Additionally, work in progress by Dr. Retzlaff shows that in monkeys, continuous single axon fibers traverse from within the sagittal suture through the dural membrane as it forms the falx cerebri, then into the brain tissue itself, and finally into the wall of the third ventricle of the brain. This continuity of innervation from suture to ventricle may represent a mechanism whereby sagittal suture function influences brain function, specifically cerebrospinal fluid production by the ventricular system (ILLUSTRATION 13-11).

Temporalis

This muscle attaches to the lateral external surfaces of the parietal bones. When abnormally contracted, it can create the aforementioned shearing tension

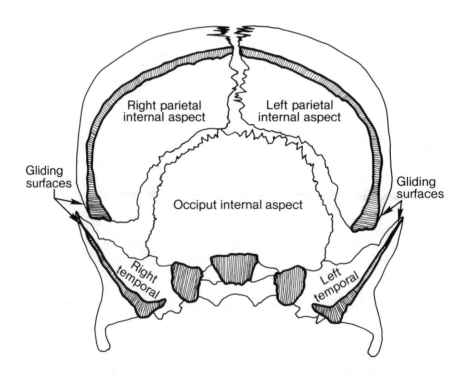

Illustration 13-10
Temporoparietal Suture Bevel

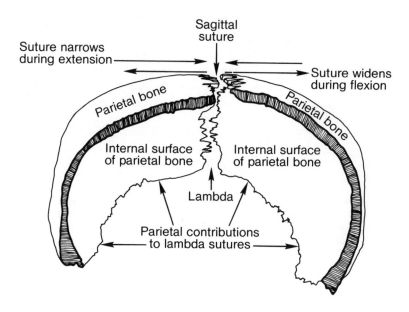

Illustration 13-11
Sagittal Suture in Flexion and Extension

across the temporoparietal suture. This shear frequently results in both local and referred pain. Many recurrent temporal headaches are caused by this mechanism, which is activated by temporalis muscle hypertonus. This hypertonic condition may be chronically caused by ongoing emotional stress or dental malocclusion.

The innervation to the temporalis muscle is from branches of the mandibular division of the trigeminal nerve (C.N. V). It normally acts to close the jaw. Its posterior fibers contribute to mandibular retraction. It arises from the whole of the temporal fossa. The muscle inserts into the coronoid process and the anterior ramus of the mandible (ILLUSTRATION 13-12).

FRONTAL BONE

The frontal bone contributes to the anterior cranial vault by its squama, and to the floor of the cranial vault (which underlies the anterior brain) by its horizontal formation. These horizontal plates also contribute to the superior aspects of the orbital cavities and to the nasal cavities. The muscular attachments to the frontal bone are rather sparse.

Temporalis

This muscle attaches to the posterior, lateral and inferior aspects of the frontal bone as it contributes bilaterally to the anterior portions of the temporal fossae. The temporalis muscle fibers which arise from the frontal bone insert into the anterior ramus of the mandible and are therefore almost vertical.

Abnormal tonus of the temporalis muscle does not interfere to any great extent with frontal motion. Our impression is that frontal bone motion is compound and includes an anterior rotation of the superior aspect about a transverse axis during

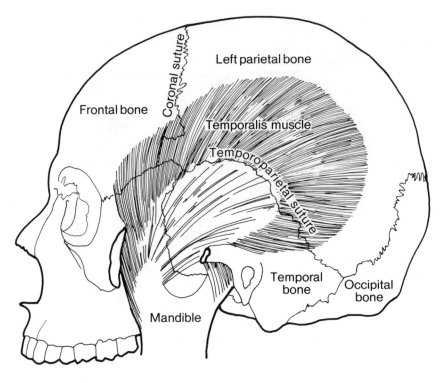

Illustration 13-12
Temporalis Muscle

the flexion phase of motion. In addition, this transverse axis translates anteriorly and inferiorly.

Frontalis

This muscle does not attach directly to the frontal bone and has minimal effect upon its motion. However, by indirect effect through the corrugator and orbicularis oculi muscles which do attach to the frontal, it can, if chronically hypertonic, inhibit the flexion phase of cranial base motion. The frontalis is innervated by temporal branches of the facial nerve (C.N. VII).

MAXILLAE

These bones powerfully influence the function of the craniosacral system via their articulations with the frontal, ethmoid, palatines (which articulate with the sphenoid), vomer and zygomatics. The maxillae also have important articulations with each other. Articulations with the lacrimals, the nasals and the inferior nasal concha have less influence on craniosacral system function but can be symptomatic when dysfunctional.

The maxillae have inconstant articulations with the orbital surfaces and the lateral pterygoid plates of the sphenoid.

Muscles which attach to the maxillae are quite numerous. Those which we consider clinically significant in maxillary function are described below.

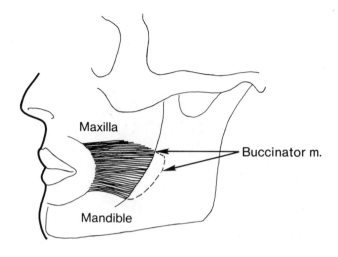

Illustration 13-13
Buccinator Muscle

Buccinator

This is the principal muscle of the cheek. It forms the lateral wall of the oral cavity. The buccinator muscle arises from the maxillary alveolar processes above, the mandibular alveolar processes below and the pterygomandibular raphe. The fibers run anteriorly and insert into the deep layer of fibers of the lips (ILLUSTRATION 13-13).

The motor innervation of the buccinator is by the buccinator branch of the facial nerve (C.N. VII). The sensory fibers are from buccal branches of the trigeminal nerve (C.N. V).

Abnormal tone of these muscles is rare in our clinical experience; however, the common origin should be kept in mind when looking for causes of temporomandibular joint disturbances and for problems involving the pterygoid process of the sphenoid. The effect on the cranial base of anterior force upon the pterygoid would be to discourage the flexion motion of the sphenoid and to encourage the extension motion as this bone participates in the normal rhythmic activity of the cranial base.

Masseter

This thick muscle consists of two portions. The larger is the superficial portion, which arises by a tendon from the zygomatic process of the maxilla and from the posterior two-thirds of the inferior border of the zygomatic arch. It inserts into the angle and inferior part of the lateral ramus of the mandible. The deep portion is smaller. It arises from the posterior third of the inferior border and from the entire medial surface of the zygomatic arch. This deep portion inserts into the superior half of the mandibular ramus and onto the lateral surface of the coronal process (ILLUSTRATION 13-14-A).

The masseter muscle is innervated by branches from the mandibular division of trigeminal nerve (C.N. V). The masseter muscle closes the jaw.

This muscle is often involved in problems with dental occlusion and in chronic jaw-clenching due to emotional problems. It contributes to ongoing temporoman-

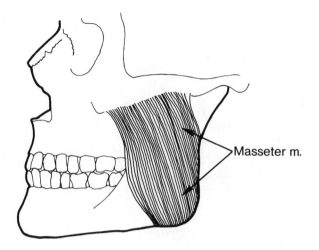

Illustration 13-14-A
Masseter Muscle

dibular joint problems and to temporal bone dysfunction, encouraging anterior and external rotation of that bone.

Pterygoideus Medialis

This thick, powerful muscle is located deep in relation to the masseter. It arises from the medial surface of the lateral pterygoid plate of the sphenoid, from the pyramidal process of the palatine bone and from the tuberosity of the maxilla. It is inserted by tendons into the mandibular ramus and the angle of the mandibular rami. It is innervated by the mandibular branch of the trigeminal nerve (C.N. V). The pterygoideus medialis closes the jaw (ILLUSTRATION 13-14-B).

Hypertonus of this muscle is often due to dental malocclusion, injury and emotional problems. Hypertonus or contracture of the medial pterygoid always results in craniosacral system dysfunction of some type.

PALATINE BONES

The palatines form the posterior fourth of the hard palate. They articulate with each other, the maxillae, vomer, inferior nasal concha, sphenoid and ethmoid bones. They occupy a key position in the osseous communication between the cranial base bones and those of the mouth, nose and face.

Tensor Veli Palatini

These muscles arise bilaterally from the scaphoid fossa at the base of the medial pterygoid plate of the sphenoid bone and from the lateral walls of the auditory tube cartilages. They insert into aponeuroses which attach to the transverse ridges of the posterior aspects of the longitudinal plates of the palatine bones.

Their innervation is from the accessory nerve (C.N. XI). The muscles tense the palate during deglutition. Contracture or hypertonus of these muscles can contribute to hearing dysfunction via their attachments to the cartilages of the auditory tubes. This abnormal hypertonus may result from sphenoid dysfunction. An ab-

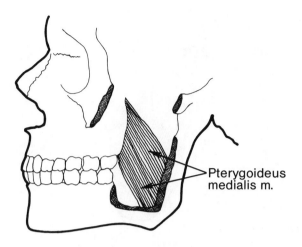

Illustration 13-14-B
Pterygoideus Medialis Muscle

normal condition of these muscles will interfere with physiological palatine bone motion. The palatines are small and light. They are not often regarded as significant levers which interfere with craniosacral system function; however, severe and painful dysfunction may develop from immobility of the palatine bones. Most often, palatine bone lesion is the result of trauma and is an osseous lesion, but contribution to the lesion pattern by the tensor veli palatini may be significant.

Pterygoideus Medialis

These muscles arise partially from the grooved surfaces of the pyramidal processes of the palatine bones. Another slip arises from the lateral surfaces of these bones. This second slip lies superficial to the pterygoideus lateralis while the first slip lies deep to it. The insertion is by tendon into the ramus and angle of the mandible. These muscles are closely related to the tensor veli palatini and to the superior pharyngeal constrictors.

The pterygoideus medialis muscles close the jaw. They are innervated by the medial pterygoid nerve from the mandibular division of the trigeminal nerve (C.N. V). Hypertonus or contracture of these muscles can strongly impair the physiological motion and function of the palatine bones and thus contribute to pain syndromes which involve the palatine bones and, via the tensor veli palatini muscles, to syndromes which involve the auditory tubes.

ZYGOMATIC BONES

These bones form the prominences of the cheeks. They contribute to the lateral walls and floors of the orbits and to parts of the temporal and infratemporal fossae (ILLUSTRATION 13-15). The only clinically significant muscle attachment which the zygomatic bones afford is partial origin for the masseter muscle. These muscle fibers insert into the mandible. Masseter innervation is from the mandibular division of the trigeminal nerve (C.N. V). The masseter closes the jaw. Hypertonus or contracture of the masseters will cause zygomatic dysfunction. This may result in

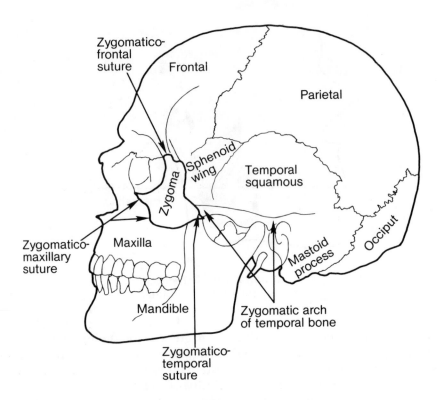

Illustration 13-15
Relationships of the Zygoma

facial or orbital pain and a drag upon the free motion of the maxillae and temporals. Depressed cheekbones are often a sign of zygomatic bone dysfunction.

MANDIBLE

This is the bone of the lower jaw and it carries the lower teeth. It consists of a horizontal body and two vertical or perpendicular rami. It has bilateral articulation with the temporal bones. The mandible is a frequent cause of craniosacral system dysfunction, transmitted via the temporal bones into the osseous cranial vault, then into the intracranial membranous system via the tentorium cerebelli.

There are numerous muscular attachments to the mandible. All the muscles of mastication affect or are affected by imbalanced tensions which involve the lower jawbone. There are many clinical problems which relate to temporomandibular joint dysfunction. Although the temporomandibular joint is often considered separately, the contribution of the muscles of mastication to the etiology of temporomandibular joint problems cannot be taken lightly. We regard the mandible as an unstable anchoring system for the soft tissues which attach to it. The articulations of the mandible with the temporal bones are very unstable. They are, therefore, extremely vulnerable to imbalanced tensions which tend to move the mandible from the midline.

The muscles which attach to the mandible are discussed below.

Platysma

This muscle arises from the fascia which covers the superior aspects of the deltoid and pectoralis major muscles. It inserts into the inferior parts of the body of the mandible. The innervation of the muscle is by branches of the facial nerve (C.N. VII).

We are unaware of any cases of platysma hypertonicity which have contributed to craniosacral system dysfunction. However, from a strictly mechanical point of view, the possibility exists that a relatively strong platysma in a state of chronic hypertonus would cause antagonistic hypertonus of those muscles which close the jaw. This situation could theoretically result in temporomandibular joint dysfunction or cause a drag upon the free motion of the craniosacral system. The muscles which close the jaw attach to the temporals, maxillae, zygomatics, parietals, sphenoid and frontal. A constant hypertonicity of these muscles, even at a low level, would indeed cause the craniosacral system to expend an increased amount of energy in order to function normally. This increased demand may be reflected in the general health of the patient.

Mylohyoideus

This muscle arises from the whole length of the mylohyoid line of the mandible. It inserts into the hyoid bone. The muscle is innervated by the mylohyoid nerve, which arises from the inferior alveolar branch of the mandibular branch of the trigeminal nerve (C.N. V). The mylohyoid muscle raises the hyoid bone during mastication, deglutition, sucking and blowing.

The effects of chronic hypertonicity of this muscle will be felt not only upon the mandible, but also upon the infrahyoid muscles. Once the hyoid has been stabilized by the antagonistic action of the infrahyoid muscles, the mandible will be subjected to a force which tends to open it. This force will be counteracted by the muscles which close the jaw. These muscles attach to the bones of the cranial vault and to the maxillae and zygomatics. It is by this mechanism that the mylohyoid may interfere with the function of the craniosacral system and contribute to temporomandibular joint dysfunction.

Digastricus

This muscle has been considered under the discussion of the muscles which attach to the temporal bones. The posterior belly of the muscle arises from the mastoid notch of the temporal. The anterior belly arises from the inferior border in a depression on the inner side of the mandible. Both bellies end in a tendon which passes through a fibrous loop attached to the side and cornua of the hyoid bone. Many dysfunctions of the temporal bone and the mandible are produced via this muscle. The digastricus can act as a transmitter of tension from the hyoid bone, or it may be in a state of abnormal contraction itself. Frequently, we have found the infrahyoid muscles to be the cause of temporal and mandibular dysfunction transmitted from the hyoid to these bones by the digastricus.

The innervation of the digastricus is by the mylohyoid nerve, which is a branch of the mandibular division of the trigeminal nerve (C.N. V); and from branches of the facial nerve (C.N. VII). The muscle normally raises the hyoid and assists in opening the jaw. The anterior belly from the mandible draws the hyoid up and forward. The posterior belly draws the hyoid up and backwards (ILLUSTRATION 13-16).

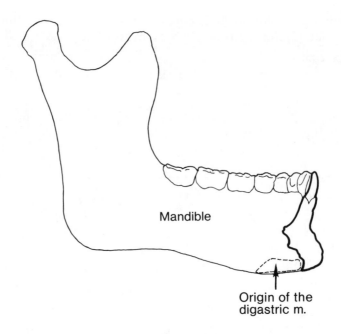

Illustration 13-16
Sagittal Section of Mandible

Pterygoideus Medialis

This muscle arises from the lateral pterygoid plate of the sphenoid, the pyramidal process of the palatine bone and the tuberosity of the maxilla. It inserts into the inferior and posterior part of the medial surface of the ramus and angle of the mandible. It is innervated by the pterygoid nerve from the mandibular division of the trigeminal nerve (C.N. V). This muscle closes the jaw.

The pterygoideus medialis muscle frequently causes dysfunction of the craniosacral system and temporomandibular joint problems. Hypertonicity results in dysfunction of the sphenoid-palatine-maxilla complex. It tends to immobilize the temporal bones through its effect on the mandible. It also tends to immobilize the sphenoid and maxillae, thus creating a considerable drag upon the whole craniosacral system.

Abnormal tonus of the medial pterygoideus is often the result of dental malocclusion or trauma to the jaw. The pathological condition of the muscle often persists long after the trauma has been forgotten.

Pterygoideus Lateralis

This muscle arises from the inferior part of the lateral surface of the great wing of the sphenoid, the infratemporal crest and the lateral surface of the lateral pterygoid plate. It inserts into a depression in the anterior part of the neck of the condyle of the mandible, and into the anterior margin of the articular disc of the temporomandibular joint. It is innervated by the lateral pterygoid nerve, which arises from the mandibular division of the trigeminal nerve (C.N. V). This muscle opens the jaw, protrudes the mandible and helps move it from side to side. It frequently contributes to chronic and acute craniosacral system dysfunction and to temporomandibular joint dysfunction. Its hypertonicity is usually caused by trauma, dental malocclusion and chronic hyperemotional states such as anger, anxiety, tension or stress.

Masseter

This muscle arises from the zygomatic process of the maxilla and from the zygomatic arch. It inserts into the angle and the ramus of the mandible, and into the lateral surface of the coronoid process. It is innervated by the masseter branch of the mandibular division of the trigeminal nerve (C.N. V). This muscle closes the jaw.

Clinical conditions which contribute to abnormal tonus of the masseter muscles include dental malocclusion, chronic hyperemotional states and trauma. Hypertonus of the masseter muscle contributes to ongoing temporomandibular joint dysfunction. It encourages anterior and external rotation of the temporal bone around an axis which is approximately through the ear canal.

Temporalis

This muscle arises from the whole of the temporal fossa, which includes the temporal, parietal, frontal and sphenoid bones. It inserts into the mandible at its anterior coronoid process and into its anterior ramus, almost as far forward as the last molar tooth. The temporalis is innervated by the temporal nerves which arise from the mandibular division of the trigeminal nerve (C.N. V). This muscle closes the jaw and retracts the mandible.

The clinical significance of the temporalis muscle is great. Chronic hypertonicity of one or both temporalis muscles can be caused by temporomandibular joint problems, dental malocclusion, chronic hyperemotional states and physical trauma. Temporalis muscle hypertonicity can underlie temporoparietal suture dysfunction, pterion dysfunction and temporal bone dysfunction. The results are always dural membrane tension patterns as well as osseous and sutural problems. Temporal bone dysfunction may be responsible for many chronic, recurrent neck, shoulder and arm pain syndromes.

Buccinator

This muscle arises from the outer surfaces of the alveolar processes of the maxillae, the mandible and the pterygomandibular raphe. It inserts into the deep layers of the muscle fibers of the lips. It derives motor innervation from the facial nerve (C.N. VII), and sensory innervation from the trigeminal nerve (C.N. V). The buccinator compresses the cheek in mastication.

In our experience, this muscle has not contributed significantly to craniosacral system dysfunction, probably because it has no firm insertional anchoring place.

Constrictor Pharyngeus Superior

This muscle arises from the inferior third of the posterior margin of the medial pterygoid plate, the pterygomandibular raphe, the alveolar process of the mandible and the side of the tongue. It inserts into the median raphe by an aponeurosis to the pharyngeal spine in the basilar part of the occiput. This muscle is innervated by branches of the pharyngeal plexus. It assists in deglutition.

The anatomical relationships of this muscle would suggest that in a hypertonic state it might significantly contribute to sphenobasilar flexion and compression dysfunction. However, in our own clinical experience, we have found little to support this idea.

Hyoid Bone

Although the hyoid bone is not strictly a part of the craniosacral system, it has such generous muscular and fascial attachments to the cranium that it cannot be omitted from consideration as a part of that system.

The hyoid acts like a floating sea-anchor, connected by muscle and fascia to parts below it, and offering attachment for muscles of the cranium above it (ILLUSTRATION 13-17).

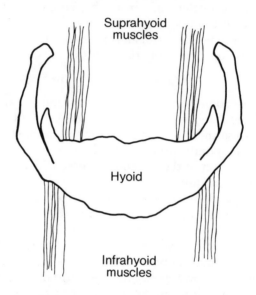

Illustration 13-17
Suspension of Hyoid Bone

The hyoid bone consists of a body, two greater cornua and two lesser cornua. Two major ligaments are attached to it. First is the stylohyoid ligament, which runs from the tip of the styloid process of the temporal bone to the lesser cornua. The second ligament, which attaches to the hyoid base, is the lateral thyrohyoid ligament. This ligament runs from the tip of the superior cornua of the thyroid cartilage to the extremity of the greater cornua of the hyoid bone. It is a round, elastic ligament which forms the posterior border of the thyrohyoid membrane.

The muscles which offer attachment of the hyoid to the cranium are discussed below.

Geniohyoideus

This muscle arises from the inferior mental spine on the inner surface of the symphysis menti of the mandible. It inserts into the anterior surface of the hyoid. The geniohyoid muscle is innervated by branches of the 1st cervical nerve via the hypoglossal nerve (C.N. XII). Contraction of the geniohyoid muscle draws the tongue and the hyoid bone anteriorly. It aids in sucking and deglutition. When the hyoid is fixed, the geniohyoid depresses the mandible.

Chronic hypertonus of this muscle is related to the tightness of the throat which is experienced in many emotional reactions, and in some somatic dysfunctions of the atlas.

Digastricus

This muscle arises as two bellies. The anterior belly arises from the inner side of the inferior border of the mandible; the posterior belly arises from the mastoid notch of the temporal bone. Both bellies insert into a tendon which connects the two bellies and passes through a fibrous loop that arises from the greater cornua of the hyoid bone.

The anterior belly of the digastricus is innervated by the mandibular division of the trigeminal nerve (C.N. V). The posterior belly is innervated by a branch of the facial nerve (C.N. VII).

The digastricus muscle raises the hyoid bone and assists in opening the jaws. The anterior belly draws the hyoid forward and the posterior belly draws it backward.

Stylohyoideus

This muscle arises from the posterior and lateral surfaces of the styloid process of the temporal bone. It inserts into the hyoid body at its junction with the greater cornua. It is innervated by a branch of the facial nerve (C.N. VII). It draws the hyoid superiorly and posteriorly.

Mylohyoideus

This muscle arises from the whole length of the mylohyoid line of the mandible and inserts into the body of the hyoid bone. It is innervated by branches of the mandibular division of the trigeminal nerve (C.N. V). This muscle raises the hyoid and the tongue, and assists in mastication, deglutition, sucking and blowing.

Problems with the mandibular division of the trigeminal nerve (C.N. V) or with the appropriate branches of the facial nerve (C.N. VII) can produce symptoms referrable to the hyoid bone. Craniosacral system dysfunction frequently manifests itself as an abnormal tension of the hyoid bone referred down from above. In order to balance this abnormal tension, the fixing muscles from below the hyoid must react by becoming hypertonic. The result is tightening of the throat which is usually attributed to hysteria and anxiety, but which can be the result of craniosacral system dysfunction.

The muscles which fix the hyoid bone from below are described below.

Sternohyoideus

This muscle arises from the posterior surface of the medial end of the clavicle, the manubrium sterni and the posterior sternoclavicular ligament. It inserts into the inferior body of the hyoid. This muscle stabilizes the hyoid against the suprahyoid muscles and draws the hyoid inferiorly. It is innervated by branches of the 1st, 2nd and 3rd cervical nerve roots via the ansa cervicalis.

Thyrohyoideus

This muscle arises from the oblique line of the lamina of the thyroid cartilage. It inserts into the inferior border of the greater cornua of the hyoid bone. Functionally, it seems to be an extension of the sternothyroideus muscle, which arises from the dorsal surface of the manubrium sterni (dorsal to the origin of the sternohyoideus) and from the cartilage of the 1st and sometimes the 2nd ribs. The thyrohyoideus draws the hyoid inferiorly or the thyroid cartilage superiorly, depending upon the relative degree of fixation of these two structures. It offers, with the sternothyroideus muscle, direct connection between the craniosacral system, via the hyoid bone, and the 1st (and sometimes the 2nd) ribs. We have found this to be a clinically significant continuity.

This muscle is innervated by fibers of the 1st, and sometimes the 2nd, cervical nerve roots.

Omohyoideus

This muscle contains inferior and superior bellies, which are united by a central tendon. The inferior belly arises from the cranial border of the scapula. This inferior belly is bound to the clavicle by a fibrous band, then passes deep to the sternocleidomastoid muscle. The inferior belly then inserts into the central tendon and changes its direction to angle more cephalad. The tendon ends in the superior belly which passes towards the cranium and inserts into the posterior border of the hyoid body. It is innervated by 2nd and 3rd cervical nerve root branches via the ansa cervicalis.

The omohyoid draws the hyoid inferiorly. It offers further connection between the cranium via the hyoid to the clavicle and then on to the scapula. It provides a mechanism whereby craniosacral dysfunction can influence thoracic inlet function, and vice versa. This connection is a frequent clinical finding which often may be due to abnormal tonus of the omohyoid muscle.

We have devoted attention to the hyoid bone and its relationships to the craniosacral system in order to emphasize its importance in many clinical syndromes which seem rather bizarre until one considers the pertinent anatomy. Many craniosacral-hyoid, thyroid-thoracic inlet dysfunction syndromes are referred for psychiatric help before the functional anatomy which underlies the symptomatology has been explored and evaluated, much less treated.

SACRUM AND COCCYX

The sacrum and coccyx are the osseous structures which comprise the inferior end of the craniosacral system. The dura mater has no osseous attachment within the spinal canal between the 3rd cervical vertebra and the 2nd sacral segment. The dural attachment to the 2nd and 3rd cervical vertebrae is only at the anterior aspect of the tube; that is, the dural tube attaches only to the posterior bodies of C2 and C3. It is firmly attached about its circumference only at the foramen magnum. It attaches within the sacral canal anteriorly. It passes out of the sacral canal via the sacral hiatus as the filum terminale then contributes to the periosteum of the coccyx. This arrangement allows for gliding movement of the posterior fibers of the dural tube between the foramen magnum and the coccyx.

Since the dura mater is relatively inelastic, circumstances which place undue tension upon the sacrum and the coccyx will have a profound effect upon the function and mobility of the craniosacral system as a whole.

Muscles which attach to the sacrum and which, by abnormal tonus, may therefore cause craniosacral system dysfunction are discussed below.

Piriformis

This muscle arises bilaterally as three digitations from the anterior surface of the sacral bone between foramena from the 1st through the 4th segments, from the margin of the greater sciatic foramen and from the anterior surface of the sacro-tuberous ligament. It passes out of the pelvis via the greater sciatic foramen and inserts by a round tendon into the superior surface of the greater trochanter of the femur (ILLUSTRATION 13-18). Its insertion is posterior to, and may partially blend with the common tendon of the obturator internus and gemelii muscles. The piriformis is innervated by branches from the 2nd sacral nerve, and inconsistently by the 1st sacral nerve. This muscle serves to externally rotate and abduct the thigh.

In our experience, the piriformis muscle is a common cause of craniosacral

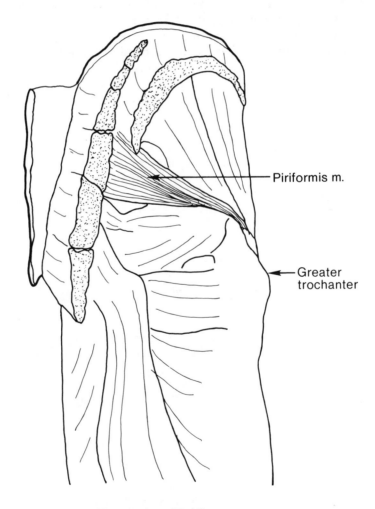

Piriformis m.

Greater trochanter

Illustration 13-18
Piriformis Muscle

system dysfunction. When in a state of hypertonus, it tends to sidebend and torsion the sacrum. It may immobilize this vertebral unit. When this occurs, it causes concurrent sidebending and torsional tendencies at the occiput, and then at the sphenobasilar joint. Recurrent cranial base motion distortions often are due to tension imbalance of the paired piriformi. This results in compromised sacral mobility which reflects up the dural tube to the cranial base.

Iliacus

This is a flat, triangular muscle which arises from the superior two-thirds of the iliac fossa, the inner lip of the iliac crest, the anterior sacroiliac and iliolumbar ligaments and the base of the sacrum. After converging, its fibers insert into the lateral aspect of the tendon of the psoas major muscle and onto the femur (ILLUSTRATION 13-19). It is innervated by fibers of the femoral nerve derived from the 2nd and 3rd lumbar spinal nerves.

The iliacus muscle flexes the thigh. Hypertonus of this muscle directly affects the craniosacral system by causing forward-flexion of the sacral base. Bilateral hypertonus will therefore contribute to dysfunction (extension lesion) of the cranial base. Unilateral iliacus muscle hypertonus will cause torsion dysfunction of the craniosacral system.

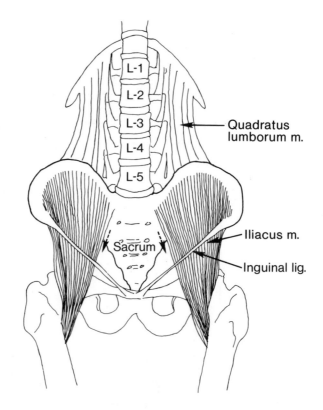

Illustration 13-19
Iliacus Muscle (Arrows Indicate How This Muscle
Can Interfere with Free Sacral Mobility)

Gluteus Maximus

This is the most superficial of the muscles of the gluteal region. It arises from the posterior gluteal line of the ilium, from the radial portion of that bone (including the crest), from the lower posterior part of the sacrum, the coccyx, the aponeurosis of the sacrospinatus muscle, the sacrotuberous ligament and the fascia over the gluteus medius. It inserts into the iliotibial band of the fascia lata and the gluteal tuberosity between the vastus lateralis and the adductor longus muscles (ILLUS-TRATION 13-20). The gluteus maximus is innervated by fibers derived from the 5th

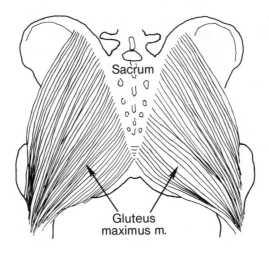

Illustration 13-20
Gluteus Maximus Muscle

lumbar and 1st and 2nd sacral spinal nerves. These fibers are passed to their destination via the inferior gluteal nerves.

This muscle extends and laterally rotates the thigh. Hypertonus of the gluteus maximus causes a reduction of sacral mobility. Unilateral hypertonus causes a side-bending and torsional dysfunction of the sacral base. Bilateral hypertonus causes a reduction of sacral base mobility in the position of flexion. These interferences with sacral mobility are transmitted to the cranial base via the dural tube.

Multifidus

This muscle consists of several tendinous fasciculi which lie in the vertical grooves on both sides of the spinous processes from sacrum to axis. In the sacral region, these fasciculi arise from the posterior sacrum from the 4th segment upward, and insert into the vertebral spinous processes two to four segments above. That is, multifidus fasciculi which arise from the level of the 4th sacral segment generally insert into the spinous process of the 5th lumbar vertebra, and those which arise from the 3rd sacral segment usually insert into the spinous process of the 4th lumbar vertebra, and so on up to the axis.

Since the multifidus fasciculi arise laterally and travel medially as they ascend, unilateral contraction produces a rotation with a tendency towards extension backwards of the involved vertebrae. Bilateral contraction of the multifidus produces spinal backwardbending.

At the lumbosacral junction, bilateral multifidus hypertonus produces backward extension between the lower lumbar and sacral vertebrae. This condition results in a compression of these vertebrae posterior to the bodies and discs. The articular surfaces seem to become impacted or "jammed" together. This situation frequently results in compression of the atlantooccipital joints and in membranous sphenobasilar joint compression. The clinical result is lower back pain, upper cervical and head pain, plus the mental changes of depression. This depression is often considered to be endogenous and is blamed for the head, neck and low back pain. Successful decompression of the lumbosacral junction, the atlanto-occipital region and the sphenobasilar joint usually produces remarkable and dramatic mood changes, as well as relief of pain. A marked improvement in the quality and range of craniosacral system motion is easily detected immediately.

Unilateral lumbosacral region multifidus contracture results in less severe craniosacral system dysfunction. The usual result is one of cranial base torsion dysfunction. If this is the case, the cranial base torsion dysfunction will often correct spontaneously when abnormal lumbosacral junction mechanics are corrected.

Coccygeus and Levator Ani

These contribute the muscular parts of the pelvic diaphragm. This diaphragm is pierced by the urethra, vagina and anal canal. It stretches across the pelvic cavity like a hammock. Both of these muscles have generous attachment to the coccyx.

When the pelvic diaphragm is in a state of hypertonus or contracture for any reason, the coccyx is pulled into anterior flexion. This condition of anterior malposition transmits tension up the dural tube from the coccyx (which has dural contribution to its periosteum) to the occiput. Such tension causes occipital compression with the atlas and often results in head pain in addition to the pelvic and low back dysfunction produced by the abnormally hypertonic pelvic diaphragm.

We have relieved many head pains and restored normal craniosacral system function simply by gently relieving the pelvic diaphragm tension and then moving the coccyx posteriorly.

LIGAMENTS

An extremely complex system of ligaments is present both within and without the craniosacral system. Both sets of ligaments have powerful effects upon the structures of the craniosacral system. These structures move in order to accommodate the rhythmic rise and fall of cerebrospinal fluid pressure within the dural membrane system.

In this section we will only consider those ligaments which are extrinsic to the system. When puzzling things happen to the normal symmetry of craniosacral system motion, one should always consider an imbalance of ligamentous tension due to injury, inflammation, stressful voluntary demands or postural problems.

The styloid processes of the temporal bones offer attachment for the stylohyoid ligaments, which connect these processes with the lesser cornua of the hyoid bone bilaterally; and for the stylomandibular ligaments, which connect these pro-

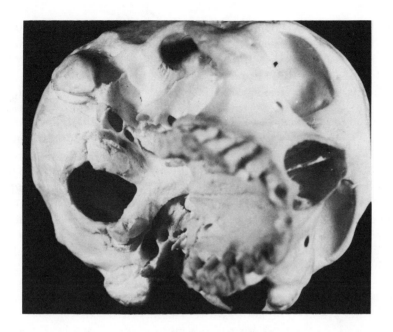

Illustration 13-21
Styloid Processes of the Temporal Bones

cesses with the angles of the mandible (ILLUSTRATION 13-21). Imbalanced tension of these ligaments will interfere with normal temporal bone motion. The styloid processes serve as levers which affect temporal bone motion. A slight tension upon the lever has an exaggerated effect upon the motion of the whole bone.

The sphenomandibular ligament connects the spine of the sphenoid bone to the lingula of the mandibular foramen. Imbalanced tension from the mandible can therefore cause dysfunction of the sphenoid bone as it moves in response to the urging of the craniosacral system.

Ligaments which, when imbalanced or under abnormal tension, interfere with normal occipital motion include the ligamentum nuchae, the fibrous raphe of the pharynx, the lateral atlantooccipital ligaments and the occipitoaxial ligaments, which pass through the foramen magnum.

There are also numerous ligaments which can easily impair the free mobility of the sacrum as it participates in the motion of the craniosacral system. These ligaments include the anterior and posterior longitudinal ligaments which connect occiput to sacrum. The intervertebral disc between L5 and S1 may be considered a ligament and can certainly impair the sacrum's ability to move. The ligamentum flava connects the lamina of L5 and S1. Imbalance of tension in these ligaments is most likely to produce a sidebending or torsional craniosacral system dysfunction pattern. The articular capsules which connect the articular processes of L5 and S1 can likewise interfere with free sacral motion when these capsules become inflamed or stiffened for any reason.

One must also consider the iliolumbar ligaments, which connect the sacral base to the transverse processes of L5; the interspinal and supraspinal ligaments; the ligaments of the sacroiliac articulation (ventral, dorsal and interosseous); the ligaments which connect the sacrum and the ischium, usually the sacrotuberous and sacrospinous; the sacrococcygeal ligaments (ventral, dorsal and lateral); the interposed fibrocartilage; and the interarticular ligaments. Postural imbalances, athletic stresses, injuries and the like will cause tension imbalances in these ligamentous structures. These imbalances are manifested as abnormality of motion in the craniosacral system; bizarre syndromes are frequently the result.

FASCIA

Fascia is a connective tissue which is derived embryologically from mesoderm. It is composed primarily of collagenous and elastic fibers. Fibroblasts and fibrocytes are always present. *Fascia exists in dynamic equilibrium.*

Collagen fibers are glistening white. They are composed of reticular fibrils which are visible with the electron microscope. These collagenous fibers form the bulk of fascia, tendon and ligament. Collagenous fibers are pliable and extremely tough, with little extensibility.

Elastic fibers are stretchable. They vary in length and thickness depending upon the tension placed upon them. They are not known to be composed of smaller fibrils but rather are homogeneous proteinaceous material.

Electron miscroscopy suggests that a unit (which we shall call the "elastocollagenous complex") may account for the contractibility of fascia. This unit is innervated. It may serve as the mechanism by which fascia exhibits the ability to contract and relax. It may also relate to fascial "trigger points." In our proposed "elastocollagenous unit" the elastic fiber is the core. The collagenous material is coiled around the elastic fibers. The collagen and elastic fibers have common attachments at the extremes of the "elastocollagenous complex" (ILLUSTRATION 13-22).

Innervation of the "elastocollagenous complex" is both sensory and motor. As the complex reaches its limit of expansion, stretch stimuli produce a reflex elastic contraction as well as the subjective sensation of pain.

There is also a ground substance present in fascia which may vary in constituency from fluid to solid. This substance transports metabolic materials throughout the body. (We refer here to both anabolic and catabolic materials.)

Our research, both independently and in conjunction with Dr. Zvi Karni, Professor of Biological Engineering at the Technion Institute in Haifa, Israel, suggests that fascia may serve in an electrical conduction capacity and therefore that fascial contraction may interfere with its electrical conductivity coefficient. Local-

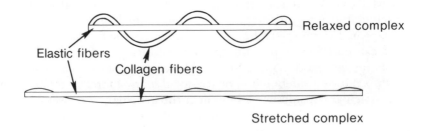

Illustration 13-22
"Elastocollagenous Complex"

ized pain and tissue devitalization may be produced as a result.

Fascia may vary in character from predominantly dense and fibrous (which may be organized or disorganized) to loose-fibrous, fibroelastic, areolar or reticular. The organized dense fibrous tissues in the extreme are the aponeuroses, ligaments and tendons. These tissues are largely inelastic; they can withstand great unidirectional stretching and tensile strains while still remaining pliable. The disorganized dense fibrous tissues have their collagen fibers arranged in an interwoven manner, rather than in parallel bundles like the organized tissues of aponeuroses, ligaments and tendons. The disorganized dense fibrous tissues form most of the fascial membranes, the dermis of the skin, the capsules of organs and the periosteum of bone. These tissues can resist strong stretching tensions in any direction. In this characteristic they differ from the organized dense fibrous tissues, which best resist stretching in only one direction. The latter tissues easily tear when stretched at right angles to their direction of fiber orientation.

Some membranes, such as the dura mater, have their bundles of collagen arranged in layers rather than in interwoven networks. Continuous abnormal tension on these tissues in a given direction will cause the fibers to organize. Fiber orientation is parallel to the direction of maximum tension to which the membrane is subjected (ILLUSTRATION 13-23). Microscopic study of fiber orientation patterns in normally disorganized fascia and the dural membrane may indicate the presence of abnormal fiber patterns.

From a functional point of view, the body fascia may be regarded as a single and continuous laminated sheet of connective tissue. This laminated sheet extends without interruption from the top of the head to the tips of the toes. It contains

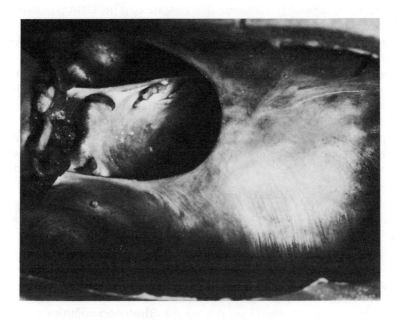

Illustration 13-23
Orientation of Dural Membrane Fibers
in Response to Stress

pockets which allow for the presence of the viscera, the visceral cavities, the muscles and skeletal structures. It also contains concentrically placed tubes which allow for the passage of the central nervous system, the vertebral column and related structures. The fascia varies in character in response to the demands placed upon it by the body which it serves.

The pia mater invests the brain and spinal cord. It is a delicate fascial membrane which carries a rich vascular network. Its tiny blood vessels serve the nervous tissue to which it adheres throughout the majority of its expanse. The fibers of the pia mater contribute to the perineurium of the nerves which exit from the brain and spinal cord. The pia mater blends with the dura mater at the exits of these nerves from the dural compartment. Its outer surface blends with the arachnoid membrane as the projections of the arachnoid villae come into intimate contact with it. The pia mater is the most central tube of fascia, as it follows the brain fissures and actually contributes to the lining of the ventricular system of the brain. It travels with the brain and spinal cord as they develop embryologically.

External to the pia mater and separated by the subarachnoid space, where the pia and arachnoid membranes are not blended or adherent, is the arachnoid membrane. The subarachnoid space is filled with cerebrospinal fluid. Communication with the pial and dural membranes is prominent at the cauda equina and at the projections of the denticulate ligament. The arachnoid membrane is delicate and avascular; it is separated from the dura mater by the subdural space, which contains a thin layer of lubricating fluid. There is functionally significant independent mobility between the dura mater, the arachnoid membrane and the pia mater. The arachnoid trabeculae, where blending with the pia mater occurs, do not restrict a small degree of motion between these two membranes. At the base of the brain the subarachnoid space enlarges considerably to form the cisternae. The cisternae are filled with cerebrospinal fluid and are named for their anatomical locations.

The dura mater is the outermost of the three concentric tubes of fascia which invest the brain. It is dense, fibrous connective tissue composed of collagenous bundles arranged in interlacing layers. It has two layers, an inner meningeal layer and an outer periosteal layer. These layers are blended into continuity at the foramen magnum, the intervertebral foramena, as the dural layers invest the cauda equina and finally as they blend with the periosteum of the coccyx. The cranial dura forms the endosteum of the vault bones of the skull. It is continuous with the periosteum of the external surfaces of the skull bones by transversing the *uncalcified and mobile* sutures.

The cervical region is an excellent example of these concepts of concentric tubes and fascial continuity. These three concentric tubes of fascia (the meningeal membranes) within the spinal canal are contained, together with the vertebral column and intervertebral discs, within yet another tube of fascia, the vertebral fascia. This fascia invests the vertebral column and its contents, in addition to the related muscles. It connects the head with the thorax and makes many important connections with the upper extremities.

The prevertebral fascia, which is the anterior part of the larger complex of vertebral fascia, is continuous from the skull to the coccyx. It invests the anterior surfaces of the longus colli and capitis muscles, the rectus capitis anterior and lateralis muscles, and attaches to the tips of the vertebral transverse processes. It extends over the scalene muscles and becomes the fascia of the thoracic wall.

Sibson's fascia, which arches over the cupula of each lung, is continuous with the fascia on the deep side of the scalenes. This fascia is actually reinforced by striate muscle fibers on occasion. It is continuous with the carotid sheath.

The carotid sheath contains the carotid artery, the internal jugular vein and the vagus nerve (C.N. X). Medially, it is continuous with the visceral fascia, which invests the esophagus and trachea. Posteriorly, it is continuous with the prevertebral fascia. Laterally, it is continuous with the fascia of the sternocleidomastoid muscle.

The carotid sheath attaches to the skull at the carotid foramen. At the base of the neck the carotid sheath adheres to the sternum and to the 1st rib. It fuses with the fascia of the scalenes. It is continuous with the pericardium below.

The cervical sympathetic neural tissue is imbedded in the posterior wall of the carotid sheath; therefore, tension on the carotid sheath affects autonomic function. The fibrous pericardium is continuous with the carotid sheath, which descends from the cranial base. Below, many of its fibers penetrate the diaphragm and contribute to the fascia of the inferior surface of the diaphragm. We have traced these same fibers down the crura of the diaphragm where they become blended with the prevertebral fascia and with the fascia of the iliopsoas muscles. Thus, we have fascial continuity from skull to pelvis, with powerful effects upon sympathetic nerve function in between. There are hundreds of similar examples in the human body which illustrate the continuity of fascia from head to toe.

One may regard the fascial organ as a maze which allows travel from any one place in the body to any other place without ever leaving fascia. At the superior end, many lamina of fascia attach to the skull. Muscles pulling upon fascia therefore affect the function of the craniosacral system.

Through fascial continuity, an injury which results in fascial contracture or edema may affect the craniosacral system. This may cause dysfunction of the central nervous system, which, in turn, can produce bizarre and virtually "impossible" clinical results.

Our approach is based on the concept of fascial continuity and slight mobility. The fascial lamina are normally mobile throughout the body and should respond to gentle traction. Areas of injury or clinically significant change produce fascial immobility. One must carefully search for these areas of immobility to locate causes of biological dysfunction. Fascial immobility, which we call "fascial drag," will *almost* always appear as an asymmetry or labored quality of motion in the craniosacral system. We have yet to find an exception to this rule but feel compelled to use the word "almost" because we do not subscribe to dogmatic and absolute concepts.

The lessons to be learned with respect to fascia are these: that it is continuous; that each viscera has carried its own fascia with it during embryologic development; that it is a slightly mobile connective tissue organ; that dysfunction or injury reduces localized fascial mobility; and that such loss of fascial mobility produces a drag upon the fascial system which manifests as abnormal alteration in craniosacral physiological motion. This alteration can be used in diagnosis, treatment and prognosis. Specific technique is discussed in Chapter 14.

CICATRIX

Experience has shown us that cicatricial tissue, whether it be clean, post-surgical scarring or post-traumatic scarring which was less than sterile, can create longstanding problems in fascial mobility.

Drag upon fascial mobility, which is induced by cicatricial formation, may result in craniosacral system dysfunction. The resulting clinical syndrome may only be traced to the fascial problem as you observe a successful therapeutic result. One of the best examples of this rather bizarre and far-fetched idea was the case of a 36-year old woman whose migraine headaches of 20 years' duration were ended when her appendectomy scar was mobilized. The appendectomy was performed when the patient was 12 years of age. The menarche occured at age 13. The headaches began at age 16. This patient had visited several clinics of good reputation, exhausted most other therapeutic modalities and was in the process of accepting her incapacitating problem as the result of a deep-seated, psychoneurotic disorder. Examination of fascial system motion integrated with craniosacral system motion led us to the appendectomy scar. Deep pressure medially on the scar produced the headache; deep pressure laterally caused relief of the headache. Mobilization of the scar was performed by sustained and deep but gentle pressure. At this writing, there have been no headaches for approximately 18 months. Spontaneous relief of low back pain, menstrual disorders and chronic and recurrent cervical somatic dysfunction also occured following cicatrix mobilization.

We have found similar, apparently bizarre relationships between headache and suspension of a right kidney, surgical removal of a right medial knee cartilage, coccygectomy and ganglionectomy of the left wrist. We have seen dysautonomia as a result of craniosacral system dysfunction which arose from surgical procedures. We have also observed the relief of "endogenous depression" as the result of mobilizing scar tissue which caused cranial base compression.

We believe that scars which significantly contribute to craniosacral system dysfunction are most easily found by the blind evaluation of craniosacral motion, both within the craniosacral system and as it is reflected throughout the total body fascia. We search for the locus of immobility while the patient is dressed in loose clothing. Only after we find the locus do we look for the presence of a scar. The movements under investigation are so subtle that we do not wish to have the visual observation of a scar or cicatrix suggest the locus of immobility. We feel much too suggestible to accept the approach of a prior visual observation or verbal history from the patient. Palpation is used first, followed by confirmation upon direct observation and patient history.

ARTICULAR SOMATIC DYSFUNCTION

Somatic dysfunction of the spinal column anywhere throughout its length will result in craniosacral system dysfunction. This probably occurs through several mechanisms:

1. Somatic dysfunction which reflects at one or more intervertebral foramena may cause tension or abnormal change in the character of the dural sleeve, which follows the spinal nerve root out to the affected foramen. This condition may produce a "dural drag" upon the free motion of the craniosacral system. Functionally, the sacral hiatus may be regarded as another foramen which has a similar effect of "dragging" upon the free mobility of the craniosacral system; therefore, any articular dysfunction of the sacrum will produce a change in the craniosacral system.
2. Facilitated spinal segments are almost always detectable by examination of the craniosacral system. This may be due to a neural mechanism from that segment

which produces craniosacral dysfunction.

3. Somatic dysfunction usually adversely affects the craniosacral system by way of its effect on fascial mobility and muscle tonus. It is very rare when these conditions cannot be detected by their effect on the free mobility of the craniosacral system.

Many muscles and connective tissues external to the craniosacral system can have a deleterious effect on that system. This chapter has taken you on a short tour of these tissues and described the possible mechanisms of their adverse effects. We hope that you will keep these possibilities in mind whenever you diagnose or treat craniosacral dysfunction, as this attitude will definitely enhance your therapeutic abilities.

Chapter 14
Diagnosis by Evaluation of Craniosacral System Function and Whole Body Response

The inherent rhythmic motions of the human body can be used quite effectively in physical diagnosis. In this chapter, our attention will be focused primarily upon the craniosacral system rhythm, the mobility of this system, and the response of the rest of the body to this rhythmic motion. Because we are focusing attention upon this system does not mean that we believe the craniosacral rhythm is the most significant body rhythm. (It *is* probably the most neglected.) It does mean that we have explored the use of this body rhythm and mobility more than any of the other known body rhythms.

Why the use of body rhythms and mobility have been so neglected in the art and science of physical diagnosis is a mystery. It would seem that we physicians have neglected the development of the use of our hands as diagnostic instruments even though they are connected to that reasoning computer we call a brain. We have allowed ourselves to be swayed by our present infatuation with scientific and technological gadgetry. This is not a criticism of scientific technology, but a plea for a balance between what our hands can tell us about patients and what sophisticated instruments and biochemical analyses can tell us. Like any other manual skill, the effective use of one's hands as diagnostic instruments requires practice. Pianists, sculptors, typists and physical diagnosticians must all develop and practice skills.

All of the minutes which you spend palpating or placing your hands on various patients' bodies are recorded in your memory at some level of consciousness. As you accumulate and correlate perceptions with known facts about these patients, more and more useful information will be gained by the touch of your examining hands upon another human body. It's a cost-free approach to diagnosis. Experience and knowledge are gained every time you touch a patient. Your learning laboratory is composed of all the people whom you contact and touch on a day-to-day basis. Additionally, if you are working in the healing areas, your patients or clients will respond positively to your increased touching. Rapport will improve quickly and dramatically.

As a professor in a college of osteopathic medicine, and as a teacher of some allopathic medical students, I (Upledger) have been astounded by the observation that many 3rd and 4th year allopathic and osteopathic medical students are reticent to touch another human being during an examination procedure. It seems untenable that a health care professional may carry a neurotic aversion to touching another human being. After overcoming the aversion to touching (which we do by touching), you can begin to obtain information about the patient with your hands. Use them. The cost of health care can decrease considerably if "touching skills" are developed and used by health care professionals (APPENDIX K).

Accurate diagnosis by the use of craniosacral system motion requires that you accumulate examination/touching experiences with many healthy and many less-than-healthy human beings. As you accumulate a data base of experience, you will be surprised, if not amazed, at the diagnostic insights you can receive from your hands. You will notice the person-to-person variations in quality, symmetry, rate, rhythm, restriction, etc., of the craniosacral motion.

The methods we have developed for use in palpatory diagnosis are described below.

QUALITY OF CRANIOSACRAL MOTION

Very gently apply your hands to the patient's body. The application of your hands can be anywhere on the body. We suggest the vault hold, the thoracic inlet, the respiratory diaphragm, the pelvis, the thighs and the feet as good "listening stations" for starters. Your touch should be too light to stimulate a perceptible body response. Note the quality of the motion which you perceive. Is it free and easy, as in good health? Is it labored, as in a rigid container fighting against its boundaries? Is the motion lethargic and lacking in inherent energy, as in states of physical or mental exhaustion? Correlate your impression of the quality of motion with other information about the patient. Keep this in your memory for future recall and comparison.

SYMMETRY OF CRANIOSACRAL MOTION

Is the motion symmetrical on the head? At the various "listening stations" listed above? Is there a lack of symmetry? Where is that lack of symmetry most pronounced? Where is the restriction that produces it?

RATE OF CRANIOSACRAL MOTION

Is the rate normal (between 6 and 12 cycles per minute)? If the rate is high, you may suspect an acute problem against which the patient is fighting very hard. Hyperkinetic children present with elevated rates. (For those of you interested in traditional Chinese medicine, an elevated rate suggests a Yang malady.) If the rate is below normal, it suggests a chronic, debilitating (Yin) problem against which the bodily defenses are failing. Resistance is flagging. This could be due to emotional exhaustion, malnutrition, metastatic malignancy or anything in between.

CRANIOSACRAL SYSTEM MOBILITY ABOVE AND BELOW THE
FORAMEN MAGNUM

Any lesion or dysfunction may place a drag on dural membrane mobility. Lesions which affect the occiput and above will interfere markedly with the free mobility of the intracranial membrane system. These lesions are either intracranial, or they directly affect the bones of the cranium and in turn have maximum effect upon the intracranial dural membrane system.

Lesions below the occiput which affect the dural tube or any of its sleeves including the filum terminale are reflected maximally as a drag upon the free mobility of the dural tube within the spinal canal. The dural tube is constructed so that it can glide longitudinally within the spinal canal. Restriction to this free gliding motion can be imposed by spinal or paravertebral somatic dysfunction, by membrane fixations within the spinal canal, by compression of the filum terminale, by problems which affect the dural sleeves, by arachnoiditis or edema and by post-operative membrane adhesions.

The examination for dural membrane mobility will not tell you what the cause of the problem is, but it will tell you where it is.

In order to determine the presence of a restriction within the total dural system, place one examining hand under the patient's sacrum and the other on top of the head over the parietal or frontal bones. Is the motion free and easy between your two hands? Next, place the cephalad hand under the occipital squama. How does the quality of the motion of the spinal dural tube compare with that of the whole system? Then place one hand under the occipital squama and one on the frontal. How does the motion between your two hands compare with that of the whole system? How does the motion of the intracranial membrane system compare with the motion of the spinal dural tube? The division of the system (intracranial or intraspinal) which moves with least ease is the one you should further examine to more precisely locate the problem.

INTRACRANIAL MEMBRANE RESTRICTION LOCALIZATION

In order to localize the restriction found within the cranial dural membrane system, apply the vault hold. Do not do anything to modify the inherent motion patterns; your touch must be very light. Look for asymmetry of motion within the cranial vault. In order to localize the asymmetry, visualize a three-dimensional globe (cranial vault) and intracranial membrane system. Answer the question, "Where is the pivot point of the motion which I am perceiving?" A lack of symmetry means that the pivot point is not on the midline; where is it? Your hands are following the motions of the surface of the cranium as though describing arcs on the surface of a globe. Try to visualize where the radii of these arcs would intersect (ILLUSTRATION 14-1). The intersection point of these arcs is the locus of the lesion. You may move your hands to an infinite number of positions upon the surface of the cranial vault in order to discover the various arcs and their radii. Occasionally, dual lesions will be involved. The arcs will change according to the proximity of your hands to each lesion, and its relative severity. This circumstance can be quite confusing until you realize that you are perceiving two or more separate lesions, each with its own focus of motion restriction. As the lesions are corrected, the cranial vault will begin to move more symmetrically.

Another difficult to diagnose circumstance is presented by the midline lesion. Here, the motion restriction is located on the midsagittal plane. The cranial motion is symmetrical, but of smaller amplitude than that of the spinal dural tube. Also, there may be a displacement of the normal fulcrum about which the reciprocal membrane system moves.

To localize this lesion, place your fingers along the median line of the patient's

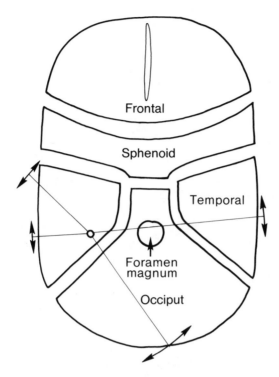

Illustraion 14-1
Cranial Base with Examples of Arcs
Secondary to a Point Restriction

head from the glabella to the external occipital protuberance. Be sure your fingers are spaced out along this median sagittal line. Rest them very lightly so as not to impede the inherent motion. The system should be moving in flexion and extension about a moving fulcrum located in the anterior straight sinus region. If the fulcrum (or axis) is immobile or fixed, where is the fixation point? The lesion is located at this point (ILLUSTRATION 14-2). If the arcing is around the normal pivot point in the straight sinus, but is not mobile, the problem is in the straight sinus. The key is the loss of normal mobility of the pivot point which moves rhythmically back and forth along the intersection of the falx cerebri and the tentorium cerebelli (the straight sinus).

Practice in locating the intersection point of the radii of the arcs which your hands describe will pay large diagnostic dividends. The resolution of the abnormal arcing during the healing process is a valuable prognostic indicator.

LOCALIZATION OF RESTRICTIONS OF THE SPINAL DURAL TUBE

Probably the most difficult techniques to describe are those which we use to localize restrictions imposed upon the spinal dural tube. The techniques are not difficult once you have experienced them, but they are nonetheless difficult to describe. It is somewhat like trying to talk about how you know which direction a sound is coming from; you have stereophonic hearing, but how do you know that a sound is coming from 5 o'clock over your right shoulder?

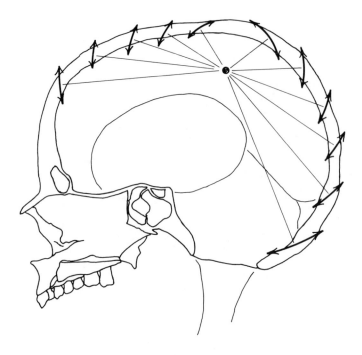

Illustration 14-2
Localization of Midline Point Restriction

We have used two separate techniques to localize dural tube restrictions. The first is very passive monitoring, and the second is very light traction. We continually change back and forth between these two approaches in deciding the location of the restriction.

Perform the passive technique after clearing any restrictions of the cranial base and the other transverse diaphragms. Gently rest the patient's occiput in your hands. A clear, unrestricted dural tube will give the impression that its longitudinal movements are free of impediment. The occiput easily rotates with the phases of craniosacral system motion (ILLUSTRATION 14-3). The two squama of the occiput feel like handles attached to the superior end of the dural tube. The handles and the tube should move freely and easily in synchrony. If they do not, there is a restriction somewhere. Often, there are minor restrictions which clear up after a few cycles of motion, so you should monitor 10 to 12 cycles before making a decision about the presence of restriction. You are monitoring the normal inherent craniosacral system motion as it manifests in the spinal dural tube. Pretend your fingers extend all the way down the tube; experience what these imaginary prolongations of your fingers are doing and what they encounter.

The traction phase of this examination is performed by gently applying a cephalad or superiorly directed traction upon the occiput so that you are causing the mobile dural tube to glide gently toward you. When you meet a restriction to the free glide of the tube, try to answer the question, "How far down the tube was my traction effect when I felt the restriction?" With practice, you will be able to answer this question.

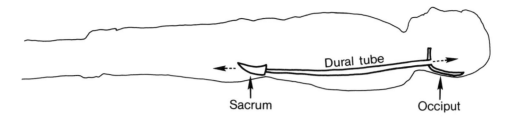

Illustration 14-3
Dural Tube Continuity
(Easy Motion Should Follow Traction from Either End)

The very light traction first affects the dural tube closest to you, the upper cervical. As the force of the traction is gently and slowly increased, you can move down the tube (caudad) almost one segment at a time. Often your patient will be able to tell you where the effect is being felt. This is most valuable feedback training. You are learning a most fascinating and potentially constructive game. The cost of error is essentially nil.

The same approach is effectively applied from the sacrum, with the patient lying supine on your hand.

A little traction first affects the filum terminale; then, as your traction force is gradually increased, the effect moves cephalad. At what level do you meet resistance?

An effective training method which we use to sharpen perception of the location of restriction in terms of distance from you is performed with polyethylene film, or Saran Wrap (ILLUSTRATION 14-4). Flatten a long sheet of the film on top of a smooth, clean table. The adhesion of the polyethylene film to the table top will offer some resistance to its movement across the table top. Gently pull on the film towards you to get a feeling for the amount of traction which you must use to move the film. Once you have this perception, place an object (such as a water glass) on the sheet of film so that the resistance to your traction is increased by the weight of the object. Move the object about on the film to several different locations. Perceive how it feels when the film's response to your traction is restricted in a given locus. Begin using lighter objects; then use multiple objects. Once you are familiar with the "feel" of the film's response to your traction, and the effect of the various objects placed in different locations, try it blind-folded. Have a friend place the objects for you. Reach out and try to touch the object after you have done your testing with manual traction. You will be surprised how quickly you can develop accuracy at touching the object which offers the restriction to your traction while you are blind-folded.

RESTRICTIONS TO THE FREE MOBILITY OF FASCIA

The fascia of the human body is continuous from head to toe. You can travel from the top of your head to your liver, spleen or right medial malleolus without ever leaving fascia. All viscera during embryological development migrate and carry their fasciae with them. Fascia possesses some limited mobility. It glides easily when subjected to gentle traction. Inflammation, adhesion, postural stress and somatic

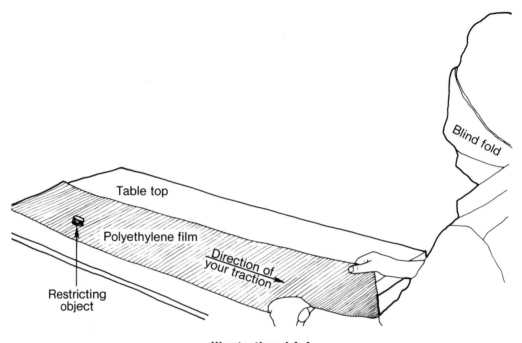

Illustration 14-4
Training Method for Localization of Restrictions

dysfunctions all interfere with the free gliding of the fasciae. Use the same principles for body fascia which we have described above for testing the mobility of the dural tube. You can practice with the polyethylene film on the table top to develop your skills. The only difference now is that you are attempting to localize extradural problems by the use of gentle fascial traction, rather than by traction directed at the spinal dural tube.

Apply gentle traction. As your force is gradually increased, the effect moves further away from you. We apply the traction at several places because the closer you are to the restriction, the more apparent it becomes. We usually begin with the upper cervical region and direct the traction cephalad. From the neck, you can usually sense as far down as the pelvis. You can then use the heels. Gently pick the extended legs up from the table and apply traction directed pedad. From the heels, you can generally sense as high as the respiratory diaphragm.

When you wish to clarify your impressions, symmetrical placement of the examining hand upon the thighs, abdomen and thorax is helpful. Fascial planes of both the anterior and posterior regions of the body are used. Improvise and locate the restriction.

Palpating Denervated Muscle Activity

While I was a visiting professor at the Technion Institute in Haifa, Israel, I was asked to perform examination of several neurological patients at the Loewenstein Neurological Institute in Ra'ana, Israel (APPENDIX B). I had no clinical knowledge of the patients except that they were all neurological cases and had longstanding problems. Cases of both coma and paralysis were included. Normal muscle moves with the craniosacral system rhythmic activity at a rate of 6-12 cycles per minute. This motion can be palpated anywhere on the body. While working with the director of the Institute, Professor Nachansohn, I discovered the fact that denervated muscle moves at about 25 cycles per minute. The character of the motion is about the same, but the rate is significantly increased (not necessarily twice the cranial rate). This muscle activity is palpable in the paravertebral musculature. We found that I could locate the level of spinal cord injury on all of the patients examined (15) by determining the level at which the rate of craniosacral rhythm, as manifested in the paravertebral muscles, elevated from the patient's cephalad norm to the more rapid rate of approximately 25 cycles per minute. The spinal cord problem was always about 2 segments above the vertebral level at which the paravertebral muscle motion rate changed. Included in these cases were quadriplegias and paraplegias due to spinal cord lesions. There was one case of poliomyelitis and one case of Guillian-Barre.

We also examined several cases of post-anoxic coma and found the cranial rhythm to be reduced to 3 or 4 cycles per minute. In cases of hemiplegia due to cerebrovascular accident, the muscle response to the craniosacral system rhythm was normal on the unaffected side of the body, and elevated on the paralyzed side. Further, the cranial rhythmic activity in the unaffected side of the head was usually normal, while it was rapid and chaotic on the affected side. Further work along these lines is definitely indicated.

THE INTERFERENCE WAVES OF INJURY AND DISEASE

This technique makes use of the whole body motion as it responds to the craniosacral system rhythm. A normal body will move into internal and external rotation in synchrony with the craniosacral rhythm. Injury and disease areas seem to set up interference waves like those that occur when one drops a pebble into a quiet pond. If you can see the interference waves created by the pebble you can tell exactly where the pebble entered the water; the waves form arcs, the radii of which intersect at exactly the point of the pebble's entry into the pond. The same is true of the wave activity which you perceive in the human body. You are using your hands to perceive the natural, symmetrical wave motion of the body. A restriction lesion sets up an interference wave pattern which superimposes itself upon the normal physiological and inherent body motion. When you can locate manually where the interference waves are coming from, you have found the source of the problem.

To locate the source of the restriction or interference waves, gently place your hands in turn symmetrically on the head, thoracic inlet, inferior costal margins, pelvis, thighs and feet of the patient. At each locus of examination allow your hands to passively move with the inherent body motion of the patient. If the arcs your hands describe are symmetrical, there is no problem. If the arcs described are not symmetrical, envision the radii of the arcs. Determine the position of their intersection. That point is the location of the restriction or lesion.

To locate the problem precisely, place your hands in as many positions as you need to make the decision. It is as if there were an infinite number of concentric globes around the lesion, each vibrating and describing arcs. Where is the center of all the concentric globes? As you get closer, the arcs get smaller. You can place one hand on the anterior surface and one on the posterior surface of the patient's body.

Your two hands will describe arcs. Where is the intersection of the arcs? The location of this intersection gives you the depth of the lesion (ILLUSTRATION 14-5).

Practice makes perfect. Using this method, we have been able to locate many obscure problems, the secondary consequences of which had been unsuccessfully treated by many physicians for years.

If there are two restrictive lesions, they seem to interfere in proportion to proximity and severity. Where there are two lesions of equal severity, the one

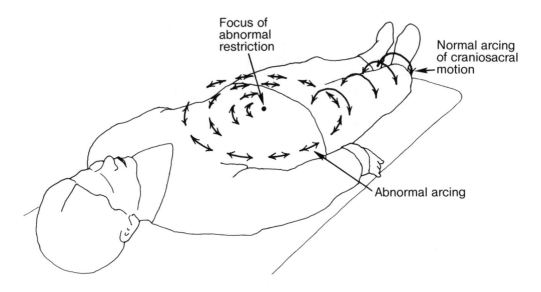

Illustration 14-5
Use of Arcs in Diagnosis

nearest the examiner's hands will be most pronounced. For example, if there are lesions of equal severity in the lower pericardium and right ovary, you will probably find the pericardial lesion but be unaware of the ovarian problem if you examine from the head. However, if you examine from the feet you will probably find the ovarian problem but not the pericardial one. On the other hand, if the pericardial problem is much more severe than the ovarian problem you might find the pericardial problem from the feet as well as from the head. You might experience some confusion from the right ovarian problem and discover it only during palpation of pelvic motion. Or, you may only find the ovarian lesion later as the pericardial problem is resolved and the intensity of its interference waves are diminished. We conceptualize this situation as an inverse relationship between distance and severity.

$$\text{Degree of abnormal motion} \quad \propto \quad \frac{\text{Severity of lesion}}{\text{Distance of lesion from examination site}}$$

SOMATOEMOTIONAL RECALL AND RELEASE

Another phenomenon which we have observed and used quite successfully in our therapeutic armamentarium we have called somatoemotional recall and release.

From our experience, it would seem that body tissues (especially connective tissues) possess a memory. When an injuring force occurs, the tissue which receives the force is changed. Perhaps it retains the energy of impact. A level of increased kinetic activity or higher entropy is set up in the impaired area. The human body then either dissipates that energy and returns to normal; or the body somehow localizes the impact energy and walls it off, much as it walls off the tubercle bacillus during the inactive state of the disease. After the energy of the injury has been effectively isolated, the body adapts to this area. Energy (electrical, magnetic, *prana*, *Qi* or your own personal preference) is then forced to move around this area rather than through it.

In some cases the cost of adaptation is so small that it produces no clinical symptoms. In other cases the cost of adaptation, or of energy detour if you will, is so great that clinical problems develop. The relationship between the original injury and the resulting clinical syndromes is often very bizarre and, for us, usually impossible to discover by reason, given our present body of knowledge. It does seem, however, that given the chance, the patient's body will lead you to the original injury which underlies the presenting chief complaint. When the original injury is discovered, the repressed emotional components of the somatic injury frequently and concurrently release. The injury may have occurred, for example, during a skiing accident which was accompanied by panic and hysteria. When you discover the original injury, the patient will usually tell you. They may also relive the panic and hysteria which accompanied the incident. Once this is done, the injury will no longer require adaptational energy and the related clinical syndrome will disappear permanently.

The technique of somatoemotional recall and release (also know as "unwinding") begins quite simply and the patient takes over very quickly. You must stay with it until the release occurs. This may take five minutes or it may take an hour. If your schedule is tight and you believe your patient may benefit from this technique, reschedule an appointment for when you have adequate time.

With the patient seated, we usually begin with one hand on the parietal region of the head and the other on the upper thoracic region posteriorly (ILLUSTRATION 14-6).

A slight, inferiorly-directed compressive force is exerted upon the parietals so that the cervical and upper thoracic vertebra are gently compressed caudally. When the effect of the pressure on top of the head is felt by your other hand in the upper thoracic region, maintain that amount of pressure and allow the patient's body to do whatever it seems to want to do. The only limit which you place on the body is to prevent it from retracing its steps. That is, once it has made a particular movement it may do anything it wants except to go back the way it has come. If it tries, you gently resist. The body may assume various positions of flexion, extension, sidebending, rotation or any combination of these positions. It is very important that the patient be relaxed throughout the procedure. If not, it is extremely difficult to follow the body's inherent direction as the willed motion or resistance of the muscles will interfere. To attain this state of relaxation, not only must the patient be in an appropriate frame of mind, but the body must be properly supported so that no fear of falling is generated. Sometimes more than one therapist is necessary to properly support the body. The releases will be multiple, and can be monitored on the parietals. As you reach a position in which an injury occurred, the parietal bone movement will reduce. As the body works the injury pattern loose, the parietals will

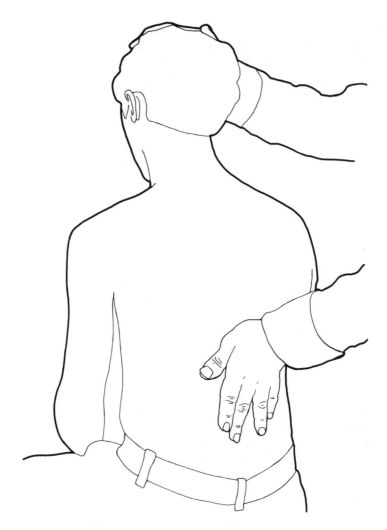

Illustration 14-6
Seated Position for Beginning
Somatoemotional Recall and Release

move into a free and easy motion pattern. If an emotional component is involved with the somatic problems it will appear before the parietal release is perceived. Try to follow wherever the patient's body leads you.

As releases occur, new balance points will present themselves. Each release seems to facilitate the next; things move more and more rapidly. Be alert. Do not inhibit your patient by dragging on their body movements. The only exception to this rule is when the body gets into a rut of continually repeating a pattern of movement, usually circular. This repetition may continue for an interminably long time. A very slight, nonspecific drag placed on the motion by the therapist will reveal an exit point where the motion will take a new direction. From this point, the motion is followed again without external drag. This is a dynamic process, and the movement to movement events and changes are unpredictable. What is predictable is the benefit your patient will experience. When the treatment session is over the patient will relax significantly. No further autonomous body movements will occur when you attempt to resume the session. But if an arm goes up into the air during the session, gently grasp it and follow. Significant restrictions may be localized in the extremities, as the first example below demonstrates.

Another method we frequently use is to gently touch the anterior ilia of the standing patient and compress slightly medially until the patient's own body movements begin. Then follow through, release after release (ILLUSTRATION 14-7). The

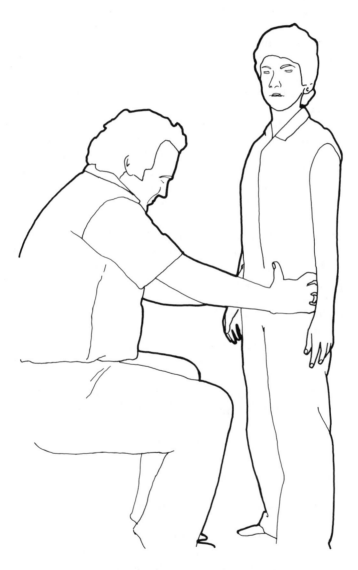

Illustration 14-7
Standing Position for Beginning
Somatoemotional Recall and Release

process can also be started with the patient lying supine. In this case, the ankles are grasped and a slight traction or compressive force introduced to start the release process. Each release which occurs during any of these techniques is like another layer of an onion you are peeling away to discover what is in the center.

Remember, the patient will finally assume the body posture in which the injury occured. You will know when this posture is correct because the craniosacral system will shut down. Often the patient will spontaneously comment that "this is exactly the position I was in when a specific accident occurred." All you have to do then is to hold that posture and wait until the complete release has occurred. Remember, release is a process which requires time to complete. Completion is signaled by the patient's body relaxation, breathing change, cessation of emotional outpouring, patient awareness of completion of the release process and a smoother, more even and higher-amplitude craniosacral system rhythmic motion.

We could describe at least a hundred examples in which difficult problems have been solved in this way. The presenting complaint may not seem at all related to the origin of the problem, but when it is illuminated the patient can almost invariably explain the connections for you.

We cannot resist citing one or two examples to illustrate both the concept and the "feel" of what we are discussing. A 42-year-old woman was diagnosed and treated successfully in this manner in about one hour. Her chief complaint was headache and neck pain of about 12 years' duration. She had had a radical mastectomy about 15 years prior. She blamed the mastectomy for the head and neck pain, as did most of the physicians she had consulted. She had been treated by neurologists, osteopaths, physiotherapists, psychiatrists and most recently by Rolfing. All treatment modalities resulted in temporary relief, but none lasted beyond days or weeks. She was treated by the somatoemotional recall and release method described above, and after about 20 minutes she was on the floor. I (Upledger) was holding only her left wrist and she yelled, screamed and flopped around on the floor like a fish on a line; the fishing line was her left arm. She did not, however, try to remove her left wrist from my grasp, although the uninformed observer would have been sure that this woman wanted nothing more than to escape. As the treatment continued, she began to sound more and more like a little child having a temper tantrum. Finally she stopped and totally relaxed. The craniosacral rhythm became smooth and easy. She then told me that her recall was of an incident, when she was about 2½ years old, in which her mother had sprained the girl's left wrist by using it to pull her up off the floor rather forcefully. Her mother had made her a dress which the girl did not like and she had found scissors and proceeded to cut the dress to pieces. When she was discovered, her mother yanked her up by her wrist, yelling and admonishing her severely. (Coincidentally, perhaps, it was the left breast which was removed due to malignancy.) She has been relatively symptom-free during the two years since this treatment.

Another example is of a 45-year-old man with normal ECG and stress tests who continued to experience chest pain. Multiple recurrent upper thoracic and rib somatic dysfunctions were present. He had undergone extensive osteopathic manipulative treatment for some years. He was controlled but not cured by this approach. The upper thoracic and rib problems were thought to result from an injury suffered about 10 years prior when he fell from an 18-foot scaffolding. Several of the scaffolding planks fell on his head when he hit the ground.

During the somatoemotional recall and release session he relived a football injury which had occurred at age 16. He had been unconscious for about 45 minutes after the injury. Until this treatment session he had amnesia for the events just before and after the injury had occurred. He had assumed that the unconsciousness was due to the blow to the head. During the treatment session he went into extreme backward bending of the head, neck and upper thorax. He actually felt the blow in the frontal region. As this position was maintained his body began to release, the craniosacral system became freer and his pain disappeared. In the year since his initial treatment, he has had little chest pain. The thoracic somatic dysfunctions have responded favorably and lastingly to treatment. He can breathe more deeply and freely. He says he is much more relaxed and easy going.

As these examples demonstrate, you should be prepared for the unexpected when using these techniques of somatoemotional recall and release. Don't panic, but persist until the patient signals you that the session is over. The most reliable signal is total body relaxation. When this has been attained, you will know that the body has given up all the restrictions it is going to yield for the day. Recheck from the listening posts. You will notice a remarkable change.

Diagnosis by whole body response, and treatment by somatoemotional recall and release are integral components of craniosacral therapy. Many patients will present with problems that have puzzled all the therapists they have seen. These methods will often unlock those puzzles and enable you to more efficiently help your patients.

Chapter 15
Newborns, Infants and Children

Newborns, infants and children present special craniosacral system problems.* As the newly-delivered child develops, the character of the cartilage, membrane and bone which comprise the cranial vault undergoes considerable modification. Under normal conditions, the skull of the term fetus is truly a membranous sac filled with cerebrospinal fluid. This fluid contributes an internal pressure to the semiclosed system. An hydraulic system is thus created which obeys all of the physical laws applicable to a semiclosed hydraulic system. Inside the membrane boundaries of the system are the visceral structures: the brain, the pituitary gland, a complex vascular system, the brain's ventricular system and innumerable others.

The bony developments in the fetal and infant skull may be thought of as "hard places" in the membrane; they contribute to its shape and functional integrity. As maturation occurs, the distances between these bony hard places are reduced. The ratio of flexible membranous cranial vault to more rigid osseous cranial vault changes in favor of the latter (ILLUSTRATION 15-1). It is therefore easy to understand how the misconception arose that the adult skull eventually becomes totally rigid.

Due to the extreme flexibility of the newborn skull, the techniques for examination and treatment of the newborn craniosacral system are quite different from those applied to the adult. Thus, as the human being develops from newborn to adult, the techniques of craniosacral examination and treatment must be gradually modified.

Craniosacral system motion in the newborn and infant is more difficult to perceive than in the adult. The range and amplitude of motion are much less in the newborn. The inherent energy which drives the system also seems much less than in the adult. Moreover, the levers (cranial vault bones) with which we perceive much of the motion are significantly smaller, and the movement of the membranous regions more subtle.

---

*It is recommended that any of you who intend to work with newborns, infants and children, familiarize yourselves with the work of Beryl E. Arbuckle, D.O., F.A.C.O.P. Dr. Arbuckle, working with Angus Cathey at the Philadelphia College of Osteopathy, pioneered a great deal of work with the anatomy of the intracranial membranes of stillborns. She also worked intensively with cerebral-palsied children. Her concepts are published in *The Selected Writings of Beryl E. Arbuckle, D.O., F.A.C.O.P.* This book is available through the American Academy of Osteopathy in Colorado Springs, Colorado.

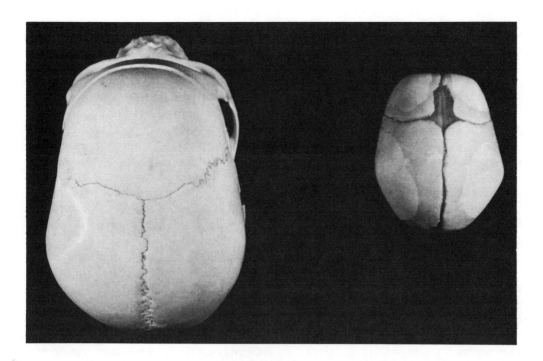

Illustration 15-1
Adult and Fetal Skulls

We suggest that in learning to examine and treat infants, you should first become very familiar with the craniosacral system activity of adults. Then extend your experience to adolescents, younger children and finally to younger and younger infants until you reach the newborn child. The developmental changes which occur are rapid in early life, but are on a continuum. You should experience many and various points along the continuum so that you are capable of adapting to the level of development of the craniosacral system at any given age.

In examining and treating newborns, we have developed a routine which we have found to be helpful and efficacious. We present it here only as a way to begin. Each of you, we hope, will develop your own individualized approach which best utilizes your particular skills.

This routine is as follows:

1. Observe the cranial vault and face for asymmetry.
2. Observe the torso, including the neck, for torsion patterns between the head and the pelvis.
3. Observe the roof of the mouth and the strength of the sucking reflex.

These observations are best made in the resting or sleeping newborn.

The examination and treatment techniques are largely inseparable and are therefore presented together.

EVALUATION OF CRANIAL BASE MOBILITY

After quickly making the above-listed observations, insert your little finger in the newborn's mouth. It is helpful to use a fingercott from which you have washed the powder, and which you have dipped in milk or glucose water. Whatever the newborn is feeding on is preferable. (We should not quibble here about mother's milk—improvise.) The cotted finger is placed in the newborn's mouth with the palmar surface of the distal phalanx facing cephalad. The child should begin to suckle on your finger. As this occurs, encourage the suckling. Place your other hand so that the activity of the external surface of the cranial vault is *gently* monitored. When the child sucks in, your finger is pressed by the sucking action against the hard palate. The hard palate is thus encouraged to move cephalad. This in turn moves the vomer. The vomer rocks the sphenoid. Mobility of the entire cranial base is thus encouraged by the suckling action. As the sucking proceeds, you should feel the rhythmic effect throughout the cranium. If you do not perceive this total head movement, *very gently* encourage the pressure on the roof of the mouth in rhythm with the child's sucking activity. Gradually, you will feel the total cranial vault begin to mobilize.

If the child does not suckle on your finger, wait long enough to be sure that this sucking will not occur, then *gradually* and *gently* begin to simulate the suckling action upon the child's hard palate.

Once you have attained mobility of the cranial vault by encouraging the movement of the cranial base, stay with the movement until it seems reasonably symmetrical. If there is an obvious sidebending or torsional distortion of the movement, try very gently to correct it by the *direct* approach. By paying attention to and gently grasping the great sphenoid wings during the course of this first technique, you can often balance the sphenoid as cranial base movement is exaggerated by your finger in the mouth. Follow several cycles of motion; with each cycle *gently* guide the movement pattern a little closer to symmetry. Releases are so subtle in infants that they are frequently missed. Just do a few cycles to *gently* correct the asymmetry, and then leave it alone. You will usually see clinical change in response to what you have done almost immediately.

Following this procedure, you may observe at least a partial correction of previously noted asymmetries of the shape of the head or face. Make a note of these changes and of the remaining asymmetries. Re-evaluation on the following day will indicate if your correction has been sucessfully made.

Decompression of Occipital Condyles

Next, decompress the occipital condyles from between the articular surfaces of the atlas. Hyperextension of the head and compression in an anteromedial direction of the condylar parts of the occiput frequently results from obstetrical deliveries which have been assisted by outlet forceps, or even by significant manual traction. This condition occurs as the obstetrical person attempts to hasten the passage of the child's body through the birth canal. These forces of hyperextension and anterior compression must be dissipated for the optimal health and development of the child. In order to do this, you must move the occiput posteriorly in relationship to the atlas.

The technique used to decompress and correct hyperextension of the occiput on the atlas is the same technique used in testing for this problem. The child's head is gently cradled between your two hands, one holding the occiput and the other the fronto-sphenoid regions. Your 3rd and 4th fingers are extended anteriorly under the occiput as far as allowed by the suboccipital and cervical tissues. The tips of these fingers are aimed at the occipital condyles. Hold the hand position *very gently* and allow the soft tissues to relax. After tissue relaxation is perceived, gently back the occiput away from the articular surfaces of the atlas. At the same time, your other hand should gently encourage the fronto-sphenoid complex to sort of "nose-dive," as though rotating anteriorly and inferiorly around a transverse axis, approximately through the anterior superior temporal squamous region.

As you feel the occiput move posteriorly, gently spread the 3rd and 4th fingers slightly away from each other. This has the effect of spreading the condylar parts of the occiput as they are decompressed. Imagine that your fingers are extended into the occipital condylar parts; your objective is to spread these parts laterally.

REMOLDING THE CRANIUM

After you have performed this technique, re-evaluate the head and face for lack of symmetry. If you still find asymmetry, gently and directly remold the shape, remembering that very light pressure is applied on the bulges, and a negative pressure is desirable on those surfaces which you wish to expand externally. You are dealing with a malleable, semi-closed hydraulic system which might be compared to a water-filled balloon, upon certain parts of which a less flexible plaster adheres. If you compress certain parts of the boundary of the hydraulic system and the remaining, non-compressed parts resist expansion, the hydraulic force inside the system is increased. In this case, the force is increased by the cerebrospinal fluid onto the brain. How much pressure would you be willing to exert upon the brain of a tiny child? Keep this in mind when you are remolding the head. Your pressure is *very small.* You can apply this very small pressure for minutes in order to achieve the desired effect. Again, remember that a very small force over a longer period of time has a much better chance of achieving an atraumatic result.

If the technique is performed correctly, you should see an immediate change in the asymmetrical shape. If the asymmetry improves and then returns a few hours or days later, you have not identified and corrected the cause of the problem. Frequently, the cause is in an abnormal torsional force in the spinal dural tube. This may be inherent in the tube itself or may be a reflection of osseous tensions, often in the sacrum and pelvis.

BALANCING THE OCCIPUT AND SACRUM

The next technique we apply to the newborn is to balance the occiput and sacrum. In order to do this, hold the occiput in the palm of one hand and the sacrum in the palm of the other. Movements of the occiput or sacrum induced at one end should freely and synchronously be expressed at the other end. If this expression of movement is inhibited or distorted, look for restrictions imposed upon the spinal dural tube, either from the sacrococcygeal complex, from one or more of the dural sleeves or from the upper cervicals as the dura attaches to the bodies of C2 and C3. All of these restrictions are mobilized by gentle, direct pressure against the restriction barriers as they are identified.

Frequently, we find a torsion of the dural tube which can be observed upon examination of the torso and pelvis for torsion. It is best perceived when you attempt to rotate the occiput in one direction and the sacrum in the other. The dural tube should allow this rotational torsion equally in both directions at both ends; if this is not the case, a gentle, direct force against the restriction barrier for a few minutes will correct the dural tube torsion.

The occiput and sacrum should be tested for sidebending in both directions, for flexion and extension in the anterior-posterior directions and for rotational torsions. All of these motions should be free, symmetrical and synchronous between the occiput and sacrum. If they are not, gentle, direct force over an extended period of a few minutes produces the correction.

BALANCING THE SACRUM AND PELVIS

The last procedure in our routine is to balance the sacrum and pelvis. Think of the iliac crests as the sides of a rectangle, the pubes and the rami as the roof and the sacrum as the floor.

The newborn child has just completed its passage through the birth canal. It has been subjected to all kinds of natural, and often unnatural forces. It does not have good control of the "guy wires," which are the ligaments and muscles responsible for pelvic symmetry. One can see how a rectangle can become a parallelogram.

Hold the child's pelvis gently, either with one hand below the sacrum and the other over the pubic symphisis, or with each thumb just lateral to the pubic symphisis and the sacrum cradled in the fingers. Test the pelvis for parallelogram shear in both directions, left and right. If you meet a restriction barrier, hold *gentle* force against it until the abnormal barrier is dissipated. The correction has been made. If the parallelogram configuration returns in a few days, explore further for an underlying cause.

Clinically, the newborn child manifests dysfunction in many ways. Symptoms we have seen include hyperirritability of the nervous system, crying to excess, poor muscle tonus (floppy baby), respiratory distress, excessive regurgitation and bowel dysfunction. We have seen many dramatic improvements within minutes following correction of the craniosacral system dynamics and function.

BEHAVIORAL AND LEARNING DISORDERS

Probably the most common problem we have found in preschool and grade school children is compression of the occipital condyles. This problem is often responsible for hyperkinetic behavior, abnormal fears and inability to concentrate for reasonable periods of time. Correction of the compression is followed by immediate and dramatic relief of symptoms. The hyperkinetic child will frequently fall asleep on the treatment table within a minute or two after the correction has been made. In our experience, a recurrence of the condylar compression problem results in a return of the hyperkinetic syndrome. Relief is again obtained by correction of the dysfunction. We have never had to correct a child more than four times to obtain a lasting result. The longest monitored case in our files is a little over five years without recurrence of either hyperkinesis or occipital condyle compression. We have treated more than fifty hyperkinetic cases to date and are presently compiling the results for publication. Further, I have trained a group of osteopaths (Society of Osteopaths) in the United Kingdom to do similar treatment for hyperkinetic children. Thus far, their results confirm our own.

It is true that some hyperkinetic behavior improves with dietary restrictions and other approaches. We would respond to this fact in two ways:
1. First, we are making no claim that craniosacral system dysfunction is the cause of *all* hyperkinetic behavioral disorder.

2. Second, if you consider the far-reaching physiological effects of the cranio-sacral system (e.g., on the vagus nerve, the pituitary gland, etc.), it seems reasonable that craniosacral system dysfunction may be the underlying cause of certain food intolerances, hypoglycemic episodes and the like. From our experience we do feel that condylar compression of the occiput is related to hyperkinetic behavior, and less frequently but significantly related to abnormal fears in children.

In any case, the treatment is innocuous; it can't hurt to try it and observe the results.

We have also treated a significant number of children suffering from reading problems, such as dyslexia. The ages in this group of patients range as high as 26 years, with an average age of about 12 years. We have found the temporal bones and occipitomastoid sutures to be dysfunctional in over half of these patients. Our present sample size is approximately 65 patients. Correction of the temporal dysfunction has been effective in about half of the treated cases. Recently, a 15-year-old boy, after four treatments and correction of internal rotation of the right temporal bone, remarked that he was enjoying reading now. He explained that he could now read whole words. This change began after the first treatment when the right temporal bone was partially mobilized. He further stated that, prior to treatment, he could only see the words in small pieces of two to four letters each. His special education teacher accompanied this boy to all of the treatment sessions and confirmed his progress.

We do not contend that all hyperkinesis, abnormal fear and dyslexia is due to craniosacral system dysfunction. We do contend that these brain function problems can and may be due to craniosacral system dysfunction. When they are, the improvement in brain function following physiological correction is usually prompt and dramatic. It leaves little doubt that there is a cause and effect relationship.

Cerebral Palsy

To date, we have treated 14 cases of spastic cerebral palsy. We use multiple therapist techniques, releasing body fascia and muscle restrictions at the same time that we release cranial restrictions. We have not failed to at least improve spasticity in all of these cases.

Three of the most dramatic cases involved almost total recovery from spastic hemiplegia. The first of these was a 3½-year-old boy whose right side was spastic and hemiplegic. His means of locomotion was to crawl about on the floor, moving sideways to his left like a fiddler crab. He could actively use his left arm and leg to drag his right side after. He would abduct the arm and leg, then adduct to move his body to the left. He had strabismus. He could not chew, so all of his food was processed in a blender. We found out later that he had constant pain in his head, right arm and leg, and in his right diaphragm area.

After the 3rd treatment, he stood up and dramatically walked. After 30 treatments, he was released with good upright locomotion and balance, good fine motor skills and coordination of all the extremities. He chews and eats regularly the same food that the rest of the family eats. He requires no more special attention. He told us that all the "men inside my body who made the pains" have gone. He shows some episodic return of strabismus of the right eye when fatigued. All of this progress has occurred in the year following the first treatment.

The key correction came from the left coronal suture, which was severely restricted and depressed inwardly. During the 3rd treatment this suture mobilized, and the depression came out. The following morning at 4:00 a.m., he awakened his mother and announced that he wanted to walk. He walked. He now rides a tricycle and is taking dancing lessons.

The second case was a 9-year-old girl. Spasticity of the right arm and hand was her most severe symptom. The right leg was spastic to a lesser degree and was smaller in length and circumference than the left. She was walking in the upright position but with difficulty. A problem with the left coronal suture similar to that noted in the previous case was found and corrected. Dramatic improvement in spasticity immediately occurred. She now has only a short and underdeveloped right leg to cope with. Her fine motor coordination of the right hand is excellent. She is under osteopathic management for pelvic dysfunction secondary to the short and underdeveloped right leg.

The third dramatic case was a 5-year-old girl who exhibited spastic quadriplegia. She was unable to creep or crawl. Release of the whole coronal suture (the frontal bone was depressed and the anterior borders of the parietal bones were overriding) produced dramatic relief of spasticity. After 8 treatments, the child was crawling and standing. She is now walking and climbing.

The other 11 cases in our files have all improved. We have strong suspicions that some of them will dramatically change when we are able to find and correct the "key lesions."

AUTISM

At the present time, we have treated 108 children who have been diagnosed as autistic by one profession or another. We have no illusion that all of these children are autistic.

Those children who are more classically autistic in the behavioral sense seem to present similar patterns of restriction in the craniosacral system. This suspicion led me (Upledger) to do an exploratory "single-blind" study of 63 children who have been called autistic and most of whose parents belong to the National Association for Parents of Autistic Children. These children whom I examined "blind" were all previously rated by Dr. Bernard Rimland, Director of the Institute for Child Behavior Research in San Diego, California. I rated the children on three scales. The first measured membranous restrictions, and the second osseous restrictions of the craniosacral system on an arbitrary scale of 0 to 10 (0 signifying no restriction and 10 extreme restriction). The third measured the inherent energy of the craniosacral system from -3 to $+3$.

Children who seem to be more "schizophrenic" in their behavior do not present the severely restricted, high energy craniosacral system. In fact, just the opposite is true: the boundaries do not seem to be restricted significantly, but there is little or no perceptible inherent craniosacral system rhythmic movement. When you actively motion-test, the system complies with your induced motions but has little inherent motion characteristic of its own. I would therefore rate what I considered to be a schizophrenic child in the lower range of membranous restriction (0, 1, etc.), and the inherent energy in the negative range (-3, -2, etc.). The more autistic child was rated as a $+9$ or $+10$ in membranous restriction, and a $+3$ in inherent motion. Other behavior disorders usually manifest as osseous restrictions and are localized.

Osseous restrictions have a firm quality. Membranous restrictions are springy or elastic and tend to give in to your exogenously applied testing force. They spring back into restriction as you reduce your force. As a result of this work, I postulate that the more classically autistic child presents with more severe membranous (dural) restriction of the craniosacral system. I also sense that these children have a very high level of inherent energy within this membranously restricted system.

The outcome of the study was that the results of Dr. Rimland's rating scale for autism and my rating of membranous restriction correlated positively at a 0.01 level of confidence. This is preliminary work and will be expanded, but the results seem quite promising.

On the basis of these preliminary results, I do not feel that schizophrenia is etiologically related to the restriction of craniosacral system function. Autism, on the other hand, may well be. Our experience in treating autism also leads us to believe that autism and schizophrenia may coexist in the same child. As the autism responds to craniosacral correction, some of our children seem to become more clearly schizophrenic.

The craniosacral system treatment series in more classically autistic children seems to follow a specific pattern of correction. The steps are as follows:

1. Find the area of the system that is moving, no matter where it is or how distorted its motion pattern. To the novice it may seem that the whole craniosacral system is locked tight. Trust us: there is motion somewhere. Expand the motion you find in the locale where you find it. Gradually, the mobile region will expand and other parts of the system will begin to move a little. (It is very helpful to work in pairs with autistic children.) Get your foot in the door and take advantage of every motion you can get.
2. Attempt cranial base anterior-posterior decompression. This may require several efforts but will eventually prove to be a fruitful endeavor.
3. Decompress the lumbosacral junction. If you are working in pairs, this can be done at the same time that the cranial base is being decompressed.
4. Balance the cranial base and sacrum. Release the diaphragms in between.

As these corrections are made, the self-abusive behavior such as head-banging or hand- or wrist-biting either abates entirely or greatly reduces in severity. This behavioral improvement is spontaneous. We postulate that long-standing, internal head pain has been relieved by the decompression. The child may well have been blocking the uncontrollable internal head pain by self-inflicted, but controllable external pain. The child may even have been stimulating endogenous opiate (endorphin) production by the self-inflicted pain, and by that means have obtained some measure of relief. The head-banging could easily represent self-inflicted pain or could be an instinctive attempt by the child to mobilize the craniosacral system.

Another change that frequently occurs at this level of correction is the cessation, partial or total, of thumbsucking. Careful observation reveals that the so-called thumbsucking is usually not sucking at all but is hard pressure upon the roof of the mouth. One need only recall the anatomy of the maxilla, palatines, vomer and sphenoid to recognize that this self-imposed pressure on the roof of the mouth may represent the child's attempt at mobilizing the cranial base.

Furthermore, once some decompression has been accomplished, autistic children will become very cooperative with the treatment. They often demonstrate a very positive attitude toward craniosacral treatment and will sometimes indicate where the therapist should place his or her hands during treatment. They are almost always correct.

5. After the anterior-posterior compression restrictions have been released and the cranial base has been reasonably balanced, it seems that we have not been able to make further progress until somatic fascial restrictions have been released. This requires the team treatment approach using body position as described in Chapter 14.

During this phase of the treatment regime, we anticipate a great deal of emotional reaction. There may be crying, laughing, screaming, or the whole gamut of emotional expression, but never yet has a child attempted to terminate or fight against this stage of the treatment. It is during this phase that we see the autistic child begin to express spontaneous emotion and creativity. Sociability may also improve considerably.

6. The next phase of treatment involves lateral decompression of the cranial base. Use the ears as your levers, and move the temporal bones laterally; then mobilize them (CHAPTER 11).

After the above corrections have been accomplished, you may treat the craniosacral system of the autistic child as you would any other. Treat what you find. It may take weekly treatments for a year to reach this level of correction.

It is important that parents and teachers are sensitive to, and understand the changes their child may pass through. As emotion begins to emerge, it must be encouraged. As creative activities appear, they must be encouraged. We don't know how far the autistic child can advance once the craniosacral system is functioning on an improved level, but our observations would lead us to believe that there is reason for hope and a need for concerted effort among parents, teachers and craniosacral therapists.

Chapter 16
Specific Clinical
Cautions and Applications

The clinical applications discussed in this chapter are those with which we have had the most experience. We can only discuss our own experiences and the functional anatomico-physiologic mechanisms which may underlie the observed responses. The list of clinical applications presented is far from exhaustive. It is not meant to limit your trials of the therapeutic techniques in various unmentioned clinical situations. Rather, it is intended to give you an area in which to start using craniosacral examination and therapy. The therapy has little, if any, serious, irreversible or long lasting side effects. It does aim at the improvement in function of a physiological system, and therefore is seldom contraindicated.

Although there may be more, we can think of only four contraindications for craniosacral treatment:

1. *Acute intracranial hemorrhage:* The manipulative approach to the craniosacral system may significantly change intracranial fluid pressure dynamics. This change is undesirable in that it may prolong the duration of hemorrhage by interrupting the tenuous progress of clot formation.
2. *Intracranial aneurysm:* The change in intracranial fluid pressure dynamics produced by craniosacral treatment may be enough to precipitate a leak or rupture of a dangerous, already present intracranial aneurysm.
3. The third contraindication is more of a caution: A very careful approach should be applied in *recent skull fracture,* lest an increase in cranial bone motion precipitate bleeding or membranous tear.
4. *Herniation of the medulla oblongata* through the foramen magnum is a life-threatening situation wherein you would not wish to alter fluid pressures within the craniosacral system by the use of manipulative techniques.

The areas in which we have rather extensive clinical experience and do consider craniosacral treatment to be efficacious and often curative are discussed below. Under no circumstances should craniosacral treatment be used exclusive of other therapeutic modalities. It should be integrated with all treatment approaches which seem appropriate in your best judgment for each individual case. A truly holistic approach is always mandatory except in clinical research settings. We should not develop loyalty to an approach or to any specific system to the exclusion of any other approach or system. Our loyalty is to the patients we treat. We must be eclectic in our selection of treatment modalities.

Acute Systemic Infectious Conditions

These respond exceedingly well to the CV-4 techniques described in Chapter 4. Two or three repetitions of the CV-4-induced "still point" will usually lower fever. Still points seem to help the patient pass through the "crisis" phase of an infectious illness. The antifebrile effect is usually seen within an hour after treatment, and is usually long-lasting. This continued effect indicates a reversal of the tide of battle between the pathogenic invader and the bodily defenses which are under attack. If the fever should return, the CV-4 technique should be repeated. The number of still points achieved during a given treatment session is determined solely by your perception of change in craniosacral system motion quality. Certainly, you should correct any other motion asymmetries you can during the treatment, but your attention should focus primarily upon the CV-4 technique.

The physiological mechanism seems to be based upon the achievement of body fluid mobility. The effect is probably very similar to the lymphatic pump, but the fluid exchange is more global through the whole body and is achieved by the patient's own autonomic nervous system.

In conjunction with antibiotic treatment and other supportive measures (e.g., bed rest, forcing fluids, etc.), the CV-4 technique will frequently move the patient from the acute onset to the recovery phase of the illness within hours.

Localized Infection

Abscesses and boils are helped a great deal by the application of the "direction of energy" techniques, as described in Chapter 9. Once again, the improvement is prompt and dramatic. You can simply direct energy from the parietal region (crown) of the patient's head to a "V-spread" formed by placing the receiving fingers on both sides of the infected area. The infected area will first begin to pulsate as the energy moves through. Then, as the beneficial effect occurs, the pulsations will reduce in amplitude. The area of involvement will soften perceptibly. The patient will usually comment upon an improved feeling or sensation, and the treatment is complete.

This treatment may be repeated once or twice daily if the improvement seems to be slipping away. We think of the dosage as being determined by which way the battle with the pathogens is going. If we see the patient's resistance beginning to wane once again, we repeat the treatment. Send reinforcements. The patient or a friend can easily perform the technique themselves with just a little instruction.

It is unfortunate that this technique is sometimes regarded as being too "far out" for a patient to accept. In those cases, we simply do it without explanation while we are pretending to do something else such as palpating the lesion, feeling the head for fever, etc. When the beneficial effect is felt by the patient, further explanation is seldom necessary, even for the skeptic. In fact, the skeptic usually will prefer not to discuss the matter, but is quite happy to accept the benefit without having to accept the challenge to their belief system. We have no problem accepting these conditions. It is, however, quite surprising how many skeptics, at a later date, bring up the subject and wish to discuss the situation which occurred.

ACUTE SPRAINS AND STRAINS

These are also amenable to the direction of energy techniques. There is better therapeutic effect when the direction of energy is combined with tissue tension-balancing techniques. Usually, the balancing of tissue tension will cause the affected part to move back chronologically through the position of injury. When this position is achieved, all craniosacral motion will stop. As the energy pattern of the injury dissipates, the tissues will release and soften locally. Craniosacral system motion will gradually return to a normal rhythm pattern. Be alert to and treat injuries which have occurred in other parts of the body at the same time. They may contribute to the severity of the more obvious problems.

CHRONIC PAIN PROBLEMS

These types of problems usually respond quite well to the integrated approach, which includes CV-4 techniques, direction of energy techniques, mobilization by gentle tissue balancing and the mobilization of the whole dural membrane system (both within the cranium and the spinal canal). The pain can be anywhere from the head to the toe. This combination of techniques plus the mobilization of any somatic dysfunction which is found will yield surprisingly beneficial results for a great number of patients who have otherwise given up.

We frequently combine the above techniques with acupuncture for pain control while performing the mobilizing corrections.

DYSFUNCTION OF VISCERA

These are secondary to autonomic nervous system dysfunctions and are very amenable to craniosacral treatment. These conditions include such things as peptic ulcer, biliary dyskinesia, the spectrum of inflammatory and ulcerative problems with the bowel, paroxysmal atrial tachycardia, asthma and numerous other complaints. For these conditions, simply make a thorough search for restriction patterns and treat what you find. Still points aid autonomic flexibility and homeostatic functions.

AUTONOMIC NERVOUS SYSTEM DYSFUNCTIONS

Dysfunctions such as Raynaud's phenomenon are often helped considerably by treating what you find after thorough examination. The CV-4 technique should be taught to the family or friends and performed on the patient *every* day.

RHEUMATOID ARTHRITIS

This is said to be amenable to daily CV-4 by a few craniosacrally-oriented physicians. We have experience with only a few such patients. One has been up and out of the wheelchair for about eight years now. The surgeons were about to operate on both hips when we began. In the beginning, this patient was not ambulatory and suffered severe pain. She had been in a Boston hospital for eight months. In keeping with our eclectic approach, we used a combination of acupuncture, traditional osteopathic manipulative treatment, craniosacral treatment and nutritional treatment. Together with the patient, we believe that the acupuncture gave pain relief early in the treatment and that the craniosacral treatment is responsible for the subsequent, near-complete remission of over seven years' duration. We have three other patients who have substantially benefited, but none as dramatically as the one described.

We feel that teaching a family member to do the CV-4 technique daily accomplishes several positive things. It is an innocuous technique, less dangerous than the administration of anti-inflammatory drugs. Among the positive aspects of the treatment are the physiological effects of mobilization, fluid exchange, improved delivery of nutrients and removal of metabolic waste products. It also gives the family a feeling of usefulness and often cements familial relationships which have been severely strained by chronic pain and invalidism.

EMOTIONAL DISORDERS

This is an area which, in our experience, is somewhat limited. We have treated a great number of emotionally disturbed children with significant success, as described in Chapter 15. In adults, we have treated a rather large number of cases of depression, which have been of varying levels of severity. Several have histories of more than one suicide attempt. Others have been institutionalized on one or more occasions, or have had electroshock treatment. Most were taking antidepressant medications. We have yet to examine a case of depression, be it endogenous or reactive, that has not shown severe anterior-posterior compression of the cranial base. Further, we have yet to see the first case which has not responded favorably and usually dramatically to successful decompression of the cranial base.

It does not seem to matter whether the depression is secondary to the death of a loved one or is "post-partum blues." The decompression technique gives dramatic relief. We wonder if perhaps the obstetrical delivery process might not result in lumbosacral compression, which migrates to the cranial base and causes depression. *Always correct the lumbosacral problem which usually accompanies cranial base compression* (CHAPTER 7).

Anxiety is the other area in which we have had major success. However, the anxious patient does not seem to present with as consistent and characteristic a craniosacral system restriction pattern as does the depressive patient. In anxiety, treat what you find. Restrictions will have a tendency to recur. Treat them again, and over a period of weeks the anxiety level seems to dissipate. Occasionally, a crisis will occur as the corrections are carried out. Be prepared to support the patient through the crisis. It usually signals the release of some repressed emotional matter which will ultimately be beneficial to the patient.

SCOLIOSIS

Among the causes of scoliosis, we should list the craniosacral system. The cranial base and the sacral base must be mobilized and balanced in all cases of scoliosis. The reasons for imbalance between these structures must then be identified and treated. The spine between the cranial base and the sacral base must also be kept mobile so that normalization of the curves can physiologically occur.

The most common causes of cranial base unleveling which we have found include facial trauma, maxillary trauma, sphenomaxillary shear or torsion, dental trauma, orthodontic braces which have immobilized one maxilla in internal rotation and the other in external rotation, vomer dysfunction due to intraosseous strain, unilateral occipital condyle compression and many extrinsic problems. Balance the cranial base and locate the cause for the imbalance.

The sacrum is frequently imbalanced due to leg length asymmetry, pelvic dysfunction, adaptive muscle tonus asymmetry (adapting to what?), trauma, spinal dysfunction due to trauma and many uniquely individualized problems.

If you find the primary lesion after stripping away the layers upon layers of adaptive dysfunction, you have a good chance of improving the scoliosis. Bones deform and reform in response to pressure; therefore, expect changes in osseous morphology, especially of the vertebral bodies as you change postural, spinal, paravertebral and craniosacral system dynamics.

VISUAL DISTURBANCES

Although these have been discussed in Chapter 6, we wish to restate for emphasis that strabismus is very amenable to the release of abnormal tension patterns of the tentorium cerebelli. Nystagmus also may respond well to release of dural membrane tensions. Visual acuity and associated problems respond well to cranial treatment; however, the site of dysfunction is not predictable. It frequently involves the atlanto-occipital region.

AUDITORY PROBLEMS

Tinnitus and recurrent middle ear problems are well treated by mobilizing and balancing the temporal bones.

CEREBRAL ISCHEMIC EPISODES

These are very favorably affected by weekly application of the parietal lift technique after thoracic inlet and cranial base restrictions have been released. We have seen marked improvement in syncopal episodes, episodic paresthesias, memory loss and the like, after only three or four weekly treatments. Of course, you treat what you find after doing the parietal lift.

We have taken you on a long journey through craniosacral therapy. The structure and function of this relatively unknown and certainly under-appreciated system have been described. Previously unfamiliar terms and a different, gentle physiological approach to treating the ailments and dysfunctions of the human body have been introduced. You have been shown how to develop and extend your sense of touch and to palpate subtle strain patterns that often hold the key to otherwise bizarre clinical presentations or stubbornly unresponsive conditions. We have tried to help you expand your understanding of the body as a unit by focusing upon the importance of the fasciae, and the integration and interdependence of the parts of the body in the concept of the craniosacral system.

If this book has helped you to understand and develop a deeper awareness and sensitivity toward your patients and their problems, it will have succeeded.

Appendices

Appendix A

The Structures of Cranial Bone Sutures

ERNEST W. RETZLAFF, Ph.D., DAVID MICHAEL, D.O., RICHARD ROPPEL, Ph.D., FRED MITCHELL, D.O.,
Department of Biomechanics, Michigan State University—College of Osteopathic Medicine, East Lansing, Michigan*

There are few studies on cranial bone sutures which have utilized modern histologic techniques. One of the most informative studies on the structure and the development of mammalian cranial sutures was done by Pritchard, Scott, and Girgis in 1956.[1] Their primary concern was the development of the suture, so there was limited discussion of the adult structure. However, this report provided us with a starting point for our investigation.

Much of the initial work on this project has been the development of suitable histologic methods. This is reported in a paper by Popevec, Biggert, and Retzlaff.

Previously reported studies on cranial bone mobility[2-4] (Eighteenth Annual National Osteopathic Research Conference, March 15-16, 1974) were based on physiological studies using the squirrel monkey, Saimiri sciureus. Histologic studies are being performed on the same animal.

It is of particular interest to note that in the 10 adult monkeys from which the bone tissue was removed there was no evidence of suture ossification.

The general pattern of the suture was similar to that reported by Pritchard et al.[1] In each sample studied the sutures displayed five distinct layers of cells and fibers between the articulating edges of the bones. The outermost layer is a zone of connective tissue which bridges the suture and is designated the sutural ligament. The next layer consists of osteogenic cells. These two layers appear to be continuous with that of the periosteum of the skull bones. This modified periosteal layer, the sutural ligament, is found on both the outer and the inner surfaces of the suture. The space between the ligaments is loosely filled with fibrous connective tissue.

The reticular connective tissue portion is seen in the space with extensions into the sutural ligament. This may provide an inner and outer binding structure which serves to hold the sutures but still permits some movement of the skull bones.

In addition to the connective tissue seen in the central space, blood vessels and nerve fibers are evident. The function of these nerve fibers is not known but it is possible that they may be involved in the physiological effects of cranial therapy.

The question whether suture obliteration, by ossification, ever occurs in man cannot be answered by this study. We do know that the sutures between the parietal bone and adjacent bones in the adult squirrel monkey show no evidence of closure in the specimens we have studied.

*Reprinted from The Journal of the American Osteopathic Association (JAOA), Vol. 75, Feb. 1976, pp. 607-608, by permission of the American Osteopathic Association, 212 E. Ohio St., Chicago, IL 60611.

273

[1]Pritchard, J.J., Scott, J.H., and Girgis, F.G.: Structure and development of cranial and facial sutures. J Anat 90:73-86, Jan 56

[2]Michael, D.K., and Retzlaff, E.W.: A preliminary study of cranial bone movement in the squirrel monkey. JAOA 74:866-9, May 75

[3]Retzlaff, E.W., Michael, D.K., and Roppel, R.M.: Cranial bone mobility. JAOA 74:869-73, May 75

[4]Michael, D.K.: The cerebrospinal fluid: Values for compliance and resistance to absorption. JAOA 74:873-6, May 75

Supported by AOA research grant #T73-91, "Cranial Motion and Intracranial Fluid Dynamics," through the AOA Bureau of Research.

Appendix B

Examination of the Cranial Rhythm in Long-Standing Coma and Chronic Neurologic Cases

Z. KARNI, J.E. UPLEDGER, J. MIZRAHI, L. HELLER, E. BECKER, AND T. NAJENSON*

INTRODUCTION

In an earlier report[1], a case of a child who had been treated with cranial therapy by Dr. J.E. Upledger, F.A.A.O. (Assoc. Professor at the Biomechanics Department, College of Osteopathic Medicine, Michigan State University, Michigan, USA, and a Visiting Professor at the Department of Biomedical Engineering, Technion—Israel Institute of Technology), during his recent summer visit to this country, was described. Here the results of a cranial examination performed by Dr. Upledger on patients in the intensive care units of the Loewenstein Neurological Institute, Ra'anana, are reported.

The purpose of the examination was to establish whether or not these patients, some of them comatose for extended periods of time, still possess a cranial rhythm and if the rhythm is substantially retarded in both amplitude and frequency in comparison with normal values. The cranial rhythm was evaluated by Dr. Upledger by means of palpation of the cranium or the extremities and the frequency counted in cycles per minutes (cpm.). Later, however, in some of the cases, a strain plethysmographic measurement[2] was carried out which correlated very closely with the values obtained by palpation for those patients.

In the following, the results of the exam-ination along with a brief description of the various cases are presented. It is, however, preceded by a short account of the nature of the cranial rhythm and the role it plays as the principal cue which directs the physician in and during cranial treatment.

THE CRANIAL RHYTHM

The cranial contents—nerves, arteries and veins, soft tissue, membranes, etc.—is in a fluid state within the enclosing membrane of the dura mater. The inner structure is compartmental[3,4] and shell like, divided into several layers. Beneath the dura mater is the subdural space bounded below by the arachnoid membrane which runs almost parallel to the dura. Further down is the subarachnoidal space between the membranes of the arachnoid and the pia mater, the latter covering the cerebral cortex. In the subarachnoidal space flows the cerebro-spinal fluid (CSF) and the subpial space contains the interstitial fluid—that extracellular fluid outside and between the nerve cells. The fluid structure is, therefore, primarily biphasic with the more viscous and quasi-stationary interstitial fluid as the inner core which is bordered externally by the lighter, almost non-viscous CSF.

The hydraulic contents are subjected to the pulsatory motions of the arterial system, the venous system and the pulmonary sys-

Reprinted with permission of the authors.

tem which transmits its effect to the dura mater through the vertebral connections along the cervical section of the spinal column. The lateral displacements which all these systems induce upon the fluid region sets the latter into motion, the nature of which depends upon the fluid properties and on the mechanical behavior of the container.[5, 6]

The classical Monro-Kellie theory[7, 8] considered the container—namely the skull bones—rigid, and the inner fluid incompressible. The immediate implication of these assumptions was that any induced motion resulted in displacement to another compartment of the body so that the total volume remained intact. While this seemed unlikely, the Monro-Kellie doctrine prevailed, at least as a first approximation of the physiology involved, for quite a while.

The incompressibility assumption was later relaxed; the fluid was assumed compressible and measurements were made to find the gross bulk modulus of the entire fluid[9] and the moduli of each of its phases, namely that of the CSF and of the interstitial fluid, separately.[10] The bulk modulus, defined as the ratio of the increment of pressure to the relative change in volume (dilatation) of a closed deformable region, was also measured in problems such as hydrocephalus.[11, 12, 13]

Even with the compressibility assumption, the values of the bulk moduli indicate that the changes in volume cannot all be "absorbed" by the compressibility of the fluid. Deformation of the outer shell of skull bones has also to be taken into account although that deformation may be small in magnitude. Thus the boundary conditions of the shell should no longer be assumed as zero lateral displacement. Instead, some displacement should occur and calculations predict that it is on the order of a few microns. This is in agreement with dial gauge measurements which, with the tips of the gauges tightly compressed against the parietal bones, yield values of 10-25 microns side displacement of these bones.[14]

There remains still a considerable gap between values of the free motion of the cranium that physicians feel during a cranial examination for mobility and those of the *constrained* motion measured by a mechanical dial gauge. The ratio of the two sets of values is about a hundred to one and this is explained by the special morphology of the cranial bones.

The geometrical arrangement of the large bones of the cranium classify it as an "open structure." Such structures, composed of a finite number of elements or of an infinite number of infinitesimal elements joined together, are characterized by having all elements contributing their small incremental motions along a common direction thus resulting, altogether, in a finite value of the integrated motion. The simplest example of an open structure is the coiled spring. Here, each infinitesimal element of the coil undergoes torsion which contributes a displacement component to the axial elongation of the spring. Each elongation is infinitesimal by itself. However, an infinite number of them are summed up along the same direction yielding, altogether, a finite value for the total elongation of the spring.

The skull bones are joined by soft-tissue sutures and the architecture of the complex is such that a small angular motion of each of the bones, which are subjected to internal pressure changes, yields a side displacement component the integral of which is noticeable and measurable. This is what the physician feels as a motion of the cranium and its rhythmicity—the cranial rhythm.

Sutherland[15] regarded the cranial rhythm as a pivot of Cranial Osteopathy. He called the cranial articular structure "a primary respiratory system" which functions "in conjunction with the brain, the ventricles, and the intracranial membranes" and considered the physiological rhythms of the respiratory and cardiovascular systems as only "secondary" to the cranial rhythm. It was further postulated that in a normal living human all skull suture articulations remained mobile throughout life. Any abnormal impairment or restricting force upon this system by any of its related structures could cause symptoms which were otherwise often considered idiopathic or the result of neurotic malady. The primary objective of the physician was to trace the impairment and try to release it thus allowing the natural physiology to be restored to its natural state of equilibrium.

The normal range of frequency of the cranial rhythm is 6-12 cycles per minute (cpm). This rate is slower than the respiratory rate in the relaxed state by almost a third. The normal amplitude, identified with the lateral displacement of the parietal bone, may reach 1-1½ mm. Changes of frequency, mostly a reduction up to 40%, have been correlated with psychiatric syndromes[16] and when the therapy restored the rhythm to its normal level the syndromes subsided and vanished.[16] Mechanical measurements of the cranial rhythm have also been carried out and found to be in good agreement with the physician's findings.[17,] [14]Of the various techniques, strain plethysmography by means of high-extension, electrical resistance strain-gauges proved more sensitive and effective and this is described elsewhere.[2]

The Loewenstein Hospital in Ra'anana, which is the country's principle center for rehabilitation, accommodates in its intensive care units severe cases of brain damage, some of which are in coma for several years. A cranial examination of the patients there offers a wide variety of cases from which comparative data can be accumulated. For that purpose, Dr. Upledger, during his recent visit, performed a cranial examination on eight patients who represented a cross section of the patient population in that hospital. The results of the examination are shown below. They are accompanied by a brief account of the patients' diagnoses and a description of their present state.

RESULTS OF CRANIAL RHYTHM EXAMINATION

I. Patient H. Sh., male, age 22. Admitted—30.11.1975. Still in hospital. Diagnosis: venomous sting of scorpion on 14.10.1975. Patient in a chronic vegetative state.

II. Patient M. Y., male, age 18. Admitted—13.11.1977. Still in hospital. Diagnosis: as a result of road accident—severe brain stem lesion. Later course: respiratory arrest; removal of left epidural hematoma and hy-

groma; tracheostomy. Patient in chronic vegetative state.

III. Patient H.S., male, age 17. Admitted—28.1.1979. Diagnosis: spastic tetraparesis, respiratory failure. Bowel and bladder incontinence, contracture of lower limbs. Connected to a Bennett respiration machine. Still in hospital.

IV. Patient A.E., male, age 11. Admitted—26.6.1979. Diagnosis: epilepsy, coma, transient tetraparesis, status post probable viral encephalitis. Had periods of ups and downs. Released August '79.

V. Patient R.J., male, age 27. A UNIFIL soldier. Admitted—10.6.1979. As a result of a gun shot wound: diffuse peritonitis; laparotomy, partial resection of liver, nephrectomy. Fracture of right femur, left olecranon and humerus. After a cardiopulmonary resuscitation—patient in anoxic coma, quadraplegia, chronic vegetative state. Released 5.10.1979 to be flown home to the Fiji Islands.

VI. Patient G.S., male, age 35. Admitted—18.7.1979. Diagnosis: weakness in the upper and lower extremities; polyneuropathy, walking difficulties, "stocking glove," sensory disturbances. Still in hospital. Improvement noticed.

VII. Patient S.H., male, age 17. Admitted—20.10.1975. Injured in a road accident. Fraction in T8, T10 and in the base of the skull. Diagnosis: sensory disturbances from T8 downward, bowel and bladder incontinence. Blindness of the right eye. Released 24.6.1977. Returned for two-week periods of hospitalization in May '78 and August '79. Services himself and independent in wheel chair.

VIII. Patient M.O., female, age 22. Admitted—12.10.1975. Fell from a balcony and fractured T8. Diagnosis: complete paraplegia with sensory disturbances from T6, 7 downwards, bowel and bladder incontinence. Independent on a wheel chair. Hospitalized for pregnancy retention (miscarriage prevention). Released 27.6.1976.

IX. Patient I.M., female, age 24. Admitted—1976, following an anasthesia for an oral surgery. Diagnosis: status post cardiac arrest with brain damage due to anoxia, coma, tracheostomy, contracture of limbs.

Patient I.M. passed away on 7.12.1979.

The above patients, except for patient I.M. (IX), were cranially examined by Dr. Upledger in August, 1979, some of them in their beds and some while sitting in their wheel chairs. The examination consisted of the count of the cranial rhythm in cpm and the estimate of the percentage ratio of the pulsatory amplitudes of the cranial rhythm to the normal values. These ratios were measured—when possible—at three places: the head, the upper extremities and lower extremities. The following table shows the results obtained:

Table — Count and amplitude ratio of cranial rhythm of patients with brain damages.

	Patient	Sex	Age	Diagnosis	Cranial Rhythm (cpm)			Amplitude Ratio (%)		
					Head	Upper extrem-ities	Lower extrem-ities	Head	Upper extrem-ities	Lower extrem-ities
I.	H.Sh.	M	22	Venomous sting of scorpion. Chronic vegetative state.	3	—	—	50	—	—
II.	M.Y.	M	18	Severe brain stem lesion. Chronic vegetative state.	4	—	—	60	—	—
III.	H.S.	M	17	Spastic tetraparesis.	2.5	2.5	NR(*)	40	10	NR
IV.	A.E.	M	11	Epilepsy. Transient tetraparesis.	2.5	6	6	30	30	30
V.	R.J.	M	27	Anoxic coma. Chronic vegetative state.	4	NR	NR	50	NR	NR
VI.	G.S.	M	35	Polyneuroapathy (Guillain-Barre).	6	6	25	70	50	30
VII.	S.H.	M	17	Paraplegia.	5	5	18	50	50	50
VIII.	M.O.	F	22	Paraplgia.	7	—	16 (Rt) 4.5 (lt)	100	—	60(Rt) 10(Lt)
IX.	I.M.	F	24	Anoxic coma. Chronic vegetative state.	—	—	—	—	—	—

(*)NR — No Rhythm detected.

Measurements were later performed on patient G.S. (VI) and patient I.M. (IX). The technique—a strain plethysmography—by means of high-extension, electrical resistance strain gauges is described elsewhere.[2] The strain gauges were applied at the upper and lower extremities and picked up the pulses, of course, superimposed on the much slower waves of the cranial rhythm. With respect to the latter, the frequency could immediately be determined. As to the amplitude ratio, it could be assessed from the ratio of the average pulse amplitude to that of the rhythm and compared with the normal values. Assuming the pulse amplitude to be practically constant with respect to the same patient, over a short period, the amplitude ratio of the cranial rhythm in reference to the normal pattern could also be assessed at least to a general approximation.

Figure 1a shows a section of the strain record measured continuously over the thumb of patient G.S. (VI).

A time indicator marked each second by a small spike of the needle and every ten seconds by a large spike. When the gain sensitivity was doubled (Fig. 1b), so did the amplitude of the cranial rhythm. The frequency count for that patient was 5-6 cycles per minute and the amplitude ratio estimated, in comparison with a normal pattern, as 40%-50%.

When the gauge was applied over the right ankle the frequency pattern changed considerably to 22-25 cycles per minute. The pulse amplitude was much weaker and a fair assessment of the amplitude ratio could not be made. When the gauge was moved to the right great toe, the pulse record was even weaker but the frequency remained in the 20-25 cpm range. If these recordings are all compared with the corresponding results in the table, the conformity is indeed striking.

Figure 2 shows a section of the strain

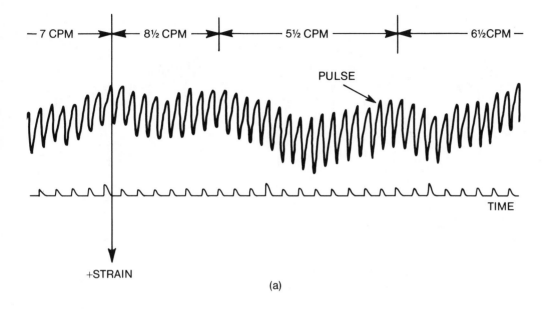

(a)

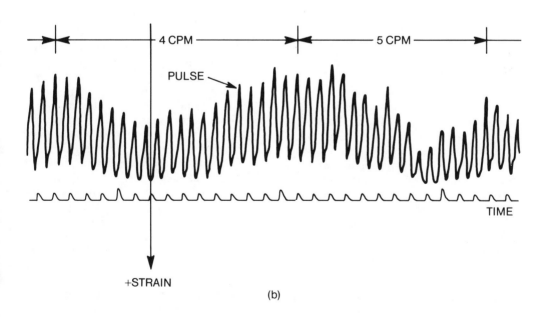

(b)

Fig. 1   *Strain-time plethysmography record over patient G.S.'s thumb, with (a) standard gain sensitivity,*
          (b) double gain sensitivity.

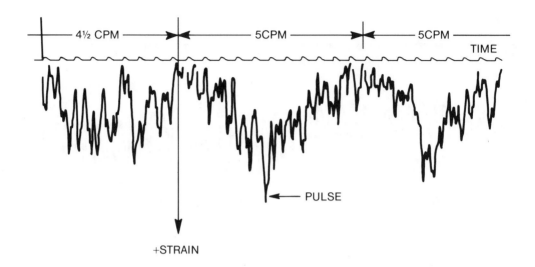

Fig. 2   *Strain-time plethysmography record over the right hand of patient I.M.*

tracing pertaining to the right hand thumb of patient I.M. (IX).

Again, the frequency of the cranial wave was around 5 cpm and the amplitude ratio assessed as 30-40%. The strain record also picked up bursts of slow spastic dilatations of the upper extremity. The patient at that time, after 3½ years in a vegetative state, was in a desperate state. She passed away a few days later.

OBSERVATIONS

No conclusive results may as yet be deduced from the cranial examination of some of the patients at the Loewenstein Hospital suffering from long-standing spinal and brain damage. Nor are the measurements sufficient to corroborate to the theories underlying cranial mobility and rhythm. However, some observations can be made which support the fundamental theories of cranial osteopathy and indicate how to proceed in further investigations.

1. A common feature of all the findings in these patients is a slow-down of the cranial rhythm to about one half of the normal level—in frequency and amplitude—when measured at the head. This level of activity is lower than the one measured in cases of psychiatric dis-

orders[16] where the rhythm was still in the range of 60-70% of the normal values.

2. The cranial rhythm is measurable all over the body and retains a constant value throughout. This conforms with a picture of a "primary respiratory system" which sustains itself to the very end of physiological life.

3. Exceptions to the constancy of the cranial rhythm were detected in some paraplegic cases. These were also the only cases where, at the lower extremities, values which *exceeded* the normal level of rhythmicity by almost 100% were measured. It should be pointed out that these patients were later released from the hospital with a fair ability to function and to move around.

4. Although cranial rhythmicity has a neurological component to its effects primarily as an amplification circuit, at both ends of input and output it is a mechanical phenomenon. As such it is also amenable to sensitive and non-invasive mechanical measurements. They, undoubtedly, will throw more light on the subject when more data is accumulated.

ACKNOWLEDGEMENT

This research has been sponsored in part

by the Julius Silver Institute of Biomedical Engineering Sciences and Grant 130-077.

REFERENCES

[1] Karni, Z. and Upledger, J.E.: Early steps of cranial therapy in Israel. Julius Silver Institute of Biomedical Engineering Sciences, Technion—Israel Institute of Technology, Haifa, Israel. Research Report 79-1979.

[2] Upledger, J.E. and Karni, Z.: Strain plethysmography and the cranial rhythm. Proc. XII Inter. Conf. on Med. and Biol. Eng. Jerusalem, Israel, August 19-24, 1979, Part IV, 69.5.

[3] Livingston, R.B., Woodbury, D.M. and Patterson, J.L., Jr.: Fluid compartment of the brain; cerebral circulation. In: Ruch, T.C. and Patton, H.D. (eds.): Physiology and Biophysics, 19th ed. W.B. Saunders, Philadelphia, 1965, 935-958.

[4] Agarwal, G.C.: Fluid flow—a special case. In: Brown, J.H.V., Jacobs, J.E. and Stark, L. (eds.): Biomedical Engineering. F.A. Davis Co., Philadelphia, 1971, 69-81.

[5] Marmarou, A., Shulman, K. and LaMorgese, J.: Compartmental analysis of compliance and outflow resistance of the cerebrospinal fluid system. J. Neurosurg. 43, 1975, 523-534.

[6] Lewer Allen, K. and Bunt, E.A.: Dysfunctioning of the fluid mechanical craniospinal systems as revealed by stress/strain diagrams. Proc. Int. Conf. on Bioengineering, Cape Town, South Africa, April 1977, 132-151.

[7] Monro: Observations on the structure and functions of the nervous system. Edinburgh, 1783.

[8] Kellie: Trans. Med. Chir. Soc. Edinburgh, 1824.

[9] Weed, L.H.: The cerebrospinal fluid. Phys. Rev. 2, 1922, 171-203.

[10] Lewer Allen, K. and Sun, H.A.: A study of the pressure of the cerebrospinal fluid in man by remote monitoring through the skull. CSIR Symposium on Biotelemetry, Pretoria, 1971.

[11] Bunt, E.A., Pastall, G., Smoliniec, J. and Lewer Allen, K.: A measurement of the effect of an enclosed volume of air on the compressibility of a stimulated cranial cavity. Med. & Biol. Eng. 14, 1976, 318-320.

[12] Haar, F.L. and Miller, C.A.: Hydrocephalus resulting from superior vena cava thrombosis in an infant. J. Neurosurgery 42, 1975, 597.

[13] Langfitt, T.W.: Increased intracranial pressure. Clinical Neurosurgery, Chap. XXI, Congress of Neurological Surgeons, Vol. 16, Williams and Wilkens, Baltimore, 1968.

[14] Frymann, V.M.: A study of the rhythmic motions of the living cranium. Jour. Amer. Osteo. Assoc. 70, 1971, 928-945.

[15] Sutherland, W.G.: The Cranial Bowl. Free Press Co., Monkato, Minn., 1939, 140 pp.

[16] Woods, J.M. and R.H.: A physical finding related to psychiatric disorders. Jour. Amer. Osteo. Assoc. 60, 1961, 988-993.

[17] Moskalenko, V.Y. and Naumenko, Y.: Cerebral pulsation in the closed cranial cavity. Izv. Akad. Nauk SSSR (Biol.) 4, 1961, 620-629.

Appendix C

Mechano-Electric Patterns During Craniosacral Osteopathic Diagnosis and Treatment

JOHN E. UPLEDGER, DO., FAAO, East Lansing, Michigan and ZVI KARNI, Ph.D., D.SC., Haifa Israel*

Cranial osteopathic manipulative diagnosis and treatment is associated with palpatory sensations perceived by the cranially oriented osteopathic physician at various locations on the patient's body. The nature of these palpatory sensations ranges from smooth, regular, and rhythmic to quick, jerky and/or irregular motion. A study of mechano-electric measurements performed on patients in an inactive state of the body shows that distinct strain gauge, electrocardiography, electromyography, and integrated-electromyography patterns correspond with each one of the palpatory sensations. This correlation far exceeds random probability.

Motions that are detectable by palpation of individual cranial bones and/or of the entire cranial vault are associated with similar palpable motions at other locations on the body.[1-3] However, the cranium and the sacrum were used in this experiment because the motion is most apparent in these two areas. The nature of the physician-perceived sensations is variable. It ranges from a smooth, rhythmic motion which ebbs and flows and occasionally ceases entirely, to a quick, jerky or vibratory motion which may be quite irregular. The motions can be represented mechanically by a single, narrow band-width amplitude (Fig. 1a), by multiple amplitudes with varying frequencies (Fig. 1b), or by a form of a step function (Dirac's function) (Fig. 1c). In the first two instances, the baseline remains unchanged; in the case of step function, a change is indicated in the baseline for a limited time period (T_c) which is attained either instantaneously (Fig. 1c) or gradually (Fig. 1d).

The purpose of this research was to determine whether there were correlations between selected mechano-electric parameters (monitored at various regions of the body) and the physician's impressions of the changes in craniosacral motion (mechanics) during craniosacral diagnosis and treatment. The results indicate that almost every perceived change in craniosacral motion (mechanics) reported "blind"** by the physician has its unique counterpart in the

** The experimental facility was physically arranged so that the physician (Dr. Upledger) was unable to visualize the recordings as they were made. All notations were made in a timely fashion on the graph by the scientific observer (Dr. Karni) as the physician's impressions were verbally communicated. The scientific observer did not offer any verbal cues to the physician. Usually, the mechano-electric pattern changes preceded the verbal communications by approximately a second. This sequence of events rules out any obscure possibility that the patients could have responded "bioelectrically" to verbal cues given by the physician as his impressions were reported.

*Reprinted from The Journal of the American Osteopathic Association, Vol. 78, July 1979, pp. 782-91, by permission of the American Osteopathic Association, 212 E. Ohio St., Chicago, IL 60611.

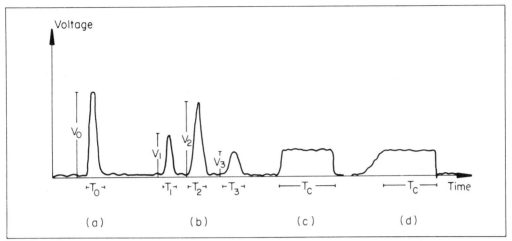

Fig. 1 *Modes of motion amplitudes: (a) single, (b) multiple, (c) step function, and (d) gradual step function.*

mechano-electric changes in patterns recorded from other locations on the patient's body.

The character of the recorded mechano-electric patterns was *not* dependent on voluntary muscle activity of the patient, nor was it attributable to changes in the contact sites on the patient's body by the physician's hands.

Unless otherwise indicated, all recordings were made with the patient in a relaxed state. However, when voluntary muscle action did occur, it was indicated on the tracings.

MATERIALS AND METHODS

The mechano-electric patterns in Figure 1 were extracted from the recorded monitoring of the time variations of mechanical strain and of electric potentials of the skin at different loci on the patient's body during the cranial diagnosis and treatment. In the preliminary experiments, six- and eight-channel tracings were recorded. Later, however, as the multi-channel record became correlated with the perceived palpatory sensation, the recording was reduced to four channels, which was easier for the observer to handle and interpret.

The four channels included at least one strain gauge, a unipolar ECG rhythm strip, and at least one I-EMG measurement. The standard arrangement was as follows: (1) a single strain gauge placed over the palpable pulse immediately below the inferior costal margin which monitored the patient's respiratory activity and the arterial pulsations; (2) a unipolar ECG rhythm strip; and (3) two EMG electrodes placed bilaterally and symmetrically on the anterior thighs. When our attention was focused upon respiratory activity, the following arrangement was used: (1) two strain gauges placed symmetrically and bilaterally just below the inferior costal margins; (2) a unipolar ECG rhythm strip; and (3) a single anterior thigh EMG. Sometimes both arrangements were applied to the same patient during a single treatment. The change from one arrangement to the other required only a few seconds.

The strain measurements were taken using Peekel electrical-resistance, high-extension rubber strain gauges type 20S.[4] These gauges possess a maximum extensibility of 20 percent and a maximum compressibility of 15 percent. Gauge specifications are as follows: overall dimensions, 46 x 17 mm. (1.80 x 0.69 inches); active length, 13 mm. (0.51 inches); electrical resistance, 119.5 ohm ± 0.2 percent; gauge factor—static extension, —0.0136 ± 2 percent; gauge factor—static compression, +0.0182 ± 2 percent. There is a negative gauge factor because of its construction; the resistance wire undergoes a compression when a positive strain (extension) is applied.

The adhesive recommended by the manufacturer for the gauge was a Peekel quick-drying adhesive type L35 which requires skin cleansing with Benzene solution. After numerous tests, it was decided that clear surgical tape was an effective adhesive for proper skin fixation. This method was used for reasons of convenience.

The strain gauges were connected to a portable Wheatstone bridge (constructed by N. St. Pierre of the Biomechanics Department). Each bridge accommodated two strain gauges and was operated either by a battery power source contained in the bridge or by drawing a 12-volt output power from the polygraph. For the more sensitive experiments, and to avoid polygraph noise, the battery source was employed.

The electromyography was recorded using silver-silver chloride electrodes (of a unity gain), preamplification units, and an "audio-oscilloscope"† Hewlett Packard EMG Unit Mark 1510B. The EMG output then was passed into an integrater (also constructed by Mr. N. St. Pierre) which converted the AC signals into their DC time-integral values. The integrater computed the area (definite integral) per unit of time between the original EMG-voltage ordinates and the time as an abscissa. The integrater also functioned as a rectifier and cut out small amplitudes below a specific threshold. Consequently, the spread of the EMG pattern was more pronounced because dominant signals were magnified and secondary redundant signals were eliminated. This is illustrated in Figure 2, which compares an ordinary one-lead ECG with its corresponding "integrated" ECG (I-ECG) recorded simultaneously over the same point on the subject's body by means of chrome plated snap electrodes. It is apparent that primarily the R-wave contributes to the time integral, and the influences of the other waves are small. Thus, in the inactive state of skeletal muscular activity, integrated electromyography (I-EMG) eli-

† In our experiments, the audio channels were completely shut off (not used at all).

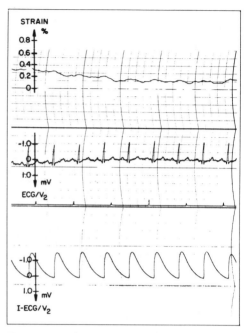

Fig. 2 *Single lead ECG and I-ECG recorded simultaneously.*

minated noise and was preferable for this research.

The strain gauge, the ECG, and the I-EMG pick-ups were all connected to a multi-channel Grass Polygraph. The highest sensitivity gain calibration was set on 0.01 mv./cm. The frequency gain settings during the experiments were 3 for the strain gauge measurements, 15 for the I-EMG, and 75 for the ECG.

RESULTS

Some typical four-channel recordings conducted during cranio-sacral manipulative procedures are shown in the following figures. Although each patient showed uniquely personalized patterns, there were repetitive features in all the tracings which allowed us to consider at least four different patterns which all patients had in common. Using the classification suggested in Application Note 700 of Hewlett Packard, 1969, we labeled these patterns as follows: (1) *Rapid oscillations.* In the strainography (SG) over the left hypochondrium, these oscillations had a relatively small amplitude of

0.02-0.1 percent strain‡ and measured frequencies of 52-96 cycles per minute (cpm). They were present throughout and, when correlated with the ECG, corresponded in a timely fashion with aortic expansion. In rare cases, the strain gauges also picked up what may have been the echo jerks of cardiac valve closures.

In the I-EMG tracings, the rapid oscillations with amplitudes of 0.1 - 0.2 mv. and measured frequencies of 52-96 cpm resulted from the fading cardiac electroactivity which was picked up on the thighs.

(2) *Transient waveforms*. These waveforms in the SG which possessed an amplitude of up to 3 percent strain and a frequency ranging from 6 to 30 cpm were in one-to-one correspondence with the respiratory rate (RR) (thoracic expansion). The average RR in the resting state ranged between 14 and 18 per minute in the majority of cases. In our study, trained athletes (karate experts) were able to voluntarily lower the RR to 6 per minute or less for 15 minutes or longer.

(3) *Rapid waveforms, or spikes*. Apart from the R-waveform in the ECG, and rarely in the SG, spikes were predominantly seen in the I-EMG. Spike amplitudes varied from 0.4 to 2.0 mv. The frequencies of spike occurrence seemed dependent upon the patient's neuromusculoskeletal pain syndrome. The appearance (frequency and amplitude) of spikes decreased with favorable response to the treatment and became a landmark of correlation between the physician's reported impressions and sensations and the patient's mechano-electric patterns.

(4) *Baseline changes*. These changes, primarily seen in I-EMG baseline, were either gradual or abrupt. Baseline changes often lasted for many seconds and then relaxed, abruptly forming the shape of a step function. They seemed to be correlated to changes in the patient's muscle tonus and/or reports of pain by the patient.

Specific terms were given to the physician-reported sensations during treatment. The following glossary was used:

‡ One percent strain means an extension of 1/100 of the original length of the gauge.

(1) *Normal rhythm (NR)*. This is a smooth regular pulsatile cranial activity in a rhythm of 8-12 cycles per minute. This rhythmic activity is in accord with the concept of a Cranial Rhythmic Impulse as put forth by Sutherland.[1,3] The sensation of the normal rhythm as perceived by the physician is that of a uniform deformation of cranial vault shape, as its dimensions *reciprocally* and rhythmically change. This rhythmic effect can be sensed by palpation anywhere on the patient's body. The cause of this deformation is at present a subject for conjecture; however, it seems related to the fact that the dural compartment represents a semi-closed hydraulic system as it extends from the cranium through the spinal canal to the sacrum. This normal rhythm was not seen on our I-EMG recordings taken during the experiments. There is, however, some strain-gauge pickup of the NR if the gauge is placed sufficiently close to the skull. (The investigators plan further work using strain gauges which will attempt to demonstrate the presence of a fluid wave motion.)

(2) *Still point (SP)*.[1,3] A still point is sensed when the normal rhythm stops temporarily. This cessation of motion might occur gradually as the rhythmic motion amplitude decreases. Or, it can take place suddenly when the zero point of the pulsatory waveform is attained, and the motion stops abruptly. On the I-EMG record over a thigh, an SP concurs with a short spike of 1.3 mv. (Fig. 3a) and with a drop to the baseline level if an absolute stop occurs (Fig. 3b).

(3) *End of still point (ESP)*.[1,3] Following an SP, the system, both skull and body, seems to expand laterally. This phenomenon usually begins with long, slow expansion which then leads to a more even and symmetric motion. The ESP correlates on the thigh I-EMG record with the *delayed* appearance of a 0.4 mv. spike signal, the delay being of the order of 1 second (Fig. 4a). Furthermore, and in contrast to the SP, an elevatd I-EMG activity takes place following the ESP (Fig. 4b).

(4) *Release (Re)*. This sensation is of a "plastic" yielding of the volumetric container in the sense that frictional resistance

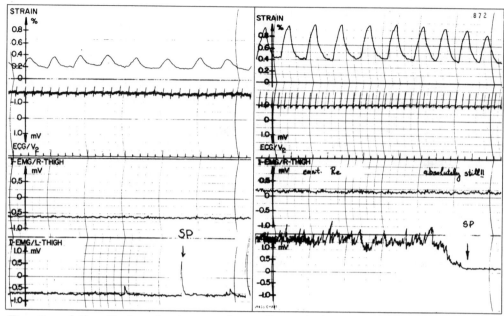

Figs. 3a and 3b. *Mechano-electric pattern for a still point (SP) as (a) spike, and (b) absolute stop.*

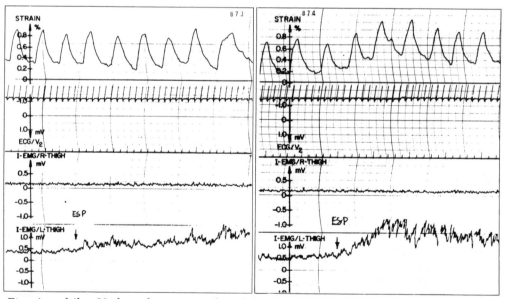

Figs. 4a and 4b   *Mechano-electric pattern for end of still point (ESP) as (a) delayed spike, and (b) before an elevated I-EMG activity.*

or obstruction to fluidity have been over-come. This relaxation of resistance is accompanied by a sharp I-EMG spike which, in magnitude, surpasses any of the previously described spike patterns. The release signals can be symmetric (Fig. 5a) or unilateral (Fig. 5b). They play a paramount role in the osteopathic treatment as landmarks for improved functional activities.

(5) *Shifting.* The impression of a tidal fluid

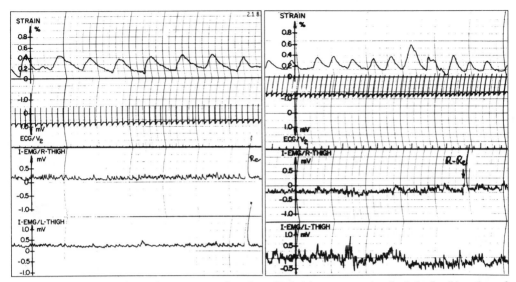

Figs. 5a and 5b   *Mechano-electric pattern for release (Re): (a) symmetrical on both thighs, (b) unilateral on one thigh.*

motion and change of direction of flow is sensed by the physician. For example, the feeling or perception could be that of an uneven lateral expansion of the skull secondary to a volumetric fluid shift. When the direction of the fluid wave changes, a mechanical change takes place in concert with it.

The pattern of the mechano-electric changes in shifting is unique and unmistakable. The I-EMG shows a clear and distinct change of the baseline in the form of a step function. This usually takes place during the peak of respiratory inhalation while the pulmonary volume is maximal. This is clearly indicated by the strain gauge records (Figs. 6a and 6b). Our correlation between the sensation of shifting and the step-function patterns was 100 percent.

(6) *Pulsating.* This is a rapid oscillatory motion of low-amplitude and high-frequency (50-80 per minute) which is most commonly perceived in a localized area of the cranium. Generally, it precedes an ESP, a release, or a shifting. It is interpreted as an indication that some important mechanical change is about to occur. Pulsating usually occurs during the resting phase of the respiratory cycle (Fig. 7).

(7) *Wobbling.* This term was used to des-cribe a low-mode (20-40 cpm), fluctuatory type of motion with amplitudes larger than those of "pulsating." Furthermore, the effect is not localized and can be felt over the body. Wobbling usually precedes a major release or shifting. The subjective impression of the physician is that of a braking mechanism which interferes with the fluid motion. The typical electromechanical pattern associated with wobbling is shown in Figure 8. This event takes place during the respiratory hold phase following inhalation.

(8) *Torsion.* ** In torsion, the impression is that of a rotational periodic motion about a longitudinal axis through the patient's body where all sections of the body are not moving in synchrony. It is an asymmetric, distortional (not volumetric) type of a motion which is manifested as asymmetric I-EMG pickups on the lower extremities. Torsion is observed in Figure 9 as a series of spikes with modest amplitudes (0.7-1.0 mv.). It does not show in the respiratory activity recordings.

A common denominator of the above physician-reported sensations is that they

---

**Torsion as used in this research is not to be confused with "torsion" as an abnormal relationship between the sphenoid and occipital bones. [1,3]

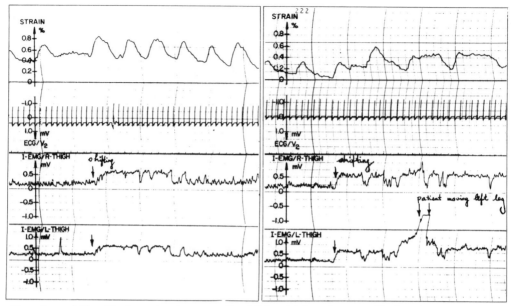

Figs. 6a and 6b   *Mechano-electric pattern for shifting: (a) long duration, (b) short duration.*

are all passive or inherent to the patient's body; they all occur when the patient is in a relaxed and inactive state and when no gross manipulative treatment is being applied. They are most easily perceived or sensed when the patient is very quiet.

DISCUSSION

It tacitly has been assumed throughout this presentation that the mechanical model underlying the impressions reported by the physician involved a fluid container composed of several physiologic compartments, each of which possessed uniquely different material properties. This container may allow for very slight changes in its volume capacity. In effect, and in accordance with the long accepted Monroe-Kellie doctrine,[5] the relatively inelastic dura mater faithfully encloses the brain and spinal cord as a continuous and connected material region,** it may represent such a container.

It is postulated that the contents of the dural container (brain, spinal cord, nerves, cerebrospinal fluid, blood, and other fluids) are very nearly incompressible.[6] As a result, the combined volume of the contents of the dural container must be very nearly constant; and the volume of any one of its compart-

ments can only be increased at the expense of the others.

** The dura mater has been described as a tough inelastic membrane which forms the endosteum of the cranial vault. It attaches firmly about the entire circumference of the occipital foramen magnum. It then passes through the entire length of the spinal canal; its most firm attachments within the canal are only to the posterior aspects of the bodies of the second and third cervical vertebrae and within the sacral canal at the level of the second segment. It is separated from the spinal canal by the epidural space which ends at the second sacral segment (S-2). Below the level of S-2, the dura closely invests the filum terminale, passes through the sacral hiatus, and descends to the coccyx where it blends with the periosteum of that bone. The dura mater is connected to the dentate ligaments within the spinal canal, to the posterior longitudinal ligament, and to its nerve root sleeves which exit from the spinal canal with the spinal nerves. The restrictions to dural motion afforded by the latter three described attachments are much less than the restrictions imposed by those attachments within the cranial vault, at the foramen magnum at C-2 and C-3, within the sacral canal, and at the coccyx. The size of volume capacity of the dural container is much greater than is required to accommodate only the neural structures and, therefore, is quite able to respond somewhat independently to the stresses and pressures to which it is subjected. When considered as the material border of a fluid container with the previously described firm attachments to bone, the influence of these bony structures upon the mechanical forces within the container becomes quite apparent.

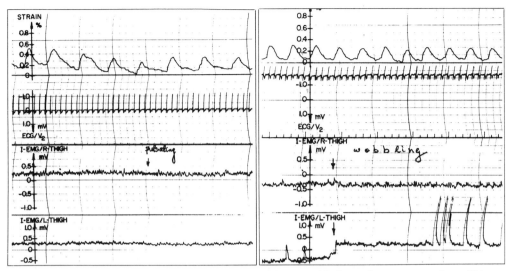

Fig. 7 *Mechano-electric pattern for pulsating.*   Fig. 8 *Mechano-electric pattern for wobbling.*

The craniosacral osteopathic doctrine considers the major skull bones to be interconnected by viscoelastic sutures,[7] acting as hinges about which a kinematic change in configuration can take place. Furthermore, because the dura mater is membranous, it is susceptible to dynamic boundary changes which correlate to the physician's impression of the rhythmic and pulsatory motions of the cranial bones. The overall picture is, therefore, that of a less than rigid mechanical model with a fluid content, the motion of which, although small, is still within the range of sensory perception for trained craniosacral osteopathic physicians.

The nature of the mechanical craniosacral effect on the neuromusculoskeletal system is, unquestionably, obscure. However, the fact that the craniosacral system does have a measurable effect on other parts of the body has been demonstrated on an input-output basis by this experiment.

CONCLUSIONS

Subjective impressions of various changes in the craniosacral mechanics which are reported by a trained craniosacral osteopathic physician are documentable by instrumental means. This documentation consists of changes in the bioelectric activity recorded by I-EMG from the lower extremi-

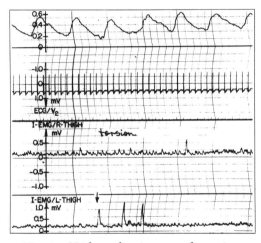

Fig. 9 *Mechano-electric pattern for torsion.*

ties, ECG, and strain-gauge recordings of respiratory activity.

Specific patterns of the monitored mechano-electric parameters correlate directly with subjective impressions of likewise specific changes in craniosacral mechanics as reported by the physician.

The range of the recorded integrated electromyographic signals is below the level of signals originating from any voluntary type of muscular activity, yet is by far larger than instrumental noise levels.

This research has been partly supported by the Department of Biomechanics, COM/MSU.

Appreciation is expressed to Drs. E. Retzlaff and R. Roppel for valuable suggestions and the use of equipment; to Mr. N. St. Pierre for technical assistance, and to Mr. J. Schulz from the Instructional Media Center, MSU, for the preparation of the figures.

[1] Sutherland, W.A.: The cranial bowl. Free Press Company, Mankato, Minnesota, 1939.

[2] Wales, A.L.: The work of William Garner Sutherland. JAOA 71:788-93, May 72.

[3] Magoun, H.I.: Osteopathy in the cranial field. Journal Printing Co., Kirksville, Missouri, 1966.

[4] Karni, Z. and Polishuk, W.Z.: Multi-strain measurement of uterine activity. Proceedings of the 24th Annual Conference in Engineering in Medicine and Biology, 101, Nov. 71.

[5] Livingston, R.B., Woodbury, D.M., and Patterson, J.L. Jr.: Fluid compartments of the brain. Cerebral circulation. In Ruch, T.C., and Patton, H.D., Eds. Physiology and biophysics, W.B. Saunders Co., Philadelphia, 1965.

[6] Agarwal, G.C.: Fluid flow. A special case. In Brown, J.H.U., Jacobs, J.E., and Stark, L. Eds.: Biomedical Engineering, F.A. Davis Co., Philadelphia, 1971.

[7] Retzlaff, E., et al.: Sutural collagenous bundles and their innervation in Saimiri sciureus. Anat Rec 187:692, Apr. 77.

Appendix D

Management of Autogenic Headache

JOHN UPLEDGER, D.O. AND JON D. VREDEVOOGD*

The functional anatomy of the head and neck supports the thesis that a significant number of headache problems are autogenic. Tissue contracture is a natural defense mechanism against injury. This defense mechanism may support the continuation of pain when it is no longer appropriate. Various mechanisms and therapeutic approaches related to headache are discussed.

Hypertonus, or contracture of the cranial or cervical soft tissue, is almost invariably a concomitant feature of headache. When it is not grossly observable, careful examination will almost always identify discrete and localized areas of abnormal tissue tonus. Often these soft-tissue tonus abnormalities persist between exacerbations of head pain. Functionally, these loci may be considered residual trigger areas. The soft-tissue change may represent either a primary or a secondary feature of the headache syndrome. In either case, soft-tissue hypertonus or contracture does contribute to chronicity and recurrence.** This may occur by a number of mechanisms. Among them are increased intracranial fluid congestion, occipital neuralgia due to soft-tissue change in or about the suboccipital triangle, spinal dural stress or tension, and cranial-suture immobility and compression. Each of these will be discussed separately.

INTRACRANIAL FLUID CONGESTION

Congestion of fluids within the cranial vault may be secondary to an obstruction to outflow at the cranial foramina that causes low-grade increases in back pressure. The most common areas for tissue contractures that increase back pressure are probably at the jugular foramina. These foramina are located just lateral to the occipital condyles (Figure 1). A somatic dysfunction in the occipitoatlantal relationship will very likely result in tissue contracture, which will increase the back pressure to cranial-vault venous outflow via these (jugular) foramina.

**The term "soft tissue," as used herein, refers to all connective tissue except bone. Frequently, "soft-tissue contracture" and "hypertonus" are used only to describe muscle conditions. Retzlaff[1] demonstrated histologically that collagen fibers are intimately related to elastic fibers. The microarchitecture of these interrelated fibers strongly suggests that collagen tissue possesses contractile ability. The same work has shown the presence of neurostructures also intimately related to the collagen-elastic-fiber complex. The presence of these nerve receptors and fibers in relationship to the collagen-elastic-fiber unit further suggests a reflexly controlled contractile function for collagen tissue. Collagen (connective) tissue may, therefore, respond to local stimuli (such as stress and tension) and to messages from higher control centers, probably triggered by pain awareness or emotional stress.

Reprinted from Osteopathic Annals, Vol. 7, No. 6, June 1979, pp. 232-41, by permission of the authors.

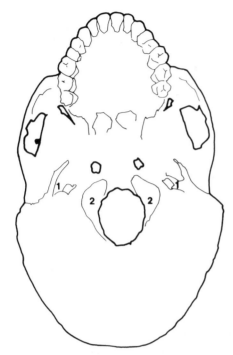

Figure 1   *Interior aspect of skull.   (1: Jugular foramen. 2: Occipital condyles.)*

The jugular foramina also afford passage to the ninth, 10th, and 11th nerves. Disturbances of these nerves may result in clinical symptoms related to cardiac rhythm, digestion, bowel function, swallowing, etc. The spinal accessory portions of the 11th cranial nerve arise from the upper five or six cervical segments. They pass cephalad through the foramen magnum into the cranial vault. They exit from the vault via the jugular foramina and provide motor fibers to the sternocleidomastoid and trapezius muscles.

On the basis of these anatomic relationships, it can be seen that tissue changes in the vicinity of the occipital condyles and jugular foramina may result in varied pain and autonomic syndromes. An effective therapeutic approach must deal with all the soft-tissue disorders that may cause obstruction to fluid outflow from the cranial vault.

THERAPEUTIC APPROACH

The cranial vault may be considered a semiclosed fluid container. The various foramina represent portals of entry and exit for this compartment. The fluid volume within the vault is maintained at a relatively constant volume by homeostatic mechanisms. Subtle changes in fluid volume and pressure may result in head pain and autonomic dysfunction. These subtle changes may be due to increased back pressure, as described above, or to a change in the fluid retention properties of the cranial vault contents. Medications may result in toxic arachnoiditis or cerebral edema; therefore, they should be used conservatively in cases of persistent or recurrent head pain and with full awareness that the clinical syndrome may be iatrogenically perpetuated and perhaps worsened. The intracranial fluid volume may also be increased by dysfunction of arterial tonus, which causes more inflow than can be accommodated by the outflow. The resultant head pain causes a neurogenic hypertonus of soft tissue, which in turn further reduces the outflow capability.

In any of these cases, effective therapy must enhance outflow capability so that intracranial fluid congestion is reduced.

Nonspecific "Thrust" Technique for the Cervicothoracic Region

This technique should be applied bilaterally. It is not directed at specific somatic dysfunction unless pain prohibits proper positioning of the patient. (It is preferable to make specific corrections later, after the generalized tissue tonus has been reduced.) The goal of the technique is the enhancement of free fluid motion from the cranial vault into the thoracic cage.

The patient should be supine, with the physician cephalad. The physician's right hand is placed so that the palm is supporting the lower cervical region. Firm contact is established between the radial side of the physician's right palm and the right cervicothoracic region of the patient. The physician's left palm is then used to support the patient's left upper cervical and occipital region. Right-side bending is extended to its extreme range of motion, using the right hand as a fulcrum. The right-side bending forces stretch the soft tissues on the left side. The patient is then asked to hold a deep inhalation as long as possible while side bending is further increased. This causes more tissue relaxation. The breathing assistance procedure is repeated until no further side bending can be introduced at the end of the held inhalation. Frequently, the physician will notice that first-rib articulations occur spontaneously during this procedure.

While side bending is maintained at its extreme, left rotation is introduced. Locking should *not* be attempted. The rotational motion affects C7 through T3 or T4. A "thrust" is then carried through the barrier to further mobilize the tissues of the cervicothoracic region. The procedure is then repeated in the opposite direction (Figure 2).

First-Rib Restrictions

Remaining restrictions of the first rib are then easily corrected by bending to the side of the restriction so that maximal tissue relaxation is obtained. With the thumb and index finger grasping the tissues in the region of the first-rib head, mobilization can usually be accomplished by the use of direct gentle pressure. If further mobilization is required, respiratory assistance (as above) may be quite helpful.

Release of Upper Cervical and Suboccipital Tissues

The patient and physician remain in the same position except for the physician's hands. These hands are approximated palms up, with the fingers flexed so that the distal phalanges are oriented at approximately 90 degrees to the longitudinal plane of the patient's cervical spine (Figure 3). The fingertips apply deep pressure in the suboccipital region bilaterally. The physician's fingertips are also used to support the patient so that the occipital region is initially suspended above the physician's palms. Fingerpad contact should be maintained with the inferior aspect of the patient's occiput. As

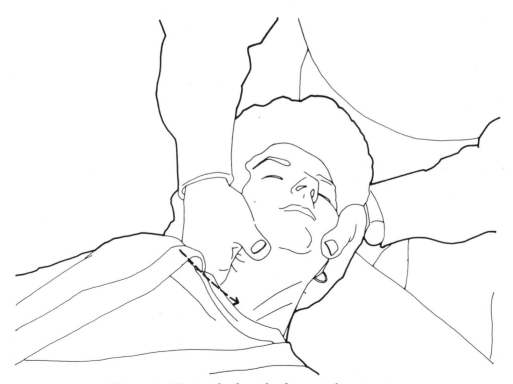

Figure 2   *Nonspecific thrust for the cervicothoracic region.*

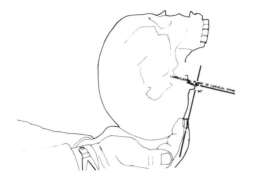

Figure 3 *Hand position for release of sub-occipital tissue.*

the suboccipital tissues relax, the occiput will gently settle into the physician's upturned palms. The firmness of bone (the atlas) will be apparent at the fingertips on completion of this technique. This is a passive and waiting technique on the part of the physician. Respiratory assistance (as above) by the patient may be employed to facilitate tissue relaxation.

As the tissues relax, a discrete area of tissue contracture may be discovered. This may be a key trigger to the pain syndrome. It should be specifically treated with further deep pressure until it is perceived to relax. This technique is aimed at releasing all tissue hypertonus that may influence outflow from the jugular foramina.

Mobilization of Occipitoatlantal and Atlantoaxial Joints

Once the relaxation of the suboccipital tissues has been obtained as outlined above, the freedom of motion of the atlas and axis should be tested by fingertip pressure as the occiput is gently supported in the physician's upturned palms. Any restriction of motion can usually be corrected with gentle direct or indirect technique in conjunction with respiratory assistance by the patient. Be gentle; do not cause tissues to reflexly contract against your palpatory intrusion.

Mobilization of the Remainder of the Cervical Spine

The entire cervical spine (segment by segment) can now be palpated by gentle

motion testing, using the fingertips to move the articular pillar regions as the occiput is supported in the upturned palms. Testing for translatory, side bending, and anterior motion usually suffices to identify remaining specific somatic dysfunctions. Those found can be gently corrected by either direct or indirect techniques with respiratory assistance.

The techniques described above are all aimed at alleviating obstruction to the outflow of fluid from the cranial vault and, therefore, favorably influencing the inflow-outflow pressure differential. This approach, in sequence, will usually effectively interrupt the autogenic nature of head pain due to intracranial fluid congestion by facilitation of outflow. The next technique (parietal lift) is aimed at *directly* alleviating intracranial fluid congestion.

Parietal Lift

The physician should be seated above the patient's head. The physician's fingertips are placed *gently* in contact with the lateral aspects of the patient's parietal bones bilaterally. The fifth-finger pads are in contact with asterion, anterior to the lambdoid sutures and just above the temporoparietal sutures. The other three fingers of each hand are placed about 1 cm. apart and must be above the patient's temporoparietal sutures (Figure 4). The physician's thumbs are now crossed upon each other above the patient's head. (They do not touch the patient's scalp.) Next, after finger placement is rechecked, *gentle* pressure is exerted to compress the lateral aspects of the parietal bones medially (Figure 5). If the temporal bones are pressured, the technique will not work and may, in fact, worsen the clinical symptoms. The amount of pressure exerted on the parietal bones is on the order of 5-10 gm. The thumbs, in contact with each other, are used to steady the physician's hands. This gentle pressure on *only* the parietal bones is held constant for several minutes. (Usually three to five minutes will suffice.) As the temporoparietal sutures disengage, it will feel to the physician as though the parietal bones are moving superiorly and spreading very slight-

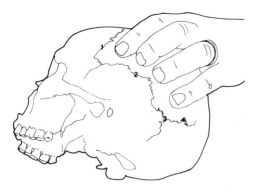

Figure 4   *Suture landmarks for parietal lift.(1: Coronal suture. 2: Temporal parietal suture. 3: Asterion. 4: Lambdoid suture.)*

ly. *Do not release your parietal pressure suddenly. Do it gradually; otherwise you may worsen the symptoms.* Usually when this release is felt, the patient will remark that "pressure" within the head has been relieved.*

Peripheral Stimulation Therapy Directed at the Alleviation of Intracranial Fluid Congestion[3]

Peripheral stimulation therapy is aimed at the activation of specific loci within the musculoskeletal system and often produces predictable therapeutic results. The activating stimulus may be a needle puncture, deep pressure, circular massage, ultrasound, or any other of a number of techniques. The important factor is that the stimulus be applied to a specific anatomic location. Only the anatomic locations that have proved useful for the achievement of the desired results are described here. The choice of the technique should be made using precautions dictated by the medical expertise of each physician.

Peripheral stimulation therapy loci, which are often effective in the reduction of tonus of the cervical musculature, are located on many areas of the body. Those given below have been the most effective in

---

*The author realizes that the presentation of this cranial technique may be controversial. However, if it is carried out with caution and sensitivity to the delicacy of the structures it affects, it can provide dramatic relief to a large number of suffering patients.[2]

my practice.

1. On the midline of the body — at the juncture of the sagittal and lambdoid sutures on the scalp, between the occiput and the atlas, between C2 and C3 (spinous processes), and between C7 and T1 (spinous processes).

2. At the juncture of the metacarpal bones of the thumb and index finger on the distal aspect of that joint capsule, about midway between its palmar and dorsal surfaces (Hoku). This locus is very reactive to needling and deep pressure (Figure 6).

3. At the midpoint of the popliteal crease bilaterally (B54). The best effect is obtained by needling (Figure 7).

4. Immediately inferior to and directly over the mastoid tips bilaterally. The best effect is obtained by transcutaneous needling or by gentle pressure and circular massage. Do not use even moderate pressure on this area, or you may induce a variety of autonomic responses. If your pressure worsens the head pain, it is too firm.

5. At the inferior aspect of the occiput on the lateral aspect of the trapezius, bilaterally. These loci are very effectively treated

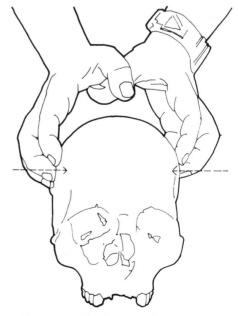

Figure 5   *Hand position for parietal lift.*

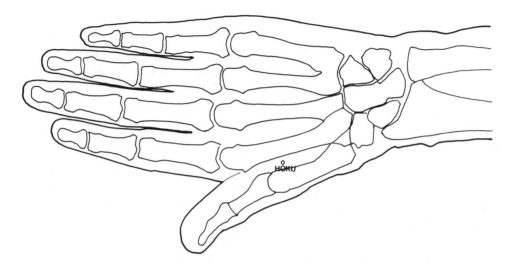

Figure 6   *Hoku peripheral stimulation point.*

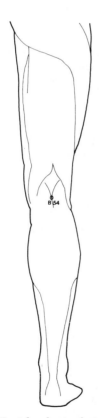

Figure 7   *Peripheral stimulation point for relaxation of cervical muscle tension.*

by needling or deep pressure.

6. About 1 inch inferior to the superior border of the trapezius, midway between the deltoid origin on top of the shoulder and the vertebral articulation of the first rib. These areas are well known to many patients as effective for the use of relaxing massage. They are very effective loci for needling to achieve cervical relaxation and to reduce intracranial fluid back pressure.[4] (Look for discrete areas of acute tenderness.)

7. The medial aspects of the scapular spines (bilaterally) frequently present effective peripheral stimulation loci, as do the medial borders of the scapulae superior to their spines.

Peripheral stimulation therapy loci, which are very useful in the reduction of intracranial fluid pressure,[5] are known in acupuncture as K1, GV24.5, and GV26. K1 is located bilaterally on the soles of the feet just proximal to the prominence of the metatarsophalangeal joints between the second and third metatarsals. These loci are very responsive to needling or deep pressure (Figure 8). The other two loci (GV24.5 and GV26) are found, respectively, on the midline between the medial aspects of the eyebrows (over the glabella) and above the mucocutaneous junction of the upper lip a third of the way towards the base of the nose. These loci are very responsive to needling or to the application of locally applied heat by contact with a warm metallic object.

All four of these areas should be stimulated within a few minutes of each other in order to achieve maximum benefit.

OCCIPITAL NEURALGIA, OCCIPITOFRONTAL CEPHALGIA, AND THE SUBOCCIPITAL TRIANGLE

The upper three cervical nerves contribute to the occipital nerves. C1 is primarily motor to the muscles of the suboccipital triangle but has some sensory fibers. C2 is the largest contributor to the greater occipital nerve, which supplies sensory fibers to the obliquus capitis inferior and to the splenius and longissimus capitis muscles. C3, the lesser or third occipital nerve, supplies sensory innervation to small portions of the occipital and mastoid scalp and to the posterior neck. It supplies motor innervation to the semispinalis capitis (Figure 9).

This brief look at the pertinent anatomy serves to illustrate the autogenic nature of head pain as tissue tension causes nerve stimulation that in turn increases tissue tension.

The therapeutic approach to occipital neuralgia and occipitofrontal neuralgia due to somatic dysfunction of the tissues of the suboccipital triangle is exactly the same as that described above for release of suboccipital tissues and upper cervical vertebrae.

The peripheral stimulation therapy loci are exactly the same as those described above for the relaxation of the cervical soft tissues.

All vertebral restrictions to motion should be treated to re-establish mobility.

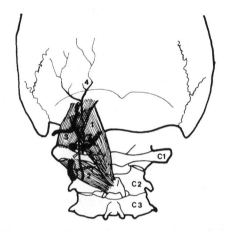

Figure 9 *Suboccipital triangle. (1: Rectus capitis posterior major. 2: Obliquus capitis inferior. 3: Obliquus capitis superior. 4: Occipital nerve.)*

SPINAL DURAL STRESS

The dural tube is a relatively inelastic and tough membrane. It attaches firmly at the foramen magnum to the posterior bodies of C2 and C3 but not again within the spinal canal until it reaches the level of S2. It becomes the filum terminale externus, passes out the sacral hiatus, and attaches to the coccyx as its periosteum.[6]

Considering the anatomic relations of the dura below the foramen magnum and the fact that it forms the endosteum of the cranial-vault bones, it becomes apparent that any continuing stress on the dura mater is capable of producing head pain.

A common situation, often ignored, is the anterior flexion of the coccyx due to trauma. The patient seldom perceives the relationship between a fall on the "posterior" and the subsequent onset of persistent

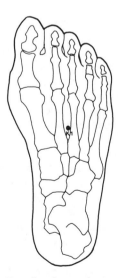

Figure 8 *Peripheral stimulation point for reduction of intracranial fluid congestion.*

head pain. Consideration of the dural osseous attachments readily illuminates a
mechanism of dural stress transmission
from the anteriorly flexed coccyx to the
foramen magnum of the occiput. This
stress, though of low grade, is continuous
and may cause recurrent occipitoatlantal
somatic dysfunction, which in turn causes
fluid outflow obstruction at the jugular
foramina and intracranial fluid congestion.
The cervical musculature becomes hypertonic in response to irritation of the motor
nerves. Visceral autonomic syndromes frequently occur. These syndromes eventually
resemble each other and become autogen-
ically perpetuated. All the techniques described above may be instituted; however,
permanent results will not be obtained until
the coccyx is mobilized.

Direct Technique

With the patient comfortably flexed in
the lateral recumbent position, the physician's gloved index finger is inserted into
the anus. The coccyx is grasped between
the index finger (in the rectum) and the
thumb (external). Anterior flexion and posterior extension motion testing is gently
carried out. Very often the patient will
comment that anterior flexion increases or
causes head pain and posterior extension
motion relieves it somewhat. These observations by the patient confirm your diagnosis. The correction is achieved by the
application of gentle direct technique
against the pathologic motion barrier with
respiratory assistance until a relaxation is
felt. This simple treatment is very effective.
It has solved some very severe and persistent headache problems.

CRANIAL SUTURAL PAIN

Quite often head pain is localized along
the course of a given suture of the cranial
vault. This condition frequently prevails as
an aftermath of the treatment of head pain
due to intracranial fluid congestion.

Retzlaff et al.[7] have illustrated histologically that the microanatomic structures
required for pain are present within the
cranial suture. Dysfunction of the suture
may therefore result in localized pain as

well as in more generalized symptoms.

Once localized sutural pain has been
identified, it may be treated quite readily by
two simple and effective methods, local
needle stimulation and the Sutherland technique of "direction of fluid."

Local Needle Stimulation

A small-diameter (27-gauge or smaller)
sterile hypodermic needle is inserted trans-
cutaneously and threaded in the subcutaneous tissues of the scalp immediately superficial and parallel to the affected sutural
region. This needle should not invade the
suture, nor should it disrupt the periosteum
of the cranial bones (Figure 10). Once in
place, the needle hub should be gently
tapped until the pain is relieved. Pain relief
usually occurs in less than three minutes.
Subjectively, it appears that this procedure
actually mobilizes the sutural restriction
(probably by stimulating nerve receptors
that are superficial to but influence intrasutural connective tissues).

Sutherland's Technique — "Directing Fluid"

This technique makes use of a mechanism that is not yet scientifically understood
but produces predictably favorable clinical
results. It is not necessary to be an experienced cranial manipulator in order to successfully employ this very effective therapeutic approach.

Place the pads of one or two fingers
gently on the scalp directly over the painful
suture area. Now, imagine a line or vector
from the painful area through the center of
the skull (using a globe as the ideational
model) and out the other side of the patient's
head so that an imaginary diameter has
been formed (Figure 11). With the other
hand, very gently palpate for a pulsation of
the scalp at the region where the vector
(diameter) would emerge from the patient's
skull. The exact location can easily be
determined in a few seconds with an extremely light palpatory touch.

Once the area of pulsation has been located, apply two or three finger pads to the
area while the fingers of the opposite hand
(in contact with the painful suture) are

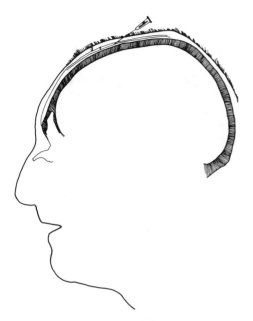

Figure 10 *Needle position for subcutaneous scalp stimulation.*

gently laid upon the scalp so that the length of two of these fingers parallel the painful suture about 0.5-1.0 cm. on either side of it (Figure 12). The painful suture will seem to begin pulsating. This pulsating will continue for a matter of minutes. As the pulsation gradually subsides, so will the pain. A very gentle spreading action by the fingers paralleling the painful suture will speed the therapeutic effect, but it is not mandatory. Remember that gentleness is absolutely necessary for the success of this technique.

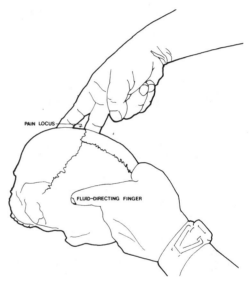

Figure 12 *Treatment of painful suture by fluid direction.*

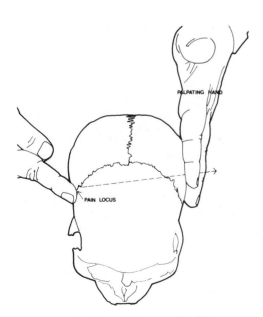

Figure 11 *Technique for locating fluid direction.*

BIBLIOGRAPHY

1. Retzlaff, E.W. Personal communication.
2. Magoun, H.I., Sr. *Osteopathy in the Cranial Field,* Second Edition. Kirksville, Mo.: Journal Printing Company, 1966, p. 179.
3. Upledger, J.E. Integration of acupuncture and manipulation. *Osteopathic Medicine* 2:7 (1977), 18.
4. Academy of Traditional Chinese Medicine. *An Outline of Chinese Acupuncture.* San Francisco: China Books & Periodicals, 1975, p. 175.
5. Frost, E. Personal communication.
6. Warwick, R., and Williams, P.L. (eds.). *Gray's Anatomy,* 35th Edition, Philadelphia: W.B. Saunders Company, 1973, pp. 806-809.
7. Retzlaff, E. W., Mitchell, F.L., Jr., Upledger, J.E., and Biggert, T. Nerve fibers and endings in cranial sutures. *J.A.O.A.* 77 (1978), 474.

Appendix E

Spontaneous Release by Positioning

LAWRENCE HUGH JONES, D.O., Ontario, Ore.*

Discovery of what appears to be a new principle of lesion production has resulted in a simple, easy method of correction without the use of force.

Undoubtedly many osteopathic physicians have observed occasional cases of spontaneous lesion correction. Probably most of them have shrugged and wished that all lesions might be corrected so easily—but that it is a one-in-a-thousand phenomenon and not worth thinking about, just a fortunate combination of influences.

Most osteopathic physicians can remember some case that was seemingly impossible; a case that resisted all their skill, diligence, and ingenuity, and continued to defy their best efforts again and again until only stubbornness kept them from admitting they were stumped. Each visit became a maddening frustration. Suppose that after months the disorder one day spontaneously corrected completely and easily before their eyes.

This background of frustration is included because it furnished the necessary inspiration for 10 years of experimentation.

The ease and effectiveness of this technique and the revolutionary concept it entails are very difficult to believe by osteopathic physicians who have accepted as necessary the use of a certain amount of force to attain a correction on hundreds of thousands of lesions in their regular practices. Yet, demonstrations in seminars in the western states have shown most of the osteopathic physicians attending that the technique is practical for them on their first or second attempt. They are convinced only after feeling it happen under their own fingers or on their own lesions.

BACKGROUND

In the original case a fortunate combination of accidents made the correction possible. A man had had a very severe and painful second lumbar lesion with psoasitis for a long period, and I had been unable to correct it despite maximal efforts. He had complained of being awakened every few minutes during the night by his pain. I was devoting an entire treatment period to finding, if possible, a position of relative comfort which he might use to secure rest without heavy sedation.

We finally found a position which achieved a high degree of comfort, but it was astonishingly extreme. It was unbelievable that such a rigid patient could tolerate, let alone enjoy, such a position. He was nearly rolled into a ball, with the pelvis rotated about 45 degrees and laterally flexed about 30 degrees.

*Reprinted from The D.O., Jan. 1964, pp. 109-116, by permission of the American Osteopathic Association, 212 E. Ohio St., Chicago, IL 60611.

The patient was so well relieved that he was propped up and left in the position while I treated another patient. When I returned and restored him to a normal position, he remained comfortable! Examination revealed an excellent correction of the lesion, with marked improvement in free mobility and two-thirds reduction in pain and tenderness. To accomplish a correction so easily in a case so desperately "impossible" was hardly believable. It was too impressive to be ignored.

Experimentation was begun on other second lumbar lesions. Many were corrected in positions similar to the one that had been effective for the first man. Most of the others responded to minor modifications of the original position. Experimentation seemed relatively safe, because no force was necessary and a position which brought immediate comfort could hardly be construed as an injury. Gradually the time of support in the position of release was reduced from 20 minutes to 10 and then to 5. Success continued down to a period of 90 seconds. Below this time, success was irregular, even though we achieved an excellent position for relief of pain and tenderness in the lesioned joint. It still appears to be the minimum, though probably some skilled technicians will be able to reduce it further.

Success with second lumbar lesions encouraged attempts on other lesions. Some results were gratifying, others disappointing, but little by little it became clear to me that all osteopathic lesions will correct spontaneously in a position of release, and that a large proportion of lesions of a given joint will follow a pattern of position common to other lesions of that joint.

During this time the position of release and comfort was found in a high percentage of the cases to be simply an exaggeration of the abnormal bony relationship found upon examination. This has occurred so consistently that I have accepted it as proof of diagnosis. On the occasions where the two do not agree, I distrust my diagnosis and rely on the position of release as both diagnosis and treatment.

SOME APPARENT PRINCIPLES

Most lesions can be corrected in exaggeration of the diagnosed abnormal bony relationship. Occasionally diagnoses are not clear. We are saved from testing aimlessly by the fact that most lesions of any given joint are likely to follow a pattern. Through the years I have been able to accumulate a list of the more common lesions. In three fourths of the lesions in which the diagnosis was not clear, disorders were found to respond to positioning according to the directions on the list, with minor variations.

This list, which will be presented later, is offered not to be blindly imitated, but as means of saving the busy physician the time-consuming experimentation needed to develop it. He must never lose sight of the principle. The techniques are successful only if they achieve the position of relief of tenderness and pain. If unsure of his diagnosis, he tries the basic positions first. Then, if necessary, he abandons them and learns the effective position by trial and error, secure in the knowledge that there is such a position for each lesioned joint. After a few weeks of practice he will not need to delay long on any lesion.

Can this simple, easy method of correction be possible? How can it be, and yet have escaped the notice of thousands of osteopathic physicians all these years? Yet the first published reference I could find to any similar work done is a statement by Dr. Ira C. Rumney of Kirksville College of Osteopathy, in January 1963.[1] In a summary of forces which can be used to re-establish normal spinal motion, he lists: "Inherent corrective forces of the body—if the patient is properly positioned, his own natural forces may restore normal motion to an area."

The phenomena demonstrated in this work indicate that the lesion formation occurred in a position much more extreme than the position in which we found the lesioned vertebrae upon examination. The patient had no pain in this extreme position. He reported, "It hurt when I started to straighten up." It hurt more as he continued to straighten. Muscles which were relatively relaxed in the extreme position tensed in an effort to splint this lesioned joint from further strain.

Is the muscular tension arranged so as to splint this joint, to prevent it from moving back into its eccentric position? *No!* The muscular tension *resists any motion away from the extreme position in which the lesioning occurred.*

Even the severest lesions will readily tolerate being returned to the position in which lesion formation originally occurred, and only to this position. When the joint is returned to this position, the muscles promptly and gratefully relax. These joints do not cause distress because they are crooked; they are paining because they are being forced to be too straight. This is the mechanism of strain. This protective muscle splinting is the "bind."

The three schematic drawings of joints in Figures 1, 2 and 3 illustrate a normal joint in normal position, a normal joint in extreme position in which lesion formation occurs but not strain, and the joint as found by the physician in lesion and in strain. Muscular tension is not the result of muscle stretching or a reflex splinting to prevent return of the joint to the extreme position. It is the opposite. It is the reflex muscle splinting which *prevents further movements away from the extreme position* where lesion formation occurred.

In Figure 3, muscle "A" is splinted in chronic contraction. Muscle "B," though stretched, is not splinted or contracted. The effect is that the joint may easily move back to the extreme position which brings relief. Any movement away from the extreme position increases the strain and is resisted by increased splinting of muscle "A." To initiate a spontaneous correction, a relaxed patient is positioned so as to return the joint to the extreme position, hold it for 90 seconds, and return the still-relaxed patient to normal.

DISCUSSION

In the light of this knowledge, what happens to some of our concepts of the osteopathic lesion? Could exaggeration of a deformity bring immediate relief to a lesion if the main factor of that lesioning were strain of ligaments or other periarticular tissues or compression of the emerging nerve? It appears likely that exaggeration of

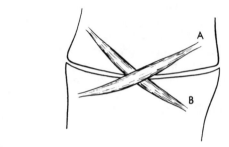

Fig. 1

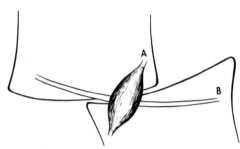

Fig. 2

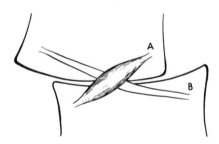

Fig. 3

the deformity would aggravate the pain in either case because of further overstretching of ligaments or compression of nerves. Local edema begins to resorb immediately upon achieving the position of release, but it requires some time. What "released," so that it could start to resorb? I still have no satisfactory explanation. Yet this new knowledge does upset many of the accepted concepts of the mechanism of producing and maintaining factors of the osteopathic lesion.

It would be a tremendous task to check each muscle and ligament involved in an osteopathic lesion to prove this theory.

However, we can reason backwards. The joint is rigid; periarticular tissues are tense. The joint seems to resist all motion. The position of greatest resistance and pain is a position opposite to that of the original abnormality. For instance, a lesion of left lateroflexion resists most violently a bend into right lateroflexion. On the other hand, even the most acute lesion will readily submit to passive movement in exaggeration of the diagnosed lesion, *and in this direction only!*

The physician palpates the tense lesioned area while moving the patient into a position of exaggeration. When he attains the optimum position, there is an almost instantaneous relaxation of tense tissues which is so marked that it is palpable by any osteopathic physician with ordinary skill. At the same time the patient if questioned will report that "you took the pressure off." Localized edema is felt to start to "melt" immediately, but it requires many seconds for the effect to be complete. This perhaps is the factor requiring the 90-second support of the joint in the position of release to effect a correction.

The concept of tissue stasis in lesions seems to be borne out, but what was the instantaneous "catch" that started it, and where? For a long time the theory of deformity of the nucleus pulposus seemed secure. Yet the principles described apply as well to all appendicular lesions as to spinal lesions. Where was the "catch" there? What have we left? Something in or around the joint is "caught."

Exactly what it is, we do not know, but it occurs in a markedly eccentric position and goes into a strain pattern when pulled away from that position. It will correct itself spontaneously if it is supported in the original eccentric position and then is returned, still relaxed, to normal. Once the physician has attained the position of release, no further effort is necessary. Happily back out of the continuous strain it has been suffering, the joint can in 90 seconds restore its own normal function again.

SPECIFIC MYOFASCIAL TRIGGERS

Many patients complain of tenderness remote from the vertebral area. Since my philosophy has always been along the lines of specific lesion for a specific pain, I have always attempted to pin down an association between a certain pain and/or area of acute sensitivity with a specific lesion. But we find that many patients are so vague about the nature and distribution of their pains that from a practicing physician's viewpoint the areas of acute sensitivity prove to be much more reliable. These are the myofascial triggers.

These triggers are a valuable aid to diagnosis for any osteopathic physician, and there are many fairly successful tricks of counterirritation used by some physicians in treatment. In this treatment by use of the position of release they are of inestimable value in eliminating guesswork.

For instance, in lower lumbar lesions it is easy to mistake paravertebral tenderness of a fourth for that of a fifth lumbar lesion; in many instances, tenderness close to the spine may be so mild as to dissuade the operator from giving either diagnosis much credence. On the other hand, their specific trigger points are inches apart and are so sharply sensitive as to remove all doubt of which lesion is the offender. Whereas the vague tension and tenderness near the spinal joint may give a relatively inconclusive manifestation of success in finding the position of release, pain at the trigger point dissolves as if it has suffered a power failure. The sudden definite release is so complete that the uninitiated patient will doubt that you are still probing the right spot. The physician knows his treatment is correct, and the patient also immediately knows.

Some of the triggers and maybe all have been known for many years. Works by Chapman, Travell, Judovich and Bates, and Yoshio Nakatani are extensive. The triggers offered here for your convenience are easily found and are *definitely specific manifestations of specific lesions.* Relief of the trigger point is accomplished only by relieving the causative lesion in the responsible joint.

Though we use the relief of tenderness in the trigger point as evidence of the correct position of release, we are treating not myofascial triggers but spinal lesions. Tension and tenderness near the spinal lesion are relieved simultaneously with relief of the trigger.

SPECIFIC TRIGGERS AND ASSOCIATED LESIONS

Right sacroiliac: Different triggers are usually relieved by different methods (see suggested techniques). The upper trigger is 1 inch from posterior spine of ilium, at 5 o'clock. The middle trigger is near the third sacral foramen, or about 2½ inches from posterior spine, at 7 o'clock. The lower trigger is just lateral to sacral cornu (associated with coccygeal pain and tenderness). The trochanter trigger is on the posterior superior surface of greater trochanter of femur. The pubic trigger is on the superior margin of pubic bone 1½ inches lateral to symphysis. (These last two are used in treating a supine patient.)

Right fifth lumbar: The upper trigger is on the medial margin of ilium near the posterior superior spine. The lower trigger is in the notch just caudad to the posterior superior spine.

Right fourth lumbar: This trigger is about ½ inch posterior to tensor fascia lata and 2 inches caudad to the rim of the ilium.

Right third lumbar: This trigger is 1 to 1½ inches caudad to the anterior superior spine of the ilium or in tensor fascial lata. The posterior third lumbar trigger is a point 2½ inches lateral to the posterior superior iliac spine and 1¾ inches caudad to the iliac crest.

Right second lumbar: One trigger is on the lateral side of the middle of the right inguinal ligament. Another is on the anterior inferior iliac spine.

Right first lumbar: This trigger is ¾ inch below and medial to the anterior superior iliac spine.

Right twelfth thoracic: This trigger is on the inner border of the iliac crest, about 2 inches from anterior superior iliac spine.

Right eleventh thoracic: This trigger is on the inner border of the crest of the ilium in the midaxillary line.

Eighth and ninth flexion lesion: This is associated with tenderness 2 or 3 inches below the xiphoid process, and often with epi-

gastric pain and ileitis. Paravertebral tenderness and pain here is often so slight as to be overlooked.

Third thoracic: This trigger is a point 2½ inches caudad to the spine of the scapula and 1 inch medial to the lateral border of the scapula.

Second thoracic: This is a point ½ inch above the spine of the scapula and 2 inches medial to the acromial process.

Second cervical: This trigger is just beneath the superior nuchal line, 1¼ inches lateral to the midline.

First cervical: The trigger is on the posterior border of the ramus of the mandible, ¾ inch above the angle.

Humerus: Affectations here appear to be actual lesions of the humeral joint, although different ones are often associated with upper thoracic lesions as indicated. Treatment is directed to a position of release in the humeral joint (see suggested techniques). (1) The first trigger is a point on the short head of the biceps 1½ inches below the coracoid process of the scapula (often associated with first thoracic lesion); second is a point about 1 inch posterior to trigger above. (2) Another trigger is at the middle of the deltoid, 1 inch beneath the acromion (usually associated with a second thoracic lesion). (3) Another is on the posterior margin of the deltoid muscle, 1½ inches from the acromial process of the scapula (often associated with third thoracic lesions). (4) Another is deep in the posterior fold of the shoulder near the tendon of the teres major (often associated with fourth thoracic lesions). (5) The circumflex nerve trigger is about 1¼ inches below the spine of the scapula and 3 inches medial to the acromion.

Elbow lesion: Elbow tenderness is on the head of the radius or in the belly of the brachioradialis muscle (tenderness on lateral epicondyle usually is a trigger from first thoracic or first rib). Tenderness on medial epicondyle usually is a trigger from the fourth thoracic or the fourth rib, or a simple extension of the ulno-humeral joint.

BASIS OF SUGGESTED TECHNIQUES

A large proportion of spinal joint lesions

will be found to follow a pattern. The majority of lesions of each joint tend to be lesioned in a position common to that joint. Though there are many atypical lesions that do not conform, the busy physician may save much time by checking out probable positions first. If successful, he has verified his positional diagnosis while making his correction.

However, he will encounter enough a-typical or less common lesions that he will continually find it necessary to abandon the hope of the typical lesion and rely upon his own diagnosis of the position of the lesion. After diagnosing it he will exaggerate the position to the position of release. Occasionally the diagnosis will not be clear, and he will need to search by trial and error. This will not discourage him when he becomes certain that every osteopathic spinal lesion has a position of release and that by finding it he can produce a correction.

Contemplation of the thousands of possible positions may seem overwhelming until we reduce the consideration of the possible positions to their three basic elements. We need to consider only the direction of rotation and/or bend and how much.

1. Rotation can be only to the right (indicated by "R") or to the left (indicated by "L"). These are described according to the direction of rotation the body of the superior vertebra in relation to the body of the inferior vertebra.

2. Bending (use of such words as flexion and extension is avoided because they mean different things to different osteopathic physicians) can be toward any one of 360 degrees, but requirements for use here are only that we bend in a direction within 30 degrees of the ideal direction. Forward or backward bending is considered simultaneously with side bending as one bend, because it is one bend and not two as we are used to thinking of it.

Then, if we imagine our patient to be standing in the center of a large clock face which has been placed face up on the floor and standing so that he faces the mark of 12 o'clock (Fig. 4), he may be considered to bend in the direction of any hour on the clock face. This will be accurate enough for

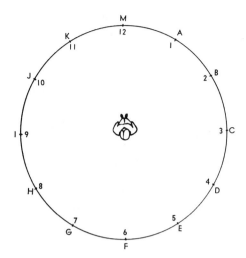

Fig. 4   *Bird's-eye view of a man standing on a clock face.*

effective practical use, though minor modifications may increase the effectiveness. For example, rather than to describe the position of a lesioned joint as right side bending and forward bending, we can say toward 2 o'clock.

To further simplify for the purpose of record keeping, we may substitute a letter for each hour and record a bend toward 2 o'clock as "B," or a bend toward 6 o'clock as "F," and so forth.

3. The amount of bend needed is quite uniform and can easily be learned with practice.

Now, since we have indicated rotation right as "R" and rotation left as "L," we can indicate a fourth lumbar lesion bent to the left side and backward and rotated to the left as "4L-HL." (Note that "M" is used at 12 o'clock rather than "L" to avoid confusion.)

Description of specific suggested techniques will include these symbols to indicate the influence brought to bear on the lesion under discussion.

In most cases the pelvis is thought of as if each side were swinging on the sacrum on a transverse axis. This does not cover oblique bends.

TECHNIQUES

High right ilium: The posterior superior

spine of right is higher cephalad than the left. The patient is prone on the table. Find the trigger point (probably the middle or upper trigger; see section on trigger points). Raise the right thigh, extending the hip; start a little abduction of the thigh, for mid-trigger relief (E). The upper trigger needs no abduction (F); the lower trigger requires a little adduction (G).

Low right ilium: The posterior superior spine is lower on the right. Treat the patient in a supine position, using the trochanter or pubic trigger. The thigh is flexed about 135 degrees on the hip; usually about a 20-degree abduction of the thigh is required, and slight medial turning in of the leg on the thigh.

Right oblique, sacroiliac: The trigger here is on right side of posterior surface of sacrum. (1) Heavy pressure (40 pounds) is applied over the base of sacrum on the left side. (2) Heavy pressure is applied near the apex of the sacrum. (3) Apply pressure as in (1), but over the right side of the base.

Right fifth lumbar: (1) This technique is for the lower trigger. The patient is prone. Find the trigger under posterior superior spine. Hang the patient's right thigh vertically off the side of the table; the doctor holds the leg a few inches below the knee and abducts the leg on thigh moderately (B). (2) For the upper fifth lumbar trigger, the technique is the same except that the pull is on the other leg and side bending is in the opposite direction (J). (See Figure 5.) (3) This technique involves simple rotation, as in fourth lumbar, R or L. (4) This technique is used in lordotic spines. The patient is prone; the doctor stands at the left and places his right foot on the near edge of the table, reaches across, and lifts the patient's right leg onto the doctor's thigh just below patient's knee (GL).

Right fourth lumbar: (1) This is similar to the fifth lumbar upper trigger technique. (2) The patient is prone; the doctor stands at the left side and reaches across to grasp the patient's anterior ilium. He rotates the patient's pelvis about 45 degrees, and leans back so that his body weight does the work (L). (3) This technique is like (4) in fifth lumbar correction.

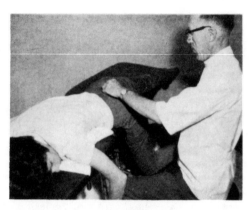

Fig. 5   *A demonstration of the technique used for the upper trigger of the fifth right lumbar vertebra (J).*

Third lumbar: (1) This is opposite of (2) for fourth lumbar (R) correction. (2) This is like (4) for fifth lumbar correction.

Third, fourth, or fifth lumbar with lordosis or definite spondylolisthesis: (1) The patient is in a prone position with the doctor at his left side. The doctor puts his right foot on the table and raises the patient's right leg up about 30 degrees and toward him, until the pelvis is rotated about 30 degrees (GL). For spondylolisthesis, repeat from the opposite side (ER).

Right second lumbar: The patient is in a supine position. Find the trigger point in front of the right ilium near middle of inguinal ligament to the lower end. Bend thighs to a little above vertical, with knees bent. Rotate the pelvis toward the left side of the patient's body, and side bend toward the left to the point of trigger relief (JR). Support the top ilium against excess adduction of the flexed thigh by a forward pull on the top of the ilium.

Right first lumbar, and eleventh and twelfth thoracic: The patient is supine, with a folded pillow beneath the lower lumbar area. In marked antexion, thighs are flexed to about a 45-degree angle with the body. Then the knees are brought slightly to the patient's right and feet slightly toward the patient's left (KL). A variation would be opposite rotation (KR) (Fig. 6).

Right tenth and eleventh thoracic: (1) With the patient prone, the doctor, at the patient's right, grasps the left anterior superior spine by reaching over the right side. He rotates the pelvis to a point of trigger release (about 45 degrees) (R). The trigger here is paravertebral. (2) This technique is like that used for correction of the seventh, eighth, and ninth thoracic, right.

Right seventh, eighth, and ninth thoracic: The patient is prone, arms hanging off the table, and the doctor is at the left side. He raises the patient's right arm up beside his head, holds the arm near the axilla, rotates the upper chest to the right, and side bends to left (RI).

Eighth and ninth flexion lesions: The patient is prone, with a large pillow folded under the lower half of the sternum. The doctor lifts up on either shoulder and rotates (BR or JL) (Fig. 7).

Right fifth and sixth thoracic: (1) This technique is as in seventh, eighth, and ninth thoracic correction. (2) The doctor is on the right side. He reaches across to left shoulder; the patient's right arm is up beside his head, or at least hanging more cephalad, and the left arm is hanging. He pulls the left shoulder back and around the caudad (JL).

Right fourth and second thoracic: The patient is prone, arms hanging. The doctor's hand is placed on the patient's chin and cheek. He bends the neck backward, to the left, and rotates slightly to the right (GR). Variations

include left rotation (GL), and right side bending (ER or EL).

Right third thoracic: Raise the patient's right arm beside the head, rotate, and side bend the head and neck toward the left, letting the head hang partly off the table in flexion of the upper thoracic area. Elevate the right shoulder in posterior direction, with the doctor's arm under the patient's axilla (JL).

Right first thoracic: Extend, side bend, and rotate to the right (DR). This is irregular; it may be necessary to side bend left (HR).

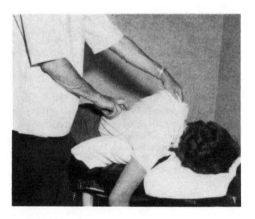

Fig. 7   *A demonstration of forward bending for right eighth and ninth thoracic correction (JL).*

Right eighth cervical: The patient is in a supine position. Mild forward bending, rotation, and side bending away from lesioned side are applied. (Palpate the transverse process in the side of the neck) (JL).

Sixth and seventh cervical: The patient is in a supine position, head off the end of the table. Back bending, side bend away and rotate toward the side of lesion or as indicated by the position of spinous process (GR). For seventh cervical lesions, rotate left (GL).

Fifth cervical: This technique is similar to that for eighth cervical correction except that more forward bending is used; it may be necessary to reverse sides (KL).

Fourth cervical: (1) This area frequently is in either back bending or spondylolisthesis. Lesions are corrected in marked backward

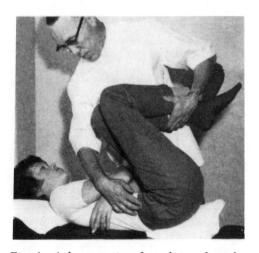

Fig. 6   *A demonstration of a technique for right twelfth thoracic correction (KR).*

bending and slight side bending as indicated. Check progress by the tender transverse process (GR). (2) Use rotation and side bending to the same side without any back bending (IL). Try the opposite if the first attempt fails (CR).

Third cervical: (1) Use side bending and rotation toward the side of the prominent tender spinous process of the second cervical vertebra, with fairly marked forward bending (AL). (2) An alternative is the same except for opposite rotation (AR).

First and second cervical: (1) Correction usually is attained with the patient in marked backward bending and with slight side bending and mild rotation as indicated by diagnosis and comfort (ER or EL) (GR or GL) (Fig. 8). (2) An alternative is marked rotation as indicated, with no bending (L) or (R).

Shoulder joint: Frozen shoulder may be eased beyond aid obtained by upper thoracic and lower cervical corrections by finding an arm position which relieves the tender spot in the shoulder (see trigger points). Shoulder stiffness with triggers 2, 3, and 4 are relieved in the prone position with the elbow behind the midline with abduction varying from 80 to 0 degrees (Fig. 9). Trigger 1 usually is relieved in a supine position with the upper arm vertical and the forearm halfway between cephalad position and across the shoulder girdle. Ten pounds of pressure are applied downward

through upper arm and shoulder. Both may be further improved by traction in a caudad direction, usually with 30-degree abduction, occasionally adducted, across chest following corrections above.

Acromio-clavicular: The upper arm is fully abducted and the forearm cephalad.

Elbow, right radial head: Usually supination is used; occasionally some abduction or adduction are necessary. (Tenderness of the lateral epicondyle indicates probably a first thoracic or first rib lesion.)

Wrist, thumb, and other fingers: All can be easily relieved by finding tender spots and locating the position of release. The thumb is usually bent backward and rotated. Tenderness is near the metacarpophalangeal joint or the carpometacarpal joint.

Knee: The medial meniscus is nearly always relieved by internal rotation of the extended leg on the thigh, usually with slight flexion and adduction (Fig. 10). The lateral meniscus usually requires external rotation.

Feet: ankle sprain: There is tenderness ½ inch below the malleolus, usually a little anteriorly. This usually is relieved by inversion of the foot with external rotation, occasionally by eversion or dorsiflexion. An ankle sprain is an osteopathic lesion and can be treated in this manner, giving much relief.

Calcaneus: There is tenderness beneath the proximal head; this usually is corrected

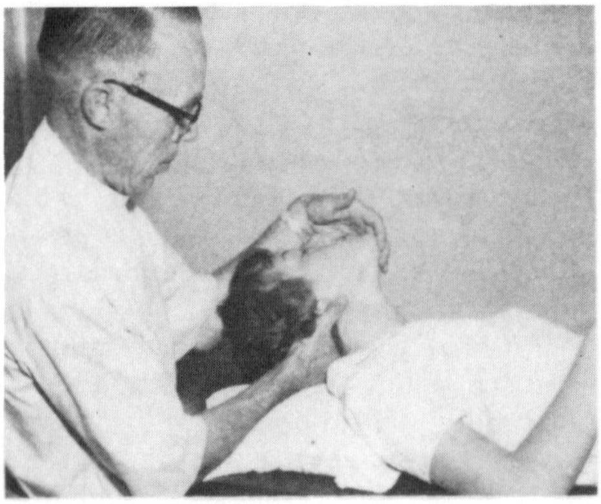

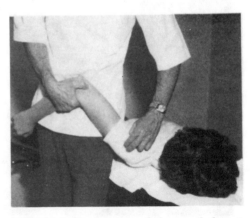

Fig. 8   *A demonstration of technique for correction of a right first cervical lesion (EL).*

Fig. 9   *A demonstration of the second thoracic shoulder reflex. The upper arm is at 8 o'clock, in 60-degree abduction, and under slight traction.*

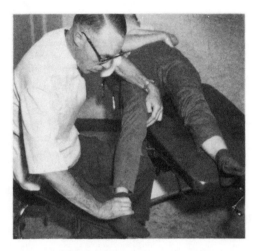

Fig. 10 *A demonstration of correction of the right medial meniscus lesion. Internal rotation, adduction, and slight flexion are applied.*

in eversion or outward rotation of heel on foot.

Cuboid: There is tenderness beneath it. There is eversion of the lateral side of the foot with moderate dorsiflexion.

Navicular: Inversion and a little internal rotation of front of foot, with some dorsiflexion.

Fibula, proximal head: (1) One method is similar to the treatment for ankle sprain. (2) It may be held forward by thumb pressure.

Bunion: There is tenderness at lateral sesamoid, which is relieved by flexion, abduction, and eversion of the great toe until sesamoid tenderness is relieved.

Right ribs: (1) The patient sits with his back to the doctor. The doctor's left foot is on the table, with a pillow on the doctor's knee. The patient drapes his left arm over the pillow, tilts his pelvis to the left, puts his feet at the right side of his hips. The position is marked right side bending, moderate forward bending, and right rotation. It takes 1 to 2 minutes to achieve the necessary relaxation. The position is (BR), or rarely, the opposite rotation (BL). (2) The patient lies on his left side, with his thighs flexed 90 degrees and his right arm hanging behind him. The doctor stands behind and holds the patient's head forward, side bent, and rotated right, and presses caudad on the right shoulder (BR).

Fifth, sixth, seventh, and eighth ribs: Use a folded pillow under left shoulder.

GENERAL RULES

1. Treat "hot" lesions first.

2. Straighten the patient out slowly enough that he can remain relaxed. He will resist and tense if rushed.

3. Check for relief of pain after correction, if only to demonstrate its absence to the patient.

4. An especially "dry" lesion will sometimes be tender after correction. A minute's traction will ease it.

5. Patients will try to help you. Don't let them.

SUMMARY

Osteopathic spinal and appendicular lesions occur in positions more eccentric than that found by the examining physician. They are in a state of strain because the natural position of the patient holds him away from the eccentric position. The strain is relieved by exaggerating the deformity found upon examination. The lesions will release and correct spontaneously if held relaxed in the exaggerated position for 1½ minutes. The correction itself is restful and comfortable.

Grateful acknowledgment is given to many who have contributed techniques or ideas, in particular: Harry Davis, D.O., deceased; G.E. Holt, D.O., Pendleton, Ore.; Hugh Barr, M.D., Penticton, B.C.; Annabelle F. Thorne, D.O., San Francisco, Calif.; Margaret W. Barnes, D.O.; Carmel, Calif.; Carl L. Fagan, D.O., Monterey, Calif.; James E. Spencer, D.O., Palo Alto, Calif.; Melvin Hennigson, D.D.S., Hayward, Calif., Rollin E. Becker, D.O., Dallas, Texas; Harold V. Hoover, D.O., Tacoma, Wash.; T.J. Ruddy, D.O., Los Angeles, Calif.; Harold S. Saita, D.O. Vancouver, B.C.; and Paul K. Theobald, D.O., Oakland, Calif.

REFERENCE

1. Rumney, I.C.: Structural diagnosis and manipulative therapy. J. Osteopathy 70:21-33, Jan. 1963; D.O. 4:135-142, Sept. 1963.

Appendix F

Self-Induction of C.R.I. Still Point Using Tandem Tennis Balls

JAMES NELSON RILEY, Ph.D.*

THE DEVICE

Two tennis balls (or racquet balls) are tethered in tandem so that they are touching one another. This can be done by putting holes through the balls on a straight line and tying them together with heavy string or leather ties. Alternatively, the two balls can be placed in the toe of a sock which is then knotted tightly. In order to assure that the balls stay in contact with each other, place the first sock inside another sock which is also tied tightly.

INSTRUCTIONS

Recline on your back, on the floor or upon a sofa or bed. Place the device under your head so that the entire weight of your head rests on the two balls. They should be symmetrical with respect to the midline. They are placed about midway "up" the back of the head in the following location: At the top of the occipital bone (but below the lambdoidal suture). This is in a slight depression in the skull just above the slight bony prominence, which is in turn just above the attachment of the main neck muscles. The level is slightly above that of the ear openings.

Allow the weight of your head to rest flexibly upon the device for 15 minutes. Relax comfortably. You may shift position slightly in order to maintain symmetry and comfort, but do so gently and gradually. *Repeat daily.*

THEORY

The craniosacral rhythmical impulse ("C.R.I.") is the rhythmical mobile activity of the craniosacral physiological system. The structures of the craniosacral system are organized around the meningeal membranes, and the craniosacral system is intimately related to the function of the nervous system (most directly the brain and spinal cord), the musculoskeletal system (most directly the cranium, spine, and pelvis), related fascia, and other systems. Induction of momentary "still points" in the craniosacral rhythmical impulse is an effective technique for mobilizing the craniosacral system's inherent self-correcting abilities, which in turn can have profound beneficial effects throughout the body.

INDICATIONS

This is a good "shotgun" technique for enhancing tissue and fluid motion, especially relaxing connective tissues throughout the body, and for restoring flexibility of autonomic nervous system response. It is beneficial for acute and chronic musculo-

---

*Reprinted with permission of the author.

skeletal lesions, including degenerative arthritis. It can lower fever as much as 4° F. It can reduce cerebral or pulmonary congestion, or dependent edema. It has been used to improve auto-immune disease, autistic behavior of children, and anxiety.

This technique can benefit most individuals to some degree, and is rarely harmful.

CONTRAINDICATIONS

The only contraindications are in situations in which even slight and transient increases in intracranial pressure are to be avoided: impending cerebrovascular aneurism or hemorrhage—as in acute stage of stroke or cranial trauma.

Appendix G

Diagnosis and Treatment of Temporoparietal Suture Head Pain

JOHN E. UPLEDGER, D.O., FAAO, Associate Professor, ERNEST W. RETZLAFF, Ph.D., Professor, Department of Biomechanics, College of Osteopathic Medicine and JON D. VREDEVOOGD, F.F.A., Assistant Professor, College of Human Ecology, Michigan State University, East Lansing, Michigan*

Recent evidence related to the microanatomy of the cranial suture offers the basis for a newly postulated mechanism for recurrent head pain and for mild to moderate cerebral dysfunction. A noncomplicated approach to the diagnosis and treatment of these problems is described.

MECHANISM AND FUNCTIONAL ANATOMY

A complete understanding of the described techniques of diagnosis and treatment requires an appreciation of the recently illuminated microarchitecture of the temporoparietal suture; a review of the gross anatomic features of the suture itself; and of the temporalis muscle, its function, and the bones to which it attaches.

Traditionally, anatomists have taught that the sutural articulations of the adult human are fused and hence immovable. Recent histologic work done by us[1,2] on adult human sutural material would contradict this view. The specimens studied were taken from living adult skulls at the time of neurosurgical craniotomy. Hence, these tissues studied resemble more closely the in vivo circumstance.

By the use of modified staining techniques[3], the authors have been able to demonstrate the presence of viable myelinated and unmyelinated nerve fibers, nerve receptor endings, a potentially functional vascular network, and collagen elastic fiber complexes within the adult human cranial suture. We have also demonstrated that these structures frequently penetrate the sutural bone margins and traverse from the diploe into the suture and vice versa. There is also evidence to suggest that some of the intrasutural vascular and neural structures may arise from the intracranial meninges (Fig. 1).

The significance of these findings is simply that now the human cranial suture may be (and in fact must be) considered as a functional anatomical complex capable, therefore, of dysfunction resultant to various unbalances, stresses, and traumas.

Since the suture is now known to possess the neural structures necessary for nerve reflex activity, sensory input into the nervous system, and motor activity, it becomes apparent that a distortion of the functional relationships between the sutural osseous boundaries may produce abnormal neurogenic activity as well as intrasutural ischemia. Either one or both of these conditions may result in local as well as referred pain. Further, our conjecture is that although evidence is scant at present, the intracranial vascular delivery system may be influenced by neurogenic reflex mechan-

Reprinted from Osteopathic Medicine, July 1978, pp. 19-26, by permission of Arthur Retlaw & Associates, Inc., Suite 570, 1000 Skokie Blvd., Wilmette, IL 60091, and by permission of the authors.

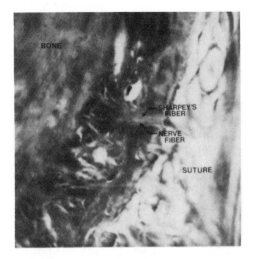 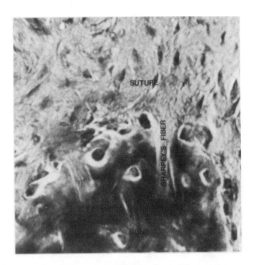

Figure 1   *Photomicrographs of human cranial bone and suture showing penetrating Sharkey's fibers. Photograph on left demonstrates how sensory nerve fibers accompany the Sharkey's fibers. Photograph on right stained by protangol silver-gelative method. Photomicrograph on left stained by Masson's acid fuscin-aniline blue connective tissue method.*

isms that possess intrasutural stimulus receptors.

In view of the aforesaid findings, it seems obvious that the restoration of sutural mobility is desirable. Several mechanisms which underlie sutural dysfunction are possible. One—which has been almost completely overlooked—is hypertonus or contracture of the temporalis muscle. This muscle is frequently and chronically contracted in situations of increased emotional stress, dental malocclusion, and/or temporomandibular joint dysfunction, among other things.

Consideration of the anatomy of the temporalis muscle shows that during its contracted state it is capable of producing compression of the temporoparietal suture.

The insertional attachments of the temporalis muscle are from the ramus of the coronoid process and from the anterior border of the ramus of the mandible. The muscle arises from the floor of the temporal fossa and from the temporal fascia. It can be seen in Figure 2 that the temporal fossa extends superior to the temporoparietal suture and, therefore, that contraction of the temporalis muscle does, in fact, cause

the parietal bone to move in an inferior direction thereby producing a compression of the temporoparietal suture contents. The potential results of this sutural compression have been discussed earlier.

The anatomy of this suture is such that temporalis muscle contraction will produce a gliding motion of the parietal bones' sutural surface inferiorly after the superior motion of the mandible is effectively resisted by the approximation of the upper against the lower molar teeth or by the surfaces of the mandibular ramus coming into opposition with the roof of the mandibular fossa of the temporal bone.

The bony surfaces of the temporoparietal suture are beveled and grooved in such a way that a sutural shearing force is generated by temporalis muscle contracture (Fig. 3).

This shear may longitudinally stress the collagen (Sharkey's) fibers that appear to be innervated. It may also reduce the crosssutural physical dimensions and, therefore, produce intrasutural pressure ischemia, as well as disrupt normal neurogenic reflex activity resulting from pressure stimulation of receptors. It may interfere with normal nerve fiber conduction as well.

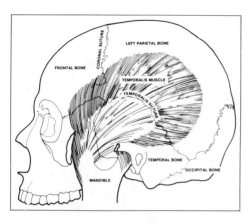

Figure 2   *Temporalis muscle attachment.*

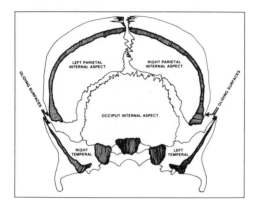

Figure 3   *Coronal section: temporoparietal suture bevel.*

DIAGNOSIS AND TREATMENT

The diagnosis of symptoms (head pain-cerebral dysfunction) resulting from dysfunction of the temporoparietal suture is usually straightforward.

Sutural compression when exaggerated, will quickly increase symptom severity if the examination is done during an exacerbation. If the patient's condition is quiescent during the examination, the symptom complex can often be produced in a matter of minutes.

The examination technique is done with the patient comfortably in the supine position. The physician should be seated above the patient's head with the forearms and elbows comfortably resting on the examin-

ation table beside and superior to the patient's head. The physician then makes finger contact with the tissues immediately overlying the inferior posterior borders of the mandibular rami bilaterally. A bilaterally equal, superiorly-directed force is then applied to the mandibular rami (Fig. 4) so that the expression of force carries through the temporomandibular joints causing the temporal bones to move slightly in a superior direction. This force stresses the temporoparietal sutures bilaterally. The force is initiated gently and is slowly increased until the patient reports either an increase in the present symptoms or the onset of their familiar symptom pattern. If this result occurs, we consider that the diagnosis is confirmed.

Next, the physician must consider the causes of temporoparietal sutural dysfunction. A visual examination of the posterior molars will offer evidence either for or against dental malocclusion. (Consultation with a dentist may be in order at this juncture.)

The tonus of the temporalis muscles should be evaluated by palpation. A fibrous texture and extraordinary tissue firmness coupled with an apparent wearing down of the molar surfaces is supportive of chronic temporalis muscle hypertonus most often resulting from emotional stress or repressed anger.

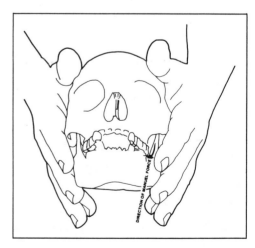

Figure 4   *Physician hand placement for technique to exacerbate symptom.*

Temporomandibular joint dysfunction is best diagnosed by palpation and observation as the mandible is put through its range of motion. Primary treatment must be directed toward the cause of the abnormal condition of the temporalis muscle be it emotional, dental, or temporomandibular joint.

Often the primary cause is no longer in existence; however, the physiologic state of the temporoparietal suture has been so disrupted by previous events that it has become immobilized in an abnormal anatomicophysiologic state of compressed immobility. In this circumstance, a simple mobilizing procedure may only require a few repetitions. If there is a continuing cause for the sutural dysfunction, temporary relief of symptoms can usually be obtained by the use of one or all of the therapeutic techniques described below.

OSTEOPATHIC MANIPULATIVE TECHNIQUE TO RELIEVE TEMPOROPARIETAL SUTURE DYSFUNCTION

After the diagnostic temporoparietal suture compression technique the gentle pressure is continued until the tissues are perceived to relax or soften. This phenomenon probably occurs because of neurogenic fatigue with secondary reduction in tissue tonus. The palms of the hands can be used to determine when temporalis muscle relaxation occurs.

After this change in tissue tonus, gentle traction is applied over the superficial surfaces of the mandibular rami bilaterally. This traction is extremely gentle and incorporates a balancing effort on the part of the physician. It is directed inferiorly following the direction of least resistance. The technique is aimed at decompressing the temporomandibular joints, the temporoparietal sutures, and at stretching the temporalis muscles by traction. Gentleness is the rule. If the physician perceives a contractile response to his traction from the tissues the efforts are too vigorous and will be self-defeating. There are limits of tractional force within which tissues can be gently stretched and which are below the contrac-

tile reflex threshold. It is within this range that this treatment technique can be effectively applied.

The same technique will effectively assist in the treatment of temporomandibular joint dysfunction.

TRANSCUTANEOUS NEEDLE STIMULATION FOR THE TREATMENT OF TEMPOROPARIETAL SUTURE DYSFUNCTION

Gentle palpation of the involved suture will usually reveal localized areas of tenderness along its course. The transcutaneous insertion of a disposable 27-gauge hypodermic needle through the scalp into the subcutaneous tissues immediately over the tender area will almost invariably normalize the sutural dysfunction. The needle should be inserted at approximately a 30° angle to the scalp surface along a line parallel to the direction of the suture. Because of the reciprocal innervation principles that seem effective in all parts of the body, these needles should always be inserted bilaterally. Aseptic techniques should, of course, be employed.

If temporomandibular joint dysfunction is present, bilateral transcutaneous needling immediately over the tender areas will prove to be a valuable adjunct. Needles should be left in place at least 5 minutes or until pain is relieved.

MANDIBULAR FULCRUM TECHNIQUE FOR TEMPOROPARIETAL SUTURE DYSFUNCTION

Another effective treatment technique makes use of two rolls of gauze or other suitable material. The rolls should be about ¼ inch to ⅜ inch in diameter. They are placed between the upper and lower teeth bilaterally at about the region of the second molar (Fig. 5). A gentle force is then applied manually in a superior direction on the anterior inferior aspect of the mandible. The gauze rolls act as fulcrums and the mandibular rami as levers which apply decompressive tractional force to the temporomandibular joints and to the temporoparietal sutures. The force applied is light

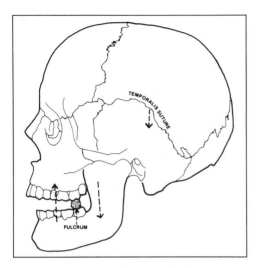

Figure 5   *Fulcrum placement for decompression of temporoparietal suture and temporomandibular joint.*

so that a contraction response is not stimulated.

Patients can be taught this technique as a method of self-help. The patient can usually learn to judge accurately the amount of force to be applied. They can easily learn to discern when their own tissues are changing from relaxed to contracted states.

REFERENCES

1. Retzlaff, E., Mitchell, F., Upledger, J., Biggert, T: Aging of cranial sutures. *Anat Rec* 190:520, 1978.
2. Retzlaff, E., Mitchell, F., Upledger, J., Biggert, T., Vredevoogd, J.: Temporalis Muscle Action in Parietotemporal Suture Compression. Presented at 22nd Annual Research Convention of American Osteopathic Association, Chicago, 1978.
3. Retzlaff, E., Fontaine, J.: Reciprocal inhibition as indicated by a differential staining reaction. *Science* 131:104-105, 1960.

Appendix H

Roentgen Findings in the Craniosacral Mechanism

PHILIP E. GREENMAN, D.O., FAAO, Kenmore, New York*

Although the craniosacral mechanism has been of great interest to the osteopathic profession, a search of the literature failed to yield many reports of the x-ray appearance of altered cranial structure. This article describes efforts to develop a method of identifying altered craniosacral mechanics and of correlating the findings with clinical observations. Good correlation was found between roentgenographic findings and clinical observations made independently by a physician schooled in the cranial concept of osteopathy.

The craniosacral mechanism has been the subject of much study, much controversy, and much interest on the part of the osteopathic profession. Since the first description of the application of osteopathic theory and technique to the cranial field by Sutherland,[1] there have been many devoted students and advocates as well as many skeptics and degraders. However, throughout the history of the osteopathic profession a dedication to the premise that body function is related to normal body structure has been axiomatic. The value of physical palpation and manipulation in diagnosis and treatment has played an important part in establishing the distinct contribution of the osteopathic profession. Throughout its history, numerous x-ray techniques have been developed to assist the clinician in detecting alterations of structure and improving his ability to return the structure to normal. The osteopathic profession can proudly acknowledge its development and use of the postural x-ray examination of the lumbar spine and pelvis in clinical practice.

My interest in the utilization of x-ray examination of the skull and lower part of the back as a diagnostic aid to the practicing clinician of the science and art of cranial osteopathy was first stimulated at the Buffalo Osteopathic Clinic in the middle 1950s. Dr. Edith Dovesmith had patients under this type of care and requested that x-ray examinations be made of the skull and lower part of the back of these patients to obtain any information possible.

A review of the osteopathic and allopathic literature yields few reports by authors who have studied the x-ray appearance of the altered structure of the cranium, although it has been intimately and intricately described by those schooled and accomplished in the cranial concept of osteopathic theory. Weaver[2-4] contributed an extensive series of papers in the middle 1930s and provided a basis for the contributions of other workers[5-7] in a symposium on the plastic basicranium, in which occasional references to series of x-ray studies were made. There was, however, no report of a

*Reprinted from The Journal of the American Osteopathic Association, Vol. 70, September 1970, pp. 24-35, by permission of the American Osteopathic Association, 212 E. Ohio St., Chicago, IL 60611.

series of cases and no description of technique utilized. White[7] stated that "special technique is required for the making of these x-ray studies" and commented:

In our second annual symposium planned to be given here next year at this time, we hope to have one paper devoted exclusively to the technique of x-ray study of the plastic base.

Unfortunately, there has been no subsequent report in the literature.

Kimberly[8] did utilize a basilar view (submentovertical) of the skull as a diagnostic aid in the treatment of the cranium in newborn and older infants. Magoun[9] raised the question of the practicability of x-ray study in confirming the position of some of the cranial structures, particularly the temporal bone.

In the past several years, I have done additional work in cooperation with Dr. Dovesmith in an attempt to develop a method of identification of altered craniosacral mechanics to substantiate the findings of the clinician and to assist the clinician in the treatment of patients afflicted with abnormalities in this mechanism. Since there are no documented guidelines for this type of study, it has been necessary to devise some new and adapt some old techniques in the roentgen study of the skull.

TERMINOLOGY OF LESION PATTERNS

The area to which maximum attention has been directed is that of the sphenoid and basioccipital bones. The terminology to be used is that developed by the proponents of the cranial osteopathic concept.[9] The abnormalities described therein, to be called lesions, are those of flexion, extension, torsion, side-bending rotation, strain or displacement (vertical or lateral), compression, and interosseous lesion. From the beginning of this work, most of the attention was directed toward four lesion patterns, namely, those of flexion, extension, torsion, and side-bending rotation. With increased experience and study, the conclusion has been reached that an occasional diagnosis of lateral and/or vertical strain and of interosseous lesion may be made.

The lesion patterns to be considered are shown in Figs. 1, 2, and 3.

X-RAY TECHNIQUE

For the purpose of this study, x-ray films of the skull, lumbar spine, and pelvis, and, in most instances, of the upper cervical spine, notably the atlas and axis, were used.

The skull was examined in the anteroposterior (AP), posteroanterior (PA), lateral, occipital (Towne), Waters, and submentovertical projections, the standard radiographic technique being used at a 36-inch target-to-film distance.

The lumbar spine and pelvis were studied in the anteroposterior and lateral projections with the patient erect. These were supplemented by oblique projections and an angle study of the sacroiliac joints. As the work progressed, it was found to be helpful also to incorporate the open-mouth projection of the atlas axis and condylar parts of the occiput in the study.

Great care was exercised in positioning the patient so that accurate projections could be obtained for purposes of measurement. A physician aware of the importance of this positioned all patients. It is possible to obtain films of satisfactory quality and detail with regard to positioning for purposes of measurement without the use of a restraining device, but, for re-evaluation of the changes in skull patterns after treatment, it would be advantageous to have a device for exact repositioning of the patient.

All studies included in this work demonstrated normal vascular and sutural markings in normal diploe with no gross organic abnormalities. The usual interpretation of the studies utilized would be "normal."

FILM MEASUREMENT

1. Angle of the base of the skull (Fig. 4). In the lateral projection, an angle is drawn between the nasion (point 1), the tuberculum sellae turcicae (point 2), and the anterior margin of the foramen magnum (point 3). The normal angle here has been variously stated, but in my experience it has been 130 ± 2 degrees. Measurement of this angle is not entirely satisfactory because of the difficulty of ascertaining accurately the

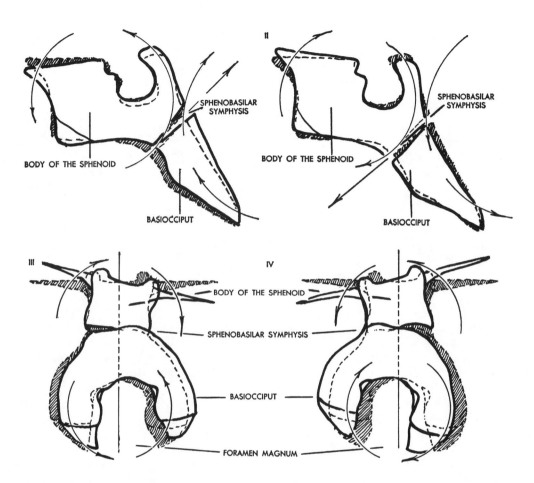

Fig. 1. *(I). Flexion. Viewed from the side, flexion of both sphenoid and occiput (increase of the dorsal convexity) results in elevation of the sphenobasilar symphysis towards the vertex. The deviation from the neutral position is shown in the shaded areas. (II). Extension of both sphenoid and occiput is just the reverse. (III). Torsion. Viewed from above, left torsion of the sphenobasilar symphysis (greater wing and basisphenoid move cephalad on the left while the basiocciput and condylar part move caudad on the same side). (IV). Right torsion of the sphenobasilar symphysis is just the opposite.*[9] (Copyright by Harold I. Magoun, Sr., D.O., Executive Vice president, Sutherland Cranial Teaching Foundation.)*

anterior margin of the foramen magnum, but it does serve as an index of the flexion or extension of the sphenobasilar junction. When the measurement is considered with the over-all appearance of the skull in its anteroposterior and superior-to-inferior diameters, a diagnosis of flexion or extension pattern of the sphenobasilar junction can be made (flexion being indicated by a more than normally acute angle and extension by a more obtuse angle). This finding is correlated with the cephalic index,[10] which

is defined as the percentage relation of the breadth to the length of the skull and can be calculated by the formula

$$CI = B/L \times 100$$

where CI is the cephalic index, B, breadth, and L, length. The skull is mesocephalic (normal) when the CI is between 75 and 80; brachycephalic (short) when it is more than 80; and dolichocephalic (long) when it is less than 75.

2. Anteroposterior measurement (Fig. 5). A midline point of reference (line *AB*) is first ob-

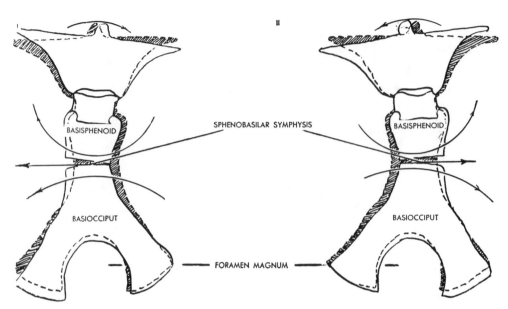

Fig. 2. *(I). Sidebending rotation viewed from above. In sidebending rotation to the left the sphenobasilar symphysis angulates to the left and moves caudad on that side. (II). In right sidebending rotation just the opposite occurs. The position of the bones in neutral is shaded.*[9] (Copyright by Harold I. Magoun, Sr., D.O., Executive Vice President, Sutherland Cranial Teaching Foundation.)

tained by drawing a line from the vertex of the skull (point 1) through the nasion (point 2) to the midpoint between the condylar parts of the occiput (point 3). This line usually carries through the odontoid process of the axis and through the spinous processes of the cervical spine, although these are not used as points of reference.

Horizontal lines are drawn across the following anatomic landmarks: the tuberculum sellae turcicae (line *CD*) (superior aspect); the horizontal base of the squama occipitalis (line *EF*), and the condylar parts of the occiput (line *GH*) (inferior aspect). These horizontal lines run approximately perpendicular to the midline of reference. Protractor measurements of the angles thus formed are made to determine if, in fact, there is variation of the horizontal lines from the true horizontal, and determination is thereby made of the declination of the structure measured. A "high" and a "low" side are recorded.

3. Side of convexity. From the midline perpendicular, measurements to contralateral points of the temporal and parietal bones

are made. The points found farthest from the midline are interpreted as being on the side of convexity. It should be noted that the overall appearance of the skull many times shows an obvious pattern. Film measurement only substantiates the diagnosis in these instances, but in many instances is necessary to establish the pattern diagnosis.

4. Atlas rotation (Fig. 6). Because observations on the relation of the atlas to the occipital condyles in varying patterns aroused interest, it was found valuable to utilize a technique of determining the rotation of the atlas.[11] Measurement is made of the relative width of each lateral mass of the atlas (*A*), to determine which is larger. Owing to the magnification factor, the wider side is the one lying anterior to its fellow. Allowance must be made for asymmetric development. In addition, the space between the medial margin of the lateral masses of the atlas and the odontoid process on each side (*B*) also is measured, and the side in which the atlas is closer to the odontoid is considered to be the anterior lateral

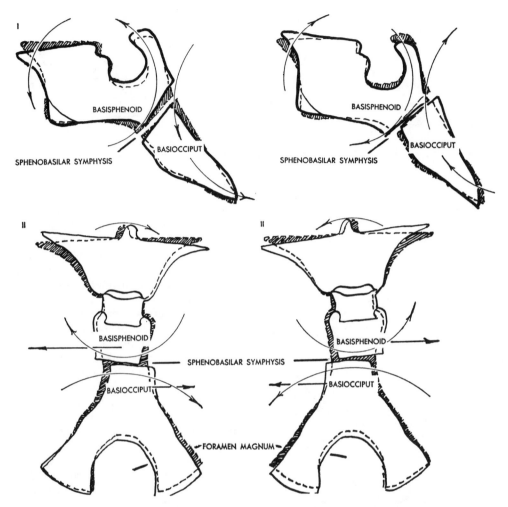

Fig. 3. *(I). Vertical strain. Viewed from the side the sphenobasilar symphysis has been strained, or displaced before ossification, with the basisphenoid moving cephalad (flexion) and the basiocciput moving caudad (extension) or vice versa. Both bones rotate about parallel transverse axes in the same direction. The lesion is named from the position of the basisphenoid: vertical strain or displacement with the sphenoid high, etc. (II). Lateral strain. Viewed from above the sphenobasilar symphysis has been strained or displaced with the basisphenoid moving to one side and the basiocciput to the other. Both bones sidebend about parallel vertical axes in the same direction. The lesion is named from the position of the basisphenoid: lateral strain with the sphenoid to the right, etc.*[9] (Copyright by Harold I. Magoun, Sr., D.O., Executive Vice President, Sutherland Cranial Teaching Foundation.)

mass of the atlas. An attempt is made to coordinate these findings with the position of the atlas demonstrated in the Waters and submentovertical views of the skull. It has been my experience that in almost all cases the atlas assumes an anterior position on the side in which the occiput of the skull is found to be low.

ROENTGEN DIAGNOSIS

By the previously described x-ray techniques, an effort was made to identify the lesions described in a preceding section.

For the determination of flexion, the diagnosis is made on the composite impression of the angle of the base of the skull, the

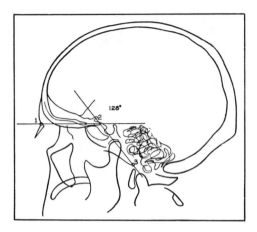

Fig. 4. *Measurement of the angle of the base of the skull.*

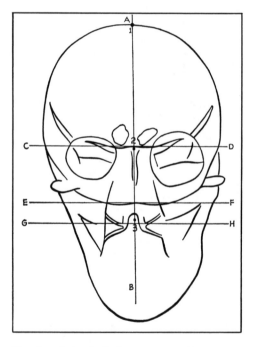

Fig. 5. *Anteroposterior measurement.*

cephalic index, and the reduction of the anteroposterior diameter of the skull. It is believed that this diagnosis can be made roentgenographically if the angle of the base of the skull is 128 degrees or less, the cephalic index is greater than 81, and the overall impression of the skull shows foreshortening of the anteroposterior diameter.

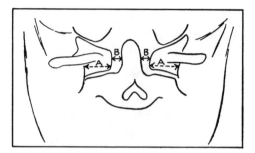

Fig. 6. *Measurement of atlas rotation.*

For the diagnosis of an extension pattern, the criteria are the opposite of those for flexion. That is, if the angle of the base of the skull is 132 degrees or more, the cephalic index is 74 or less, and the ratio of the superior-inferior diameter of the skull to the anteroposterior diameter is decreased, a diagnosis of extension is made.

For a diagnosis of sphenobasilar torsion, it is necessary to ascertain that one side of the sphenoid bone is higher than the other and that one side of the occiput is lower than the other, with a high sphenoid and a low occiput occurring on the same side. A diagnosis of sphenobasilar torsion is made on skull films, the high side of the sphenoid being demonstrated on line *CD* (Fig. 5) and the low side of the occiput demonstrated on lines *EF* and *GH*. It is unusual to find a specific side of convexity when the skull is of this particular pattern.

The side-bending pattern of the sphenobasilar junction is seen when the low side of the occiput is on the same side of the skull as the low side of the sphenoid bone. When these findings are noted on lines *CD, EF,* and *GH,* and substantiated by film measurement showing the side of convexity of the skull to be on the same side, a diagnosis of side-bending of the sphenobasilar junction is made.

It is much more difficult to demonstrate roentgenographically the criteria necessary for diagnosis of lateral strain at the sphenobasilar junction than the other lesions aforementioned. It appears, however, that this diagnosis is suggested by clear visualization of the sphenobasilar junction on the submentovertical film. The axis of the osseous sphenobasilar junction is well demonstrated in this projection. By observing the relation of the axis of the basioccipital bone and the axis of the sphenoid bone, represented on the film by the sphenoidal sinus, it may be determined whether the axes are continuous. If the axis of the sphenoid bone is demonstrated to be to one side or the other of the axis of the occiput and if it is possible to demonstrate in the same view that the skull is quadrilateral, the diagnosis of lateral strain at the sphenobasilar junction can be made. The finding of quadrilateral skull is demonstrated when the long axis of the right frontal to the left occipital bone is of different length than the axis from the left frontal to the right occipital bone. This diagnosis is difficult. It is believed, however, that these two findings will substantiate the criteria for lateral strain at the sphenobasilar junction.

To identify vertical strain at the sphenobasilar junction is extremely difficult, because on conventional lateral roentgenograms there is considerable overlapping of bones other than the sphenoid and basilar bones, and these are difficult to demonstrate in this projection. Occasionally it is possible to demonstrate well both the sphenoid and the basioccipital bone in the lateral projection, and if the long axes of each are not continuous, one might hypothesize the presence of vertical strain. This area is much easier to demonstrate in children prior to the development of the mastoid process. Tomography with a midline sagittal cut could be most helpful in identifying changes in this area. To date, no studies along this line have been attempted.

Combinations of the abnormalities just described also occur and are diagnosed when the criteria for flexion or extension are present in a skull wherein the criteria for side-bending or torsion also are present. In practice, it appears that combination patterns are as common as single lesions.

Table 1 shows the lesion patterns demonstrated in 25 consecutive patients in whom the x-ray techniques just described were carried out.

In addition, the relation of the atlas to the occiput was determined in each patient by the criteria previously described (Fig. 5). The following observations were made:

Atlas anterior on side of low occiput 10
Atlas anterior on side of high occiput 3
No atlas rotation 12

CLINICAL CORRELATION

For 10 of the 25 patients studied, it was possible to obtain an independent clinical evaluation by a physician schooled in the cranial osteopathic concept. There was correlation between clinical and x-ray diagnosis in seven of these and disagreement in three. In two of these three the lesion was diagnosed as torsion by x-ray appearance and side-bending by clinical appearance. In the third, x-ray appearance was that of left side-bending, and the clinical appearance was that of right side-bending.

Owing to the difficulty in correlating clinical and roentgen observations in the first two cases mentioned, a review of the x-ray appearance of the pattern was made, and an interesting discovery was made. In both cases, there was marked asymmetry in

TABLE 1. CRANIAL LESIONS IN 25 PATIENTS		
Flexion		2
Extension		0
Torsion		3
Left	1	
Right	2	
Side-bending		7
Left	3	
Right	4	
Side-bending & flexion		4
Left	0	
Right	4	
Side-bending & extension		1
Left	0	
Right	1	
Torsion & flexion		5
Left	2	
Right	3	
Side-bending & lateral strain		1
Side-bending, lateral strain & flexion		1
None		1

the region of the superior orbital fissure. Since the superior orbital fissure is formed by the lesser and greater wings of the sphenoid bone, asymmetry of the sphenoid must be present. From the clinical point of view, the diagnosis of sphenoid position is taken from the great wing, whereas the roentgen view of the sphenoid is taken across the tuberculum sellae turcicae (line CD) basically through the root of the lesser wing. Therefore, when there is asymmetry at the sphenoid, lack of correlation of clinical and x-ray diagnosis is to be expected. Of further interest is the fact that in embryologic development of the sphenoid, the body and lesser wings form in one part and the great wing and pterygoids develop in another part.[12] It might be hypothesized that the finding of asymmetric sphenoidal development with asymmetric superior orbital pressure might be the result of an interosseous lesion of the sphenoid prior to complete ossification.

Obviously, the correlation of roentgen and clinical observations in a much larger series of cases would be necessary to substantiate the 70 per cent correlation ratio in the cases reported here. The findings to date, however, are most encouraging.

In 23 of the 25 patients it was possible to attempt correlation of the relation of the sacral base to the cranial base as demonstrated by the occiput. According to the cranial concept, the occiput should be found low on the same side as the low side of the sacrum. In this series, there were three patients in whom the occiput was level and three in whom the sacrum was level, leaving a total of 17 in whom this evaluation might be made. In 15 of these 17, the occiput was found to be low on the same side as the sacrum. In only two was the occiput found to be high on the side on which the sacrum was low. This gave a correlation of 89 per cent.

In addition, an attempt was made to correlate the angle of the sacral base with the findings of flexion or extension in the cranium. In this series it was not possible to find any correlation between the presence of flexion, extension, or normal base of the skull with any findings of increased, decreased, or normal angle of the sacral base. Continued study of this question should be made.

ILLUSTRATIVE CASES

CASE 1

A 43-year-old woman had had intermittent right-sided headache from the occiput to the right retro-orbital area for several years. It was not associated with nausea or vomiting and apparently not related to physical activity or menstrual function. There had been no known injuries to the head or neck. Symptoms had been unresponsive to therapy, although temporary relief had been obtained with the usual analgesics. The system history and physical examination elicited no other abnormalities. Structural evaluation revealed an S-shaped spinal curvature convex to the right in the cervicodorsal area and left in the lower dorsal and lumbar area, with a pelvic tilt to the left, bilateral lumbar muscle spasm, restriction at the left sacroiliac region, and some occipital spasm bilaterally, the left occiput being low.

Roentgen examination demonstrated the sacral base plane to decline to the left with a type 1 rotary scoliosis convex to the left in the lumbar area (Fig. 7). The lumbosacral angle was 39 degrees, with normal appearance to the lumbar lordosis (Fig. 8). The left occipital bone was low, as was the left sphenoid bone (Fig. 9). The angle of the base of the skull was 128 degrees (Fig. 10). The convexity of the skull was to the left (Fig. 11), and the cephalic index was 77. There was evidence of anterior rotation of the atlas on the left side. The craniosacral diagnosis was that of left side-bending pattern of the skull and sacral base declination left, with left lumbar lordosis.

CASE 2

A 51-year-old woman had had recurrent retro-orbital and temporal headache associated with occipital pain and occasional nausea and vomiting. Symptoms were never bilateral but could be on either side. This patient had received such analgesics as Darvon, mixed tranquilizers, estrogenic

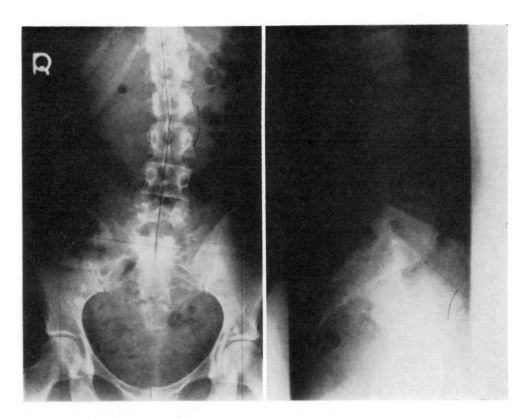

Fig. 7. *(left). Standing view of the AP/lumbar spine and pelvis demonstrates shortening of 3/16" of the left lower extremity; sacral base declination of 7/8" to the left; and rotary scoliosis of the lumbar spine convex to the left.* Fig. 8. *(right). Standing lateral projection of lumbar spine demonstrates a lumbosacral angle of 39° with normal lumbar lordosis and intervertebral disk spaces.*

substances, and Wigraine, all with no relief. Symptoms had been increasing for the preceding 2 years. Approximately 8 years previously she had had osteopathic manipulative therapy for pain in the lower part of the back, with a lift to the right shoe. This had controlled the symptom. During the period of present complaint, the patient had not been wearing the shoe lift. The remainder of the system history and physical examination showed no abnormality. Structural examination revealed an S-shaped spinal scoliosis, which was convex to the left in the cervicodorsal area and convex to the right in the lower thoracic and lumbar area. The pelvis showed tilting to the right side, and the right occipital bone was low. There was rather marked suboccipital muscular spasm

bilaterally, with restriction of atlanto-occipital motion. X-ray study showed shortening of the lower extremity by ⅜ inch, with sacral base declination to the right of ⅜ inch (Fig. 12). There was lumbar scoliosis convex to the right. The lumbosacral angle measured 39 degrees, and there was normal lumbar lordosis (Fig. 13). The skull x-rays revealed that the right occipital bone was low and the right sphenoid bone high (Fig. 14). The angle of the base of the skull was 124 degrees, with a fairly normal appearance (Fig. 15), and the cephalic index was 81 (Fig. 16). The atlas showed anterior rotation on the right. The craniosacral roentgen diagnosis was right torsion, with short right lower extremity and sacral base declination to the right.

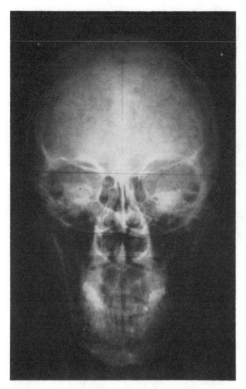

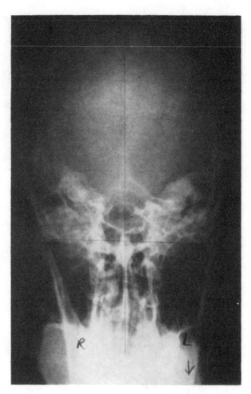

Fig. 9. *Anteroposterior view of the skull shows the sphenoid to be low on the left side. The occipital squama and conylar parts are low on the left side. The side of convexity of the skull is to the left.*

Fig. 11. *Occipital view of the skull shows the occiput to be low on the left and the side of convexity to the left.*

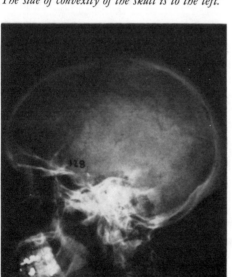

Fig. 10. *Lateral view of the skull shows the angle of the base to be 128°.*

SUMMARY AND CONCLUSIONS

An attempt has been made to develop an x-ray examination procedure and diagnostic criteria for abnormalities of cranial contour and structural relation in keeping with abnormalities described on a clinical basis by proponents of cranial osteopathy. The technique of film measurement and interpretation has been described. Two illustrative cases have been presented. Observations in the first 25 patients studied have been reported.

At present it appears that it is possible to demonstrate roentgenographically side-bending, torsion, flexion, and extension patterns of the skull. It appears also that occasionally lateral and vertical strain of the sphenobasilar junction can be demonstrated.

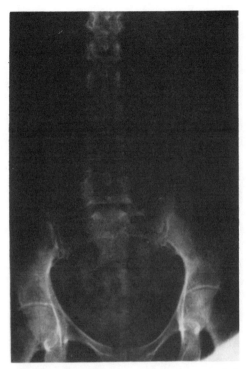

Fig. 12.   *Anteroposterior standing view of the lumbar spine and pelvis demonstrates 3/8" shortening of the right lower extremity with sacral base declination of 5/8" to the right, and lumbar scoliosis convex to the right.*

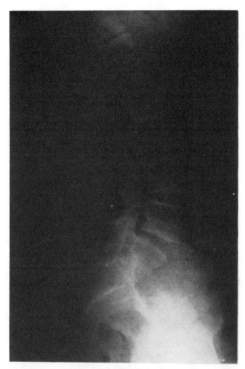

Fig. 13.   *Standing lateral view of the lumbar spine shows normal lumbar lordosis and intervertebral disk spaces. The lumbosacral angle is 39°.*

Correlation of clinical observations with the finding of low occiput on the side of the low sacrum is excellent, but that with the lumbosacral angle and the angle of the base of the skull is extremely poor. It appears that the atlas tends to rotate anteriorly on the side of the low occiput.

The correlation of the roentgen findings and independent clinical evaluation in a short series appears to be good and most encouraging. It is hoped that this work will serve as the basis for additional studies by others interested in this field. Additional areas for study might well include the use of stereoscopic and tomographic x-ray techniques.

The encouraging results to date provide a stimulus to search for increased knowledge in this intriguing field.

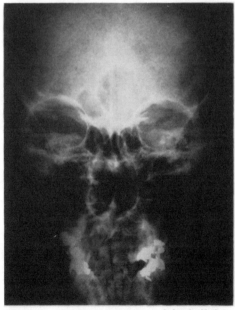

Fig. 14.   *Anteroposterior view of the skull shows the right occiput to be low and the right sphenoid to be high.*

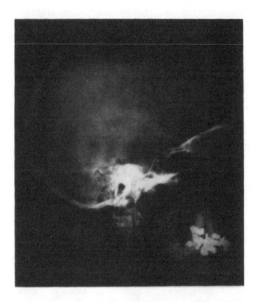

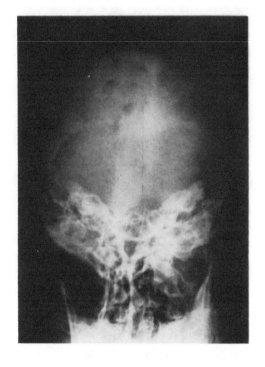

Fig. 15. *(above). A lateral film of the skull shows the angle of the base to be 124°. The anteroposterior diameter is normal. Fig. 16. (right). An occipital view of the skull shows the right occiput to be low with no particular side of convexity.*

1. Sutherland, W.G.: The cranial bowl. Treatise relating to cranial articular mobility, cranial articular lesions and cranial technic. W.G. Sutherland, Mankato, Minn., 1939
2. Weaver, C.: The cranial vertebrae. JAOA 35:328-36, Mar 36
3. Weaver, C.: The cranial vertebrae. Part II. JAOA 35:374-9, Apr 36
4. Weaver, C.: The cranial vertebrae. Part III. JAOA 35:421-4, May 36
5. Naylor, C.L.: Symposium on the plastic basicranium. I. The basicranium. JAOA 37:94-7, Nov 37
6. Sanborn, E.E.: Symposium on the plastic basicranium. II. The intracranium. JAOA 37:183-9, Jan 38
7. White, E.C.: Symposium on the plastic basicranium. III. Lesionability of the basicranium. JAOA 37:183-9, Jan 38
8. Kimberly, P.E.: Personal communication to the author
9. Magoun, H.I.: Osteopathy in the cranial field. Ed. 2. Journal Printing Co., Kirksville, Mo., 1966
10. Meschan, I: Roentgen signs in clinical diagnosis. W.B. Saunders Co., Philadelphia, 1956
11. Wortzman, G., and Dewar, F.P.: Rotary fixation of the atlantoaxial joint. Rotational atlantoaxial subluxation. Radiology 90:479-87, Mar 68
12. Gray. H.: Anatomy of the human body. Ed. 28. Edited by C.M. Goss, Lea & Febiger, Philadelphia, 1966

Shanks, S.C., and Kerley, P., editors: A textbook of x-ray diagnosis. Vol. 1, Head and neck. Ed. 4. W.B. Saunders Co., Philadelphia, 1969

Yound, B.R.: The skull, sinuses, and mastoids. A handbook of roentgen diagnoses. Year Book Publishers, Inc., Chicago, 1948

Appendix I

The Relationship of Craniosacral Examination Findings in Grade School Children with Developmental Problems

JOHN E. UPLEDGER, D.O., FAAO, East Lansing, Michigan*

A standardized craniosacral examination was conducted on a mixed sample of 203 grade school children. The probabilities calculated supported the existence of a positive relationship between elevated total craniosacral motion restriction scores and the classifications of "not normal," "behavioral problems," and "learning disabled," by school authorities, and of motion coordination problems. There was also a positive relationship between an elevated total craniosacral motion restriction score and a history of an obstetrically complicated delivery. The total quantitative craniosacral motion restriction score was most positively related to those children presenting with multiple problems.

This research was undertaken to determine if there is a relationship between restricted mobility of the craniosacral system and developmental problems in grade school children, particularly "exceptional children," those who have learning disabilities and emotional impairments.

A standardized craniosacral examination was designed and conducted on each of a mixed sample of 203 grade school children by the author. A study of interexaminer agreement for the reliability of the examination protocol was previously done by the author with three other examiners.[1]

The work and results described herein represent a part of a broader research project that is still under way. The ultimate goal of this research is an evaluation of the efficacy of craniosacral osteopathic manipulative therapy as it applies to "exceptional children." Collaborative work is presently under way by investigators in the areas of education and psychology to more clearly categorize and define the individual problems of these "exceptional children."

The ultimate goal of the investigators is to determine if significant relationships exist between specific craniosacral restriction patterns and learning and/or behavioral disorders. A significant relationship has been shown. An experimental treatment program is in progress.

The weaknesses of the present categorization methods for the children's problems are recognized. These weaknesses are being addressed at the present time.

Prior to completion of the examinations and the written recording of the results in the present study, the examiner had no knowledge of any specific problems afflicting any of the children.

THE EXAMINATION

Table 1 is the standardized examination form which was completed for each of the children.

Reprinted from The Journal of the American Osteopathic Association, Vol. 77, June 1978, pp. 738-54, by permission of the American Osteopathic Association, 212 E. Ohio St., Chicago, IL 60611.

TABLE 1. — STANDARD EXAMINATION FORM

Subject's name _____ Date _____

Age _____

Height _____ Weight _____

Cardiac pulse rate/minute _____ Cranial pulse rate/minute _____

Respiratory rate/minute _____

Cranium — obvious asymmetries (face, orbits, ears, brows, forehead, mandibular deviation — mouth open and closed)

Sutures — tissue texture abnormalities and overriding noted

Motion
Variables   Rating
 1 — Occiput — Right restriction of motion _____
 2   Left restriction of motion _____
 3 — Temporal bones — Right restriction of motion _____
 4 _____ Left restriction of motion _____
 5 — Cranial vault — Restriction toward flexion (Extension lesion*) _____
 6 _____ Restriction toward extension (Flexion lesion*) _____
 7 _____ Side bending rotation, restriction toward right (Left side bending and restriction lesion*)____
 8 _____ Side bending rotation, restriction toward left (Right side bending and restriction lesion*)____
 9 _____ Torsion, restriction toward right (Left torsion lesion*) _____
10 _____ Torsion, restriction toward left (Right torsion lesion*) _____
11 _____ Compression-decompression restriction _____
12 _____ Lateral strain, restriction toward right (Left lateral strain lesion*) _____
13 _____ Lateral strain, restriction toward left (Right lateral strain lesion*) _____
14 _____. Vertical strain, restriction toward superior motion (Inferior vertical strain lesion*) _____
15 _____ Vertical strain, restriction toward inferior motion (Superior vertical strain lesion*) _____
16 — Sacrum — Restriction toward flexion (Extension lesion*) _____
17 _____ Restriction toward extension (Flexion lesion*) _____
18 _____ Restriction toward right torsion (Left torsion lesion*) _____
19 _____ Restriction toward left torsion (Right torsion lesion*) _____
     Examiner — Name _____
                  Cardiac pulse rate/minute _____
                  Respiratory rate/minute _____
         All motion variables rated:1   = No restriction
                              1.5 =
                               2   = Moderate and transitory
                              2.5 =
                               3   = Severe restriction

*Traditional Cranial Academy terminology for "naming the lesion."

Precautions were taken to minimize the possible effect of other cues to the examiner on the conduct and reporting of the results of the craniosacral examination. A research assistant recorded the name, age, height, and weight of each child before summoning the examiner. The parents had no significant contact with the examiner prior to the examination. The initial contact between the examiner and the subject was in the examination room. Every effort was made to have the child lying quietly in the supine position on the table when the examiner entered the room.

Prior to the craniosacral motion testing, the examiner's pulse and respiratory rates were taken and recorded by the research assistant, as were the pulse, respiratory, and cranial rhythmic impulse rate of the child.[2] Obvious asymmetries noted visually and by palpation were then orally reported to the research assistant.

Next, each motion variable (Numbers 1 to 19, Table 1) of the craniosacral system was carefully tested and rated on a scale of 1 to 3. Motion variables were tested and reported in a specific sequence (Table 1) to eliminate differences which might result from varying the order of motion testing. Each motion was tested and rated in terms of restriction of response to a force applied in a given direction. In rating the restriction or resistance to a given tested examiner-induced motion, quantitative scores were assigned: a score of 1 equals no restriction; 2 equals moderate and/or transitory restriction; 3 equals severe restriction. Ratings of 1.5 and 2.5 were allowed. The resistance to (restriction against) that motion was reported and rated rather than the *"positional lesion."* This liberty was taken by the author in order to minimize conceptual error and controversy related to the cause of the restriction. It is our goal to simply note that the restriction was discovered.

In testing the types of motion, gentle movement of the head in the desired direction was initiated by the examiner. The motion was then monitored until it reached a restricted end point. Range-of-motion, bilateral equality, and ease or restriction to motion, as initiated by the examiner, were evaluated.

The exact procedure for testing each of the 19 parameters shown in Table 1 was as follows.

PARAMETERS 1 AND 2—
OCCIPUT, RIGHT AND LEFT

With the patient comfortably supine and the examiner comfortably seated at the head of the table, the examiner's hands were laid palms up on the table so that the ulnar sides of the two hands approximated each other. The fingers were flexed between 60 and 90 degrees. The fingertips were placed in contact with the patient's occipital region in a (nearly) symmetrical fashion immediately caudad to the superior nuchal line. The examiner's fingertip contact was allowed to remain passive until the soft tissues relaxed and the examiner could sense the firmness of the deeper bony structures. Once this relaxation of soft tissue occurred, gentle traction was applied in a postero-cephalad direction. As the occiput moved in compliance with this traction, a gentle laterally directed force was added to the traction by each of the examiner's hands. The resistances of the two sides of

the occiput to this examiner-induced passive motion were then rated individually on the 1 to 3 scale.

PARAMETERS 3 AND 4—
TEMPORAL BONES, RIGHT AND LEFT

For testing of restriction to motion of the temporal bones, the examiner and the patient remained in the same relative positions as aforementioned.

The patient's occiput was gently cradled in the examiner's interlaced fingers (hands palms up). The examiner's thumbs were positioned so that they were in contact with the temporal mastoid processes and tips.

First, a side-to-side motion was gently induced so that when one mastoid tip was pressed medially, the opposite tip was allowed to move freely in a lateral direction and vice versa. The motions were tested in rhythm with the cranial rhythmic impulse (CRI).* Several excursions were monitored. Then, resistance to a very minute circular motion of the temporal bones was tested. The axis of this motion can be conceptualized as running through the external auditory canal and through the petrous portion of the temporal bone. Resistance to these examiner-induced motions was rated on each side in terms of its severity. Before terminating this temporal bone testing, symmetry of motion was restored by the examiner.

PARAMETERS 5 THROUGH 15—
SPHENOBASILAR JOINT

These parameters were all tested using the "vault hold." The positions of the subject and the examiner were unchanged except for the application of the examiner's hands to the subject's head.

The "vault hold" is the descriptor for the method of application of the examiner's hands to the subject's head. This applica-

---

* The cranial rhythmic impulse (CRI) is an involuntary, physiologic, rhythmic motion which has been reported by those skilled in cranial osteopathy. It is perceived by the examiner as his hands are gently and passively placed upon the subject's head. The perceived rhythm is reportedly not in synchrony with the cardiovascular and respiratory rhythms of either the subject or the examiner.

tion was for the evaluation of the interosseous motions which are conceptualized to occur between the bones of the cranial vault. The index fingers of each hand were applied gently to the area overlying the external surfaces of the great wings of the sphenoid. The fifth fingers of each hand rested in contact with the occipital squama approximately one-half inch medio-posterior to the occipito-mastoid suture above the superior nuchal line. Some slight differences in the placement of these fingers may result if examiners have small hands, or if a head is relatively large in size, but this does not interfere with the proprioceptive cues that can be perceived.

The third and fourth fingers of each hand were not used in the motion-testing process during sphenobasilar evaluation. The thumbs did not contact the subject's head but did contact each other. They served to provide the examiner with proprioceptive and kinesthetic cues abut the equality of motion when movements in one direction were compared with reciprocal movements in the opposite direction.

The types of cranial motion tested using the vault hold were:

Parameters 5 and 6—Flexion-extension.

Parameters 7 and 8—Right and left side bending with a degree of rotation.

Parameters 9 and 10—Right and left torsion.

Parameter 11—Compression-decompression.

Parameters 12 and 13—Right and left lateral strain.

Parameters 14 and 15—Vertical strain in superior and inferior directions.

PARAMETERS 5 AND 6—
FLEXION-EXTENSION

Using the vault hold, the examiner exerted a gentle force over the occipital squama and great wings of the sphenoid concurrently. This force was directed caudad and was applied by his paired index and fifth fingers. The thumbs were in contact with each other and furnished proprioceptive and kinesthetic cues so that the examiner's force was applied as symmetrically equal as possible. After the cranium re-

sponded to the initiating force (of approximately 5.0 grams or less), the examiner became passive and followed the cranial motion to its restricted end point. This was the test for flexion. Restriction against this examiner-induced motion was then rated and reported after comparison with restriction encountered when testing for extension, next.

To test for extension, a similar bilaterally equal force was applied by the examiner in a cephalad direction. The testing was then repeated until the examiner gained a reliable impression as to the relative ease/resriction of these reciprocal motions.

PARAMETERS 7 AND 8—
SIDE BENDING-ROTATION,
RESTRICTION TOWARD RIGHT AND
LEFT, RESPECTIVELY

The vault hold was applied as aforementioned. In order to test for restriction toward side bending-rotation toward the right, the examiner's left index and fifth fingers were gently moved cephalad and medialward while slightly approximating each other. Resistance (restriction) to this examiner-induced passive motion was compared with side bending-rotation motion testing toward the left. In order to test for restriction toward the patient's left, the examiner repeated the same procedure using his right hand. Restrictions were rated on the 3 point scale, each side individually.

PARAMETERS 9 AND 10—
TORSION-RESTRICTION TOWARD THE
RIGHT AND LEFT, RESPECTIVELY

Using the vault hold, the examiner applied a gentle force with the index finger of one hand and the fifth finger of the other hand simultaneously in a superior (cephalad) direction. First, testing was completed for torsion on one side and, then, after allowing the motion to return to a position of easy neutrality, testing was completed on the opposite sides. The forces were extremely gentle. Following the initiation of motion by the examiner, the motion was monitored to its restricted end point. The restriction was rated for the side on which the great wing of the sphenoid bone resisted superior motion; if the left great sphenoid wing and the right occipital squamous moved easily in a superior direction, but the right great wing and the left squamous moved superior (cephalad) with difficulty, the restriction was rated as a 2 or 3 on the right side in reference to the right wing of the sphenoid bone offering resistance to the superior motion.

PARAMETER 11—
COMPRESSION-DECOMPRESSION
RESTRICTION

Using the vault hold, the examiner exerted a force over the great wings of the sphenoid bone with his index fingers. This force was in a frontal direction away from the fifth fingers which were gently immobilizing the areas over the occipital squama. It is essential that this force be applied as bilaterally equally as possible. The examiner's thumbs in contact with each other furnish valuable kinesthetic and proprioceptive cues during this testing procedure. Following the initiation of the motion, it was monitored to the restricted end point and rated on the 3 point scale (ease/restriction in response to the initiating force). A free anterior-posterior expansion motion (indicated by ease of motion in a frontal direction) suggested the absence of compression.

PARAMETERS 12 AND 13—
LATERAL STRAIN-RESTRICTION TOWARD
THE RIGHT AND LEFT, RESPECTIVELY

Using the vault hold, the occiput was gently held immovable by the examiner's fifth fingers. The index fingers were then used to induce motion and test restriction bilaterally on a horizontal plane in a direction at approximate right angles to the median sagittal plane of the subject's head. Restrictions toward this induced motion were rated and recorded toward the right and toward the left of the examiner.

PARAMETERS 14 AND 15—
VERTICAL STRAIN-RESTRICTION OF
SUPERIOR MOTION AND INFERIOR
MOTION, RESPECTIVELY

Using the vault hold, the occiput was gently held immovable by the examiner's fifth fingers while his index fingers (overlaying the great wings of the sphenoid bone) exerted a gentle symmetric force on a frontal plane first in a superior (or cephalad) direction, and then in an inferior (caudad) direction. As the vertical motion carries to its end point, it can be perceived that it possesses an arcing component which is directed posteriorly. Restrictions were rated as they limited the superior and/or inferior response to motion testing in those directions.

PARAMETERS 16, 17, 18, AND 19—
SACRUM

All four of these parameters were tested with the patient supine upon the upturned palm of the examiner's right hand. The spine of the sacrum rested in the space between the examiner's third and fourth fingers. The sacral apex and coccyx rested in the examiner's upturned palm. The tips of the examiner's third and fourth fingers were just lateral to the spinous processes of the fourth or fifth lumbar vertebra (depending on the patient's size). The distal aspects of the examiner's index and fifth fingers were in contact with the superior lateral aspects of the sacrum.

PARAMETER 16

The test for restriction toward sacral flexion was performed by using the examiner's palm to gently induce an anterior motion of the sacral apex.

PARAMETER 17

The test for restriction toward sacral extension was performed by inducing an anterior motion of the sacral base. Both of these motions were tested through several cycles of the CRI and the restrictions to examiner-induced motion toward both flexion and extension were rated on the 1 to 3 scale.

PARAMETERS 18 AND 19—
RESTRICTION TOWARD RIGHT AND
LEFT TORSION, RESPECTIVELY

The examiner maintained the same manual contact with the patient's sacrum as was used for testing Parameters 16 and 17. To test for restriction toward right torsion, pressure was applied in an anterior direction on the left sacral base area. Pressure on the right side was applied similarly to test for restriction toward left torsion motion. Both parameters were then rated on the 1 to 3 scale for restriction toward induced passive motion.

THE SAMPLE

Two hundred and three subjects for this study were obtained by parental response to written notices taken home by children attending Ingham County Grade Schools and by children enrolled in the MSU Motor Coordination Clinic. These notices informed parents of the objectives and protocol of the research. Cooperation and signed consent of interested parents was requested.

There was also some direct communication between a limited number of interested special educators and school nurses, and the parents of "exceptional children."

Parents who expressed a desire to have their children participate in the research (by returning the signed consent form to the cooperating agency) were then contacted by the research assistant who arranged all appointments for examinations, reviewed pertinent records, and obtained developmental and other historical data. There was no situation in which the examiner had significant contact with parent or subject prior to completion of the craniosacral examination.

Significant data were then extracted from these records and histories by the research assistant in cooperation with the statistical analysis consultant (Eric Gordon, Ph.D.). Eight categories of significant problems were then decided upon by Dr. Gordon (Table 2). Categories 1 to 4 were considered the major problem areas. Categories 5 to 8 represent factors from the history that were considered as possibly clinically significant.

The criteria for entry into one of the eight problem categories were as follows.

CATEGORY 1 NORMAL-NOT NORMAL †

A child was considered "not normal" in

this category only if one of the following criteria were met:

(1) A classroom teacher had first suspected that the child manifested a problem which would label that child as "exceptional." (The problem could have been in either the behavioral, motor coordination, and/or learning disability area.)

(2) The classroom teacher felt strongly enough about that suspicion to seek and obtain evaluation by a specialist in either psychology, motor coordination, and/or remedial education.

(3) That specialist did, in fact, concur with the classroom teacher's opinion and recommended appropriate specialized treatment or a training program for the child in question.

Children classified as "Not normal" in category 1 were *not* so classified on the basis of a teacher's opinion alone, nor was this classification made solely on the basis of the parent's opinion. Confirmation by an appropriate specialist was a required criterion. There were 164 children categorized as

TABLE 2. EIGHT PROBLEM CATEGORIES CONSIDERED SIGNIFICANT FOR DATA COLLECTION

Category	Diagnosed by
1—"Normal—Not normal"	School authorities
2—Behavioral problems	School authorities
3—Motor coordination and speech problems	School authorities Motor Coordination Clinic
4—Learning disabilities	School authorities
5—Seizure history	History obtained from parents
6—Head injury	History obtained from parents
7—Obstetrical complications	History obtained from parents
8—Ear problems (History of with or without hearing loss)	History obtained from parents

† The author recognizes that the terms "normal" and "not normal" are not truly definable. Classroom teachers, however, did use this terminology in describing the subjects examined in the project. Therefore, these descriptions have been used in reporting this research.

"Normal" and 39 children classified as "Not normal" in this category.

CATEGORY 2—
BEHAVIOR PROBLEMS

Children were placed in this category on the following bases:

(1) when a specialist in the field of psychology (usually a school psychologist) had so indicated on the school record.

(2) when the child had proven to be unmanageable to the parent so that professional evaluation (child psychologist or pediatrician) had been obtained privately and confirmed the parent's suspicion.

There were 10 subjects with positive findings in Category 2 (Table 3) wherein the parent and not the classroom teacher sought professional help for "behavioral problems." In all of these cases a professional psychologist had confirmed the problem, even though the children's school conduct was not considered exceptional by the teacher. Therefore, these subjects were considered as "normal" in category 1. All other children in this problem category (2) were considered "not normal" and to have "behavioral problems" by their teachers.

CATEGORY 3—
MOTOR COORDINATION AND
SPEECH PROBLEMS

All children in this problem category were referred from the MSU Motor Coordination Clinic, where a problem in this area of development had been confirmed. There were 19 subjects with diagnosed motor coordination problems who were considered "normal" in category 1 by the school teachers (Table 3). Therefore, they were considered as "normal" in category 1. All other motor coordination problems were noted as such by the classroom teachers.

CATEGORY 4—
LEARNING DISABILITIES

Children were considered "learning disabled" if the classroom teacher noticed the problem, obtained confirmation from a specialist, and had the child placed in a special education program.

There were four exceptions to these criteria, which were included in the data. In these cases (Table 3), the "learning disability" was noticed first by the parents who obtained private evaluations by a psychologist. The parents' suspicions were confirmed and the children were placed in private schools which specialized in remedial training of "exceptional children."

This category included problems such as dyslexia, dysgraphia, anomia, dysphasia (both receptive and expressive), and dyscalculia.

CATEGORY 5—
SEIZURE HISTORY

All children in this category had a history of at least one episode of seizure or convulsion. Most of these histories were validated by professional medical histories furnished by parents. However, if a parent reported and described the incidence of seizure or convulsion and the description of the event seemed accurate, the child was placed in this category.

The purpose of collecting these data was to uncover significant relationships between seizure history and craniosacral restrictions, as well as to illuminate this problem category as a possible contributing factor for positive findings in categories 1 to 4.

CATEGORY 6—
HEAD INJURY

Children were placed in this category on the basis of information from parents and from medical records when available. The research assistant attempted to eliminate minor "bumps" and "cuts" on the head from this category.

The unreliability of data obtained is recognized; however, only those children with history of hospitalization, "concussion," fracture and/or unconsciousness were included.

The purpose for the inclusion of this category was to search for areas which may, in fact, justify more in-depth investigation of head injuries as possible contributing factors to the problem of "exceptional children."

CATEGORY 7—
OBSTETRIC COMPLICATIONS

The criteria for classifying a delivery as obstetrically complicated were one or more of the following:

(1) Cesarean section
(2) High forceps delivery
(3) Induction of labor for reasons other than convenience
(4) Fetal distress in utero
(5) Breech delivery
(6) Prolonged labor
(7) Precipitous labor
(8) Toxemia of pregnancy
(9) Severe trauma during pregnancy which resulted in pelvic fracture

All information was obtained from the parents. Documentation was occasionally available from medical records; however, this was the exception.

Even though the validity of these data may be questionable, the investigators included the category in order to uncover tendencies toward correlation between obstetric complications as a contributing factor to problems in categories 1 to 4, and a correlation between craniosacral restriction patterns and obstetric complications. More in-depth study seems justified by these results.

CATEGORY 8—
EAR PROBLEMS

Children placed in this category had histories of myringotomy, hearing deficit, or recurrent ear infections (at least 5 repetitions) which had required treatment by a physician. Otitis externa was not included.

This category was included simply because of the frequency with which the problem occurred in the histories. The statistical analysis does not appear to justify further study.

The occurrence of problems in categories 2 through 8 for the 164 children examined who were classified as "normal" by the classroom teachers and school authorities are presented in Table 3. One hundred and thirty-five of these 164 children had no classifiable problems in categories 2, 3, and 4 (behavioral, motor-speech, and learning disabilities, respectively).

Subject children numbers 1 through 41 presented no classifiable problems within this study. Subjects 42 through 135 presented positive findings only in categories 5 through 8, which are being investigated as possible contributing factors. The occurrence of positive findings in categories 2, 3, and 4 in "normal" subjects 136 through 164 has been explained in the aforementioned paragraphs which deal with those categories.

The column on the extreme right of Table 3 indicates the quantitative total scores given each subject for the craniosacral examination.

The occurrence of other problems in categories 2 through 8 for the children who were classified as "not normal" by classroom teachers and school authorities is listed in Table 4. The total quantitative craniosacral examination score is given in the column on the extreme right of the table.

Comparison of Tables 3 and 4 provides an overview of the density of problem occurrence in categories 2, 3, and 4 when children were classified as "normal" or "not normal" in category 1. (This comparison lends support to the validity of the classroom teacher's opinions of the normalcy of the child's development.)

STATISTICAL ANALYSIS

This investigation involved three types of statistical measures:

(1) Summary descriptive statistics were used to describe the sample.

(2) Two tailed "t" tests were used to test the differences in mean scores between patient groups in the various categories.

(3) Pearson Product—Moment correlations were calculated in order to investigate the relationships between variables.

(The readers should be aware that no previously determined levels of significance [alpha] are available.)

RESULTS AND DISCUSSION

Table 5 gives the mean scores, the standard deviations, and the standard errors derived from the craniosacral examination and the probabilities that the differences in mean scores for each of the 8 categories could have occurred by chance. Categories in which the craniosacral examination score differences were considered to be significant are as follows:

Category 1 (Normal-Not Normal)—The ability of the differences in mean examination scores occurring and agreeing with the opinion of the school authorities by chance is less than 1 in 1000 (<.001).

Category 2 (Behavioral Problems)—The probability of the correlation found between school authority opinions and craniosacral examination scores occurring by chance is less than 1 in 1000 (<.001).

Category 3 (Motor Coordination Problems)—The probability of the differences in mean cranial examination scores occurring and agreeing with the Motor Coordination Clinic

Subject number	Category							Total cranio-sacral exam (Σ V) score*
	2	3	4	5	6	7	8	
			No positive findings in categories 1 through 8					
1								22.5
2								23.0
3								27.0
4								21.5
5								22.0
6								28.0
7								22.0
8								28.0
9								24.5
10								21.0
11								31.0
12								24.5
13								23.0
14								25.0
15								31.0
16								23.0
17								24.0
18								34.0
19								32.0
20								27.5
21								22.5
22								30.0
23								26.5
24								25.0
25								23.0
26								24.0
27								24.0
28								21.5
29								23.0
30								26.5
31								22.0
32								23.5
33								25.0
34								28.5
35								22.0
36								24.5
37								27.5
38								23.0
39								20.5
40								22.0
41								29.0

TABLE 3. OCCURRENCE OF OTHER PROBLEMS FOR CHILDREN CLASSIFIED AS "NORMAL" IN CATEGORY 1.

TABLE 3. (continued)

Subject number	Category							Total cranio-sacral exam (Σ V) score*
	2	3	4	5	6	7	8	
Children with no positive findings in categories 1 through 4, but with positive findings in the contributing categories 5 through 8								
42						X		26.5
43					X			22.0
44				X		X	X	27.0
45						X	X	28.5
46				X				22.0
47					X			27.0
48					X		X	23.5
49				X		X		29.5
50					X		X	25.0
51				X			X	26.0
52							X	26.5
53						X		31.0
54						X		25.0
55					X			25.5
56						X		22.0
57					X	X		24.5
58						X		23.5
59				X	X	X	X	25.5
60					X	X	X	26.5
61						X		24.5
62					X	X	X	21.5
63					X			30.5
64					X	X		28.0
65					X			24.0
66					X			24.0
67					X		X	26.5
68					X			27.5
69						X		28.0
70					X		X	24.0
71				X	X		X	19.0
72					X			23.5
73					X	X		25.5
74					X			23.5
75					X			19.0
76							X	23.5
77					X			34.5
78							X	22.5
79				X	X			24.0
80				X		.X		26.0
81					X			25.0
82					X			22.5
83					X	X		26.0
84				X	X			26.5
85						X	X	35.0
86				X	X	X		27.0
87						X		27.0
88				X			X	24.0
89						X		26.0
90					X		X	24.0
91					X	X		25.5
92					X			23.0
93					X			25.5
94				X	X			21.5
95					X			34.0
96					X			27.0

TABLE 3 (continued)

Subject number	Category							Total cranio-sacral exam (Σ V) score*
	2	3	4	5	6	7	8	
97				X				25.0
98					X			24.0
99					X	X	X	27.5
100							X	24.0
101						X		24.5
102					X	X	X	23.5
103					X			29.5
104					X			27.5
105						X		28.0
106					X		X	24.5
107							X	27.0
108					X	X	X	28.5
109				X	X			25.0
110						X		25.0
111					X			26.0
112							X	23.5
113					X	X	X	21.5
114					X			24.5
115							X	26.0
116				X				34.0
117					X			28.0
118					X		X	24.5
119					X			24.0
120					X			25.0
121						X	X	24.5
122					X	X		25.5
123					X			30.0
124					X	X	X	27.0
125							X	25.5
126					X		X	23.0
127							X	23.5
128					X		X	36.5
129					X	X	X	27.0
130				X	X		X	21.5
131					X			22.0
132						X	X	22.0
133					X		X	23.5
134					X		X	28.0
135							X	27.0
Occurrence of positive findings in categories 2, 3, and 4 in children categorized as "normal" by teachers								
136		X						24.5
137		X						24.0
138		X			X		X	22.5
139	X				X	X		27.0
140	X			X		X		27.0
141	X					X		26.0
142			X		X			34.0
143		X					X	25.5
144		X			X			28.0
145		X			X			26.0
146	X							30.0
147		X			X	X		35.0
148		X						20.0
149		X			X			34.5

Subject number	Category							Total cranio-sacral exam (Σ V) score*
	2	3	4	5	6	7	8	
150		X	X					23.5
151		X				X		29.5
152	X		X					30.0
153	X	X			X		X	29.0
154	X				X		X	39.5
155		X						21.0
156		X			X			32.0
157	X				X	X		31.5
158		X			X			29.5
159	X							22.5
160	X					X		32.5
161		X				X		37.0
162		X	X			X		28.5
163		X			X			26.5
164		X		X		X	X	28.5

TABLE 3. (continued)

*Perfect score (no restriction) = 19

diagnosis by chance is 2 in 1000 (.002).

Category 4 (Learning Disability)—The probability of the differences in mean examination scores occurring and agreeing with the opinion of the school authorities by chance is less than 1 in 1000 (<.001).

Category 7 (Obstetric Complications)—The probability of the agreement between the presence of a history of an obstetrically complicated delivery of the subject child and the elevation of the mean scores of the craniosacral examination in those children occurring by chance is less than 1 in 1000 (<.001).

The craniosacral examination appears to be valid as a test for behavioral problems, learning disabilities, obstetrically complicated deliveries, and to confirm the opinion of the child's teacher as to whether the child's progress in school is "normal" or "not normal."

Table 6 gives the correlation coefficients (r) between each singular parameter studied during the craniosacral examination and the total score derived from the motion restriction rating of the 19 parameters tested. The (r) and (p) values were computed to determine which of the parameters would most reliably predict high total numerical scores derived from the 19 motion parameters.

There is no apparent significant relationship between total motion restriction of the craniosacral system and the subject's age, height, weight, pulse rate, heart rate, or the rate of the cranial rhythmical impulse. All children were within normal ranges of height and weight.

The most reliable predictors (of the individual motion parameters measured) for the highest total scores have the highest (r) values. Motion Parameter 11 (Compression-Decompression) was the most reliable predictor of widespread restriction within the total craniosacral system as tested. All other parameters of motion were found reliable at probabilities of less than 1 chance in 1000.

The correlation coefficients (r) for all combinations of motion restriction variables (5) and Categories (C) of problems are presented individually and in summation in Table 7. All (r) values presented represent probability (p) values of less than .05 (5 chances in 100) of the correlation occurring as a random happening. Correlation coefficients (r) which are equal to or greater than .21 on the table represent probabilities of .001 (1 chance in 1000) or less of the relationship between the examination

TABLE 4. OCCURRENCE OF OTHER PROBLEMS FOR CHILDREN CLASSIFIED AS "NOT NORMAL" IN CATEGORY 1.

Subject number	2	3	4	5	6	7	8	Total craniosacral exam (Σ V) score*
165		X				X		29.5
166	X		X					27.0
167	X	X	X			X		37.5
168		X	X			X		29.5
169	X		X			X		33.5
170		X			X			25.5
171		X						20.0
172	X	X			X	X	X	29.0
173		X	X			X		39.0
174		X				X		32.0
175				X	X	X	X	34.5
176	X			X	X	X	X	34.0
177	X			X	X	X	X	28.5
178				X	X		X	28.5
179		X	X			X		27.0
180		X			X	X	X	34.0
181	X	X	X					32.0
182		X	X		X			40.0
183	X		X				X	34.0
184	X	X	X	X	X	X	X	45.0
185	X		X		X	X		32.5
186	X		X				X	28.0
187	X		X					35.5
188	X		X					33.5
189		X	X			X		28.0
190	X				X	X		35.0
191			X					27.0
192	X		X		X	X	X	47.5
193	X					X		33.5
194		X			X			26.0
195	X				X			29.0
196	X	X	X	X	X			33.5
197		X			X	X		30.0
198	X				X			26.0
199	X				X		X	21.0
200	X				X			27.0
201			X		X	X		30.0
202	X		X		X			24.0
203		X	X		X	X		29.5

*Perfect score (no restriction) = 19

score and the presence of a problem in that category having occurred by chance.

It can be seen that the total numerical score of the 19 motion parameters tested is most significantly correlated with the presence of multiple problems. The craniosacral examination would also appear to be reliable in identifying those children whom the school authorities have categorized as "not normal," and those children classified as having "behavioral problems" and/or "learning disabilities." The craniosacral examination also seems an excellent method of determining which children were the products of complicated obstetric deliveries and which children are classified as having motor coordination problems.

Study of restriction patterns as reflected by the (r) values suggests the hypothesis that specific types of problems may be related to certain interdependent motion restrictions and/or restriction patterns of the craniosacral system. Further research of this hypothesis is under way by the author.

TABLE 5. PROBABILITY OF MEAN CRANIOSACRAL MOTION EXAMINATION SCORE DIFFERENCES FOR EACH OF THE EIGHT CATEGORIZED PROBLEM TYPES.

Category	Frequency	Mean score	Standard deviation	Standard error	Probability
1—"Normal"	165 (82%)	26.05	3.704	0.288	.000
"Not normal"	38 (18%)	31.24	5.736	0.931	
2—Behavioral	32 (16%)	31.30	5.763	1.019	.000
No	171 (84%)	26.22	3.891	0.298	
3—Motor — Speech	34 (17%)	29.19	5.585	0.958	.002
No	169 (83%)	26.59	4.279	0.329	
4—Learning disability	25 (12%)	32.40	5.949	1.190	.000
No	178 (88%)	26.27	3.850	0.289	
5—Seizure history	25 (12%)	27.70	5.429	1.086	.434
No	178 (88%)	26.93	4.495	0.337	
6—Head injury	92 (45%)	27.78	5.086	0.530	.032
No	111 (55%)	26.39	4.097	0.389	
7—Obstetrical complications	67 (33%)	28.78	5.161	0.631	.000
No	136 (67%)	26.15	4.064	0.343	
8—Ear and hearing problems	55 (27%)	27.19	5.592	0.754	.752
No	148 (63%)	26.96	4.211	0.346	

TABLE 6. RELATIONSHIPS BETWEEN TOTAL SCORES AND TESTED SINGULAR VARIABLES.

Singular variable	Correlation coefficient (r)	Probability (p)	
Age	.09	.101	
Height	.08	.128	
Weight	.03	.322	
Pulse rate	.01	.415	
Resp. rate	.05	.233	
CRI. rate	.04	.305	
Motion parameters			
1	.37	< .001	Right occiput restricted
2	.38	< .001	Left occiput restricted
3	.36	< .001	Right temporal restricted
4	.40	< .001	Left temporal restricted
5	.46	< .001	Flexion, restricted toward
6	.45	< .001	Extension, restricted toward
7	.44	< .001	S.B.&R., restricted toward right
8	.42	< .001	S.B.&R., restricted toward left
9	.39	< .001	Torsion, restricted toward right
10	.37	< .001	Torsion, restricted toward left
11	.53	< .001	Compression-decompression, restriction of
12	.39	< .001	Lateral strain, restricted toward right
13	.33	< .001	Lateral strain, restricted toward left
14	.24	< .001	Vert. strain, restricted superior motion
15	.45	< .001	Vert. strain, restricted inferior motion
16	.47	< .001	Sacrum restricted toward flexion
17	.36	< .001	Sacrum restricted toward extension
18	.30	< .001	Sacrum restricted toward right torsion
19	.24	< .001	Sacrum restricted toward left torsion

TABLE 7. RELATIONSHIPS BETWEEN MOTION PARAMETERS (1-19) AND PROBLEMS FOUND IN CATEGORIES (1 THROUGH 8)—CORRELATION COEFFICIENTS (r) (N=203)

Motion restriction variables	Normal not — C-1	Behav. problems C-2	Motor-speech C-3	Learn disabilities C-4	Seizure history C-5	Head injury C-6	Obstetrical complications C-7	Ear problems C-8	Multiple problems Σ C
1-Occiput right	.1793	.1485	.2752	.1546	—	—	.1316	—	.2596
2-Occiput left	—	.1226	—	—	—	—	—	—	.1080
3-Temporal right	.2338	.1710	.1262	.1474	—	—	.2798	—	.2290
4-Temporal left	—	—	—	.1292	—	—	—	—	.0950
5-Toward flexion	.3107	.2080	—	.3052	—	—	.1798	—	.3014
6-Toward extension	.2115	.1683	—	.2336	—	—	—	—	.1515
7-S.B. & R. toward right	.2801	.1696	—	.1877	—	—	.1673	—	.2629
8-S.B. & R. toward left	.1694	.2497	.1745	.2178	—	.1362	—	—	.2571
9-Torsion toward right	.2672	.1812	.1634	.2140	.2005	.1327	.1798	—	.3513
10-Torsion toward left	.2284	.1386	—	.1784	—	—	—	—	.2135
11-Compression — decompression	.2631	.2337	—	.2020	—	.1639	—	—	.2124
12-Lat. strain toward right	—	—	—	—	—	—	.1161	—	.1184
13-Lat. strain toward left	.1676	.1399	—	.1523	—	—	—	—	.1163
14-Vert. strain toward superior	.1708	.1349	.1864	.1470	—	—	—	—	.1949
15-Vert. strain toward inferior	—	.1639	—	.1669	—	—	—	—	.1311
16-Sacrum toward flexion	.2225	.2430	—	—	—	—	.1392	—	.2413
17-Sacrum toward extension	—	—	—	—	—	—	—	—	.1461
18-Sacrum toward right torsion	—	—	—	.2413	—	—	—	—	.0876
19-Sacrum toward left torsion	.1804	.2519	—	.1538	—	—	.2268	—	.2225
Σ V Total Score	.4396	.4019	.2114	.4380	—	.1505	.2687	—	.5014

r ⩽ .21 probability is less than .001
All values given represent probabilities of less than .05.

CONCLUSIONS

1. The use of a standardized quantifiable craniosacral motion examination represents a practical approach to the study of relationships between craniosacral motion restrictions and a variety of health problems which may or may not be related to central nervous function.

2. In general, the accuracy of school authorities' opinions which classify children as "normal" or "not normal" are supported by these data (Tables 3 and 4).

3. The probabilities calculated (Tables 5 and 7) support the existence of a positive relationship between elevated total craniosacral motion restriction scores and classifications of "not normal," "behavioral problems," and "learning disabled" by school authorities, and of motor coordination problems, as diagnosed by the MSU Motor Coordination Clinic.

4. There is a positive relationship between an elevated total craniosacral motion restriction score and a history of an obstetrically complicated delivery (Tables 5 and 7).

5. The total quantitative craniosacral motion restriction score (Σ V) is most positively related to those children presenting with multiple problems (Σ C) on Table 7.

1. Upledger, J.E.: The reproducibility of craniosacral examination findings. JAOA 76:890-9, Aug 77.
2. Magoun, H.I., Sr.: Osteopathy in the cranial field. Journal Printing Co., Kirksville, Mo., 1966, pp. 313-23.

Baker, E.G.: Alteration in width of maxillary arch and its relation to sutural movement of cranial bones. JAOA 70:559-64, Feb 71.

Beter, T.R., Cragin, W.D., and Drury, F.: The mentally retarded child and his motor behavior. Charles C. Thomas, Publisher, Springfield, Ill., 1972.

Brierley, J.B.: Metabolism of the nervous system. D. Richter, Ed. Pergamon Press, New York, 1951, pp. 121-35.

Brooks, C., Kao, F.F., and Lloyd, B.B.: Cerebrospinal fluid and the regulation of ventilation. F.A. Davis Co., Philadelphia, 1965.

Davson, H.: Physiology of the cerebrospinal fluid. Churchill, London, 1967.

Dunbar, H.S., Guthrie, T.C., and Karspell, B.: A study of the cerebrospinal fluid pulse wave. Arch Neurol (Chicago) 14:624-30, Jun 66.

Frymann, V.M.: Relation of disturbances of craniosacral mechanisms to symptomatology of the newborn: Study of 1,250 infants. JAOA 65:1059-75, Jun 66.

Leusen, I.: Regulation of cerebrospinal fluid composition with reference to breathing. Physiol Rev 52:1-14, Jan 72.

Magoun, H.I., Sr.: The temporal bone. Troublemaker in the head. JAOA 73:825-35, Jun 74.

Michael, D.K.: The cerebrospinal fluid. Values for compliance and resistance to absorption. JAOA 74:873-6, May 75.

Michael, D.K., and Retzlaff, E.W.: A preliminary study of cranial bone movement in the squirrel monkey. JAOA 74:866-9, May 75.

Miller, H.C.: Head pain. JAOA 72:135-43, Oct 72.

Morris, P.R., and Whiting, H.T.A.: Motor impairment and compensatory education. G. Bell and Sons, London, 1971.

New York Academy of Science. Minimal brain dysfunction. Annals of the New York Academy of Science, vol. 205, February 28, 1973.

Pritchard, J.J., Scott, J.H., and Girgis, F.G.: The structure and development of cranial and facial sutures. J Anat 90:70-86, Jan 56.

Retzlaff, E.W., et al.: The structures of cranial bone sutures. JAOA 75:607-8, Feb 76.

Retzlaff, E.W., Michael, D.K., and Roppel, R.M.: Cranial bone mobility. JAOA 74:869-73, May 75.

Retzlaff, E.W., Roppel, R.M., and Michael, D.K.: Possible functional significance of cranial bone sutures. Association of Anatomists, 88th Session, MSU-COM, 24-27, Mar 1975.

Sutherland, W.G.: The cranial bowl. Free Press Co., Mankato, Minn., 1939.

Wales, A.L.: The work of William Garner Sutherland, JAOA 71:788-93, May 72.

Winchell, C.A.: The hyperkinetic child. Greenwood Publishers, Westport, Conn., 1975.

Woods, R.H.: Structural normalization in infants and children with particular reference to disturbances of the central nervous system. JAOA 72:903-8, May 73.

Appendix J

The Reproducibility of Craniosacral Examination Findings: A Statistical Analysis

JOHN E. UPLEDGER, D.O., FAAO, East Lansing, Michigan*

A statistical analysis of the data derived from 50 craniosacral examinations on 25 preschool children is presented. These data would seem to support the reliability and reproducibility of the examination findings when the examinations are performed by skilled examiners. During all 50 examinations, the rate of the cranial rhythmical impulse (CRI) was counted and compared with the pulse and respiratory rates of both the subject and the examiner. The results of this comparison would tend to help establish the CRI as an independent physiologic rhythm. A single-blind protocol was employed. All reasonable precautions were taken to control variables.

This study is the first part of a clinical research project currently in progress, the broad objectives of which are:

(1) To determine whether, in fact, there is a cranial rhythmical impulse (CRI)** (perceptible by a craniosacral examiner) which is different from the cardiovascular and respiratory rhythms of the subject and the examiner. (No inference is made from these data as to whether the perceived CRI may or may not be the resultant modulation of other physiologic rhythms, as has been hypothesized by some investigators and observers.)

(2) To determine whether statistically significant relationships exist between craniosacral interdependent motion system dysfunctions, on the one hand, and the "minimal brain damage/dysfunction" (MBD) syndromes of school children (for example, dyslexia, dysgraphia, hyperkinesis, hypokinesis, and motor discoordination)[1-3] on the other.

(3) To determine whether craniosacral osteopathic manipulative therapy[4-8] may modify the progress of MBD-afflicted children when added to their existing therapeutic regimen (remedial education, psychotropic drug therapy, motor coordination training, et cetera).

(4) To gather photographic evidence, which may or may not support the craniosacral examination findings.

The aim of the first part of the research project was completed to test the reproducibility of the author's craniosacral examination findings.

The recorded results of 50 craniosacral examinations performed on 25 preschool

---

**The cranial rhythmical impulse (CRI) is an involuntary, physiologic, rhythmic motion which has been reported by those skilled in cranial osteopathy. It is perceived by the examiner as his hands are gently and passively placed upon the subject's head. The perceived rhythm is reportedly not in synchrony with the cardiovascular and respiratory rhythms of either the subject or the examiner.

Reprinted from The Journal of the American Osteopathic Association, Vol. 76, August 1977, pp. 890-99, by permission of the American Osteopathic Association, 212 E. Ohio St., Chicago, IL 60611.

children were subjected to statistical analysis by an unbiased statistician. Each child was examined by the author and either Dr. Irvin Gastman (second year student at MSU-COM, trained in craniosacral techniques by the author), Dr. Fred L. Mitchell, Jr. (Department of Biomechanics, MSU-COM), or Dr. Robert C. Ward (Office of Medical Education, Research and Development, MSU-COM).

Nineteen parameters of craniosacral motion[4, 6, 9, 10] were rated on a three-point scale: 1 = easy or "normal" response to induced passive motion; 2 = moderate or transient restriction to induced passive motion; and 3 = severe or complete restriction to induced passive motion. Increments of 0.5 were allowed (table 1).

The experimental design was single blind (neither examiner had knowledge of the other's findings). As the examination progressed, the results were verbally reported by each examiner to a technician who recorded them.

The CRI[4, 5, 6, 11] was reported by the examiner at the beginning of each examination, as were the child's pulse and respiratory rates. These findings were recorded on the child's examination sheet by the technician, as were the examiner's own pulse and respiratory rates. These physiologic measures were recorded so that the CRI might be compared with other body rhythms of both the examiner and the subject.

METHOD

The methodology employed in this study is a straightforward, single-blind protocol. The examinations were done on the premises of a local day-care center in East Lansing, Michigan. The children were between the ages of 3 and 5 years.

Each child was brought into the examination area by a teacher who remained with the child throughout the two examinations (performed consecutively by the author and one of the three examiners named previously). Since each child was examined in a familiar setting with a familiar teacher present, problems of cooperation and apprehension were minimized.

After the height, weight, and age were

TABLE 1. PARAMETERS RATED BY EACH EXAMINER[4,6,8]
Occiput
1—Right (restriction of motion)
2—Left (restriction of motion)
Temporal bones
3—Right (restriction of motion)
4—Left (restriction of motion)
Sphenobasilar joint
5—Restriction toward flexion
6—Restriction toward extension
7—Sidebending rotation, restriction toward right
8—Sidebending rotation, restriction toward left
9—Torsion, restriction toward right
10—Torsion, restriction toward left
11—Compression-decompression restriction
12—Lateral strain, restriction toward right
13—Lateral strain, restriction toward left
14—Vertical strain, restriction toward superior motion
15—Vertical strain, restriction toward inferior motion
Sacrum
16—Restriction toward flexion
17—Restriction toward extension
18—Restriction toward right torsion
19—Restriction toward left torsion
The rating system employed is as follows:
1 = easy or "normal" response to induced passive motion
2 = moderate or transient restriction to induced passive motion
3 = severe or complete restriction to induced passive motion
Increments of 0.5 between 1 and 3 on the rating scale were allowed.

recorded by the technician, the child was placed in a supine position on a portable treatment table. The first examiner was seated comfortably at the head of the table. (The other examiner was away from the examination area while the first examiner reported his findings.)

Prior to the commencement of the cranial portion of the examination, the technician recorded the pulse and respiratory rates of both the examiner and the child;

these data were taken as the child was allowed to lie quietly on the table. Next, the examiner verbally reported to the technician (for recording) the CRI rate of the child as counted for one minute.

Following these initial steps, the examiner was asked by the technician to rate and report verbally the ease/restriction to examiner-induced passive motion for each of 19 parameters of craniosacral motion. These ratings were recorded on the examination sheet by the technician as they were reported. The technician attempted to elicit from the examiner the rating of each of the parameters in the sequence given below. Where examiners were hesitant or doubtful, the technician forced a rating decision.

Following the completion of the first examination, the second examiner was summoned and the examination procedure was repeated on the same child. Between examinations, the child remained quiet in the supine position on the table. The examiner sequence was such that the examiners alternated between performing first and second in order to rule out unknown variables which might be introduced by a given examiner being first or second consistently.

The author examined all 25 children. Dr. Gastman examined 11 children, Dr. Ward 8 children, and Dr. Mitchell 6 children. The data obtained by the author are compared to the other three examiners' results both as an aggregate and individually. At no time did any examiner have knowledge of the previous examiner's findings prior to the completed recording of those examination data by the technician. The examination records were then statistically analyzed for the percentage of agreement and the reliability coefficients.

RESULTS

The results of the statistical analysis of examination data follows, in tabular form (Tables 2-7).

Parameters 1 through 19 are delineated in Table 1. This system of parameter identification is carried through all data tables. Appendix A presents the mean and standard deviation values. The raw data are presented in Appendix B.

DISCUSSION

The primary objective of this study is the determination of inter-rater reliability and percentage of agreement as they relate to data derived from the craniosacral examination of preschool children.

The examination data reported by the author were compared with those data reported by three other examiners skilled in craniosacral examination techniques. Each of 25 subjects was examined consecutively by the author and one of the other three examiners. The author was first examiner for 13 subjects and second examiner for 12 subjects.

An examination protocol was devised to include the recording of the CRI rate per minute,[4, 5, 6, 11] the pulse and respiratory rate per minute of both the subject and the examiner, and 19 parameters of passively induced craniosacral motion. The rating system relates to the degree of restriction toward each passively induced motion evaluated during the examination procedure.

It should be noted that the rating of all parameters refers to restriction toward the named motion rather than the naming of the "lesion" of the craniosacral mechanism.[4, 6] This modification in nomenclature was made to minimize "lesion" conceptualization as a source of error.

A second objective of the study was the comparison of CRI rate per minute with other body rhythms of both the subject and the examiner.

Tables 2, 3, and 4 give the reliability coefficients and the percentage of agreement of the author's data as compared with each of the other three examiners individually. Table 5 compares the author's data with all other examiners' data as an aggregate.

The appearance of a low reliability coefficient where percentage of agreement is high is due to the lack of variance from normal of a given parameter, for example, restriction toward induced passive flexion of the sphenobasilar joint.[4, 6] The author rated all 11 subjects as 1 (no restriction to flexion). Dr. Gastman gave 1 ratings to 10 of these children and 1.5 to 1 child. These data suggest that none of the 11 children

TABLE 2. AUTHOR'S EXAMINATION RESULTS COMPARED WITH DR. GASTMAN'S RESULTS (N = 11).

Parameter	Reliability coefficient	Percentage of agreement between examiners Rating variance allowed (%)*				Total percentage of agreement achieved allowing up to 0.5 rating variance
		±0	±0.5	±1.0	± > 1.0	
1	.41	82	0	18	0	82
2	.39	73	9	18	0	82
3	.57	64	18	18	0	82
4	.47	73	18	9	0	91
5	0	91	9	0	0	100
6	.67	91	9	0	0	100
7	.95	91	9	0	0	100
8	.73	73	18	9	0	91
9	.29	55	27	18	0	82
10	.75	73	27	0	0	100
11	.92	73	27	0	0	100
12	.88	82	18	0	0	100
13	.66	36	55	9	0	91
14	.44	55	27	18	0	82
15	.87	55	27	18	0	82
16	0	82	18	0	0	100
17	0	82	18	0	0	100
18	.77	64	36	0	0	100
19	.36	64	18	18	0	82

*Rating scale of restriction to induced passive motion:
1 = no restriction; 1.5 = mild restriction; 2.0 = moderate restriction;
2.5 = moderately severe restriction; 3 = severe to absolute restriction.

TABLE 3. AUTHOR'S EXAMINATION RESULTS COMPARED WITH DR. WARD'S RESULTS (N = 8).

Parameter	Reliability coefficient	Percentage of agreement between examiners Rating variance allowed (%)*				Total percentage of agreement achieved allowing up to 0.5 rating variance
		±0	±0.5	±1.0	± > 1.0	
1	.71	75	2	25	0	75
2	.76	63	25	13	0	88
3	.49	75	0	25	0	75
4	.50	75	0	25	0	75
5	1.00	100	0	0	0	100
6	.96	88	12	0	0	100
7	.87	75	13	12	0	88
8	.98	88	12	0	0	100
9	1.00	100	0	0	0	100
10	.61	50	25	25	0	75
11	.95	75	25	0	0	100
12	.98	75	25	0	0	100
13	.71	88	12	0	0	100
14	.54	75	13	12	0	88
15	0	88	12	0	0	100
16	.24	13	25	62	0	38
17	0	88	12	0	0	100
18	.44	88	0	12	0	88
19	.60	75	0	25	0	75

*Rating scale of restriction to induced passive motion:
1 = no restriction; 1.5 = mild restriction; 2.0 = moderate restriction;
2.5 = moderately severe restriction; 3 = severe to absolute restriction.

TABLE 4. AUTHOR'S EXAMINATION RESULTS COMPARED WITH DR. MITCHELL'S RESULTS (N = 6).

Parameter	Reliability coefficient	Percentage of agreement between examiners Rating variance allowed (%)*				Total percentage of agreement achieved allowing up to 0.5 rating variance
		±0	±0.5	±1.0	± > 1.0	
1	.77	83	0	17	0	83
2	1.00	100	0	0	0	100
3	0	50	17	33	0	67
4	.82	50	33	17	0	83
5	.70	67	0	33	0	67
6	.88	83	0	17	0	83
7	.53	67	0	17	16	67
8	.63	83	0	17	0	83
9	.70	50	17	33	0	67
10	0	67	0	33	0	67
11	.61	50	33	17	0	83
12	1.00	100	0	0	0	100
13	0	83	0	17	0	83
14	.53	83	17	0	0	100
15	.65	50	17	33	0	67
16	0	50	17	17	16	67
17	0	0	17	50	33	17
18	0	50	0	50	0	50
19	.63	67	0	17	16	67

*Rating scale of restriction to induced passive motion:
1 = no restriction; 1.5 = mild restriction; 2.0 = moderate restriction;
2.5 = moderately severe restriction; 3 = severe to absolute restriction.

TABLE 5. AUTHOR'S EXAMINATION RESULTS COMPARED WITH RESULTS OF ALL OTHER EXAMINER'S RESULTS AS AN AGGREGATE (N = 25).

Parameter	Reliability coefficient	Percentage of agreement between examiners (total) Rating variance allowed (%)*				Total percentage of agreement achieved allowing up to 0.5 rating variance
		±0	±0.5	±1.0	± > 1.0	
1	.72	80	0	20	0	80
2	.77	76	12	12	0	88
3	.56	64	12	24	0	76
4	.75	68	16	16	0	84
5	.88	88	4	8	0	92
6	.91	88	8	4	0	96
7	.70	80	8	8	4	88
8	.87	80	12	8	0	92
9	.78	68	16	16	0	84
10	.54	64	20	16	0	84
11	.91	68	28	4	0	96
12	.97	84	16	0	0	100
13	.85	64	28	8	0	92
14	.85	68	20	12	0	88
15	.88	64	20	16	0	84
16	.38	52	20	24	4	74
17	.16	64	16	12	8	80
18	.67	68	20	12	0	88
19	.46	68	8	20	4	76

*Rating scale of restriction to induced passive motion:
1 = no restriction; 1.5 = mild restriction; 2.0 = moderate restriction;
2.5 = moderately severe restriction; 3 = severe to absolute restriction.

TABLE 6. PERCENTAGE OF AGREEMENT BETWEEN THE AUTHOR AND OTHER EXAMINERS ON TOTAL EXAMINATION.				
Rating variance allowed	Dr. Gastman (N = 11)	Dr. Ward (N = 8)	Dr. Mitchell (N = 6)	Aggregate (N = 25)
0	72%	77%	65%	71%
±0.5	92%	88%	74%	86%

displayed even moderate restriction toward flexion. Both examiners are in 100 percent agreement regarding this finding. Since the agreement is so high, the probability that these particular children did not manifest restriction toward flexion is also very high. However, since the variance of findings from normal is practically zero, the reliability coefficient is zero. This appearance of unreliability is quite misleading, since both examiners working blind arrived at similar conclusions. (Low reliability coefficients coupled with high percentage of agreement may also occur when neither physician actually examines the parameter but simply rates it as normal, and when the test is insensitive, parameters offer testimony against this possibility.) Similar situations to the one described prevail wherever the reader observes a low reliability coefficient coupled with a high percentage of agreement on the same parameter. The frequency of this happening is related to the fact that most of these somewhat randomly selected preschool children may be thought of as reasonably "normal," and, therefore, the examiners agreed that there was little or no restriction of motion.

When the reliability coefficient and the percentage of agreement are both high, this indicates that an abnormal rating was reported similarly by both examiners. For example, in Table 2, parameter 7, the reliability coefficient is .95 and the percentage of agreement is 100 percent if one allows ±0.5 motion restriction rating variance (91 percent if one allows 0 rating variance). This parameter is a measure of restriction toward induced passive right sidebending-rotation motion.[4-6] The data reflect that there were indeed restrictions noted and that the rating of the abnormal restrictions was both highly reliable and reproducible.

Another example of a highly reproducible and reliable rating is seen in Table 3, parameter 9 (restriction toward induced passive right torsion of the sphenobasilar joint[4,6]). The author and Dr. Ward achieved a reliability coefficient of 1.00 and 100 percent agreement. The range of ratings was 1-3 and the mean rating for both examiners was 1.750. This indicates that both the author and Dr. Ward found the same restriction under blind conditions on the same patients every time. The variances from a 1 rating are such that a perfect coefficient of reliability was achieved as well as a perfect percentage of agreement.

Parameters that show a low reliability coefficient and a low percentage of agreement indicate that abnormal restrictions were found but that agreement between examiners as to the degree of restriction was poor. Such is the case for parameter 17 of Table 4, with the author and Dr. Mitchell in rather marked disagreement. (Parameter 17 rates induced passive motion of the sacrum toward extension.[4,6]) In this instance, the author rated all subjects between 1 and 2, with a mean rating of 1.5. Dr. Mitchell's range of rating was 1-3, with a mean of 1.92. This disagreement indicates that the two examiners are either measuring different things, or that they are interpreting their findings differently.

It is interesting to note the data derived from the examination of the sacrum (parameters 16-19). Considering only the percentage of agreement, the author and Dr. Gastman achieved 100 percent agreement (allowing ± 0.5) on parameters 16, 17, and 18, and 82 percent on parameter 19. Since Dr. Gastman was trained in craniosacral technique by the author, it would indicate that both examiners are using similar meth-

TABLE 7. COMPARISON OF CRI RATE WITH PULSE AND RESPIRATORY RATES OF EXAMINER AND SUBJECT.

Patient No.	Patient			Examiner	
	Pulse/minute	Resp./minute	CRI/minute	Pulse/minute	Resp./minute
1	84	18	12	80	18
	84	24	15	68	18
2	84	22	12	74	18
	84	22	15	80	16
3	96	18	9	84	16
	88	22	8	76	18
4	96	24	8	76	18
	84	34	8	72	16
5	84	30	12	90	20
	120	28	14	84	28
6	92	22	14	72	16
	88	20	16	70	20
7	92	24	16	86	22
	88	24	14	76	18
8	80	24	12	94	16
	100	26	16	76	20
9	100	22	12	90	18
	96	24	14	98	22
10	96	24	12	74	18
	96	24	13	80	16
11	84	20	12	78	20
	100	28	12	72	18
12	90	24	16	84	16
	96	24	16	62	10
13	110	24	12	76	16
	120	36	12	66	16
14	96	20	10	74	16
	84	24	14	60	14
15	92	20	12	80	16
	82	36	13	60	12
16	92	20	10	80	14
	82	20	12	72	16
17	96	24	13	82	16
	96	24	12	72	14
18	90	24	10	78	16
	96	36	13	66	14
19	120	24	12	82	16
	92	40	12	64	14
20	88	28	11	84	18
	100	20	10	76	16
21	90	24	12	90	20
	88	22	10	80	14
22	82	22	10	74	18
	124	24	10	76	22
23	76	16	10	88	16
	80	16	9	76	16
24	88	18	12	80	16
	84	20	10	74	16
25	82	24	11	82	18
	80	28	8	80	15

ods and techniques which then result in similar interpretations and ratings.

Agreement achieved between the author and Dr. Ward indicate only 38 percent agreement in evaluation of sacral flexion,[4,6] but 100 percent agreement in the evaluation of sacral extension.[4,6] The reverse is true of the results of achieved percentage of agreement with Dr. Mitchell. The author and Dr. Mitchell reached 67 percent agree-

APPENDIX A1				
Parameter number	Minimum value	Maximum value	Mean	Standard deviation
Upledger				
1	1.00	2.00	1.23	.410100
2	1.00	2.00	1.32	.462208
3	1.00	2.00	1.73	.467099
4	1.00	2.00	1.18	.404520
5	1.00	1.00	1.00	.000000
6	1.00	1.50	1.05	.150756
7	1.00	2.00	1.41	.490825
8	1.00	2.50	1.27	.517863
9	1.00	2.00	1.27	.410100
10	1.00	2.00	1.18	.404520
11	1.00	3.00	1.41	.664010
12	1.00	2.00	1.27	.410100
13	1.00	3.00	1.95	.471940
14	1.00	2.00	1.23	.343776
15	1.00	3.00	1.32	.643146
16	1.00	1.00	1.00	.000000
17	1.00	1.50	1.05	.150756
18	1.00	2.00	1.36	.393123
19	1.00	2.00	1.27	.410100
Gastman				
1	1.00	2.00	1.23	.410100
2	1.00	2.00	1.18	.337100
3	1.00	3.00	1.59	.664010
4	1.00	2.00	1.18	.337100
5	1.00	1.50	1.05	.150756
6	1.00	1.50	1.09	.202260
7	1.00	2.00	1.36	.452267
8	1.00	2.00	1.36	.504525
9	1.00	2.00	1.32	.462202
10	1.00	2.00	1.23	.343776
11	1.00	2.50	1.36	.551856
12	1.00	2.00	1.18	.404920
13	1.00	3.00	1.77	.606780
14	1.00	2.00	1.32	.462208
15	1.00	3.00	1.59	.700649
16	1.00	1.50	1.09	.202260
17	1.00	1.50	1.05	.150756
18	1.00	2.00	1.32	.404520
19	1.00	2.00	1.27	.467099

APPENDIX A2 MEAN TABLE.				
Parameter number	Minimum value	Maximum value	Mean	Standard deviation
Upledger				
1	1.00	3.00	1.75	.707107
2	1.00	3.00	1.94	.863444
3	2.00	3.00	2.19	.372012
4	1.00	2.00	1.50	.534522
5	1.00	3.00	1.50	.755929
6	1.00	2.00	1.50	.534522
7	1.00	3.00	1.56	.728869
8	1.00	3.00	1.88	.834523
9	1.00	3.00	1.75	.707107
10	1.00	3.00	1.44	.728869
11	1.00	3.00	2.00	.755929
12	1.00	3.00	1.69	.798995
13	1.00	3.00	1.63	.744024
14	1.00	3.00	1.38	.744024
15	1.00	3.00	1.44	.728869
16	1.00	3.00	1.50	.707107
17	1.00	2.50	1.31	.593867
18	1.00	3.00	1.75	.707107
19	1.00	2.00	1.38	.517549
Ward				
1	1.00	3.00	1.75	.707107
2	1.00	3.00	1.88	.640870
3	1.00	3.00	2.13	.640870
4	1.00	2.00	1.50	.534522
5	1.00	3.00	1.50	.755929
6	1.00	2.50	1.56	.623212
7	1.00	3.00	1.38	.744024
8	1.00	3.00	1.81	.752970
9	1.00	3.00	1.75	.707107
10	1.00	2.00	1.56	.495516
11	1.00	3.00	2.13	.694365
12	1.00	2.50	1.56	.623212
13	1.00	2.50	1.56	.623212
14	1.00	2.50	1.44	.623212
15	1.00	3.00	1.50	.755929
16	1.00	2.00	1.75	.462910
17	1.00	2.00	1.25	.462910
18	1.00	3.00	1.63	.744024
19	1.00	2.00	1.63	.517549

ment on sacral flexion, but only 17 percent agreement on sacral extension. Further, it may be noted that the percentage of agreement achieved between the author and Dr. Mitchell on the cranial portion of the examination is much higher than that achieved on the sacral motion testing. The reader should be aware that the author and Drs. Ward and Mitchell did not discuss or practice craniosacral technique with each other prior to embarking upon this study. (The author merely asked these two examiners to familiarize themselves with the examination protocol and then to adhere to it as strictly as possible.)

Table 5 presents the data on all 25 subjects for comparison of the author with the other three examiners as an aggregate. These data are more strictly a statistical evaluation of the reproducibility of the author's examination results. This analysis was carried out because this study is essentially an attempt to determine the reliability and reproducibility of the author's

APPENDIX A3. MEAN TABLE.				
Parameter number	Minimum value	Maximum value	Mean	Standard deviation
Upledger				
1	1.00	2.00	1.83	.408248
2	1.00	2.00	1.17	.408248
3	2.00	2.00	2.00	.000000
4	1.00	3.00	2.00	.894427
5	1.00	3.00	1.67	.816497
6	1.00	3.00	1.33	.816497
7	1.00	3.00	1.50	.836660
8	1.00	2.00	1.17	.408248
9	1.00	3.00	1.92	.801041
10	1.00	2.00	1.17	.408248
11	2.00	3.00	2.25	.418330
12	1.00	3.00	2.33	1.032796
13	1.00	3.00	1.67	1.032796
14	1.00	3.00	2.08	.801041
15	1.00	3.00	1.75	.758288
16	1.00	2.00	1.50	.547723
17	1.00	2.00	1.50	.547723
18	1.00	2.00	1.17	.408248
19	1.00	2.00	1.17	.408248
Mitchell				
1	1.00	3.00	2.00	.632456
2	1.00	2.00	1.17	.408248
3	1.00	2.00	1.58	.491596
4	1.00	3.00	2.00	.948683
5	1.00	3.00	1.67	.816497
6	1.00	3.00	1.50	.836660
7	1.00	3.00	2.00	.894427
8	1.00	2.00	1.33	.516398
9	1.00	3.00	2.00	.894427
10	1.00	2.00	1.17	.408248
11	2.00	3.00	2.58	.491596
12	1.00	3.00	2.33	1.032796
13	1.00	3.00	1.83	.983192
14	1.00	3.00	2.17	.752773
15	1.00	3.00	2.17	.752773
16	1.00	3.00	1.92	.917424
17	1.00	3.00	1.92	.917424
18	1.00	2.00	1.33	.516398
19	1.00	3.00	1.67	1.032796

APPENDIX A4. MEAN TABLE.				
Parameter number	Minimum value	Maximum value	Mean	Standard deviation
Upledger				
1	1.00	3.00	1.54	.575905
2	1.00	3.00	1.48	.668954
3	1.00	3.00	1.94	.416333
4	1.00	3.00	1.48	.653197
5	1.00	3.00	1.32	.627163
6	1.00	3.00	1.26	.522813
7	1.00	3.00	1.48	.637050
8	1.00	3.00	1.44	.666458
9	1.00	3.00	1.58	.656379
10	1.00	3.00	1.26	.522813
11	1.00	3.00	1.80	.721688
12	1.00	3.00	1.66	.812917
13	1.00	3.00	1.78	.708284
14	1.00	3.00	1.48	.684349
15	1.00	3.00	1.46	.691014
16	1.00	3.00	1.28	.522015
17	1.00	2.50	1.24	.459166
18	1.00	3.00	1.44	.546199
19	1.00	2.00	1.28	.434933
Aggregate				
1	1.00	3.00	1.58	.640312
2	1.00	3.00	1.40	.559017
3	1.00	3.00	1.76	.647431
4	1.00	3.00	1.48	.653197
5	1.00	3.00	1.34	.624500
6	1.00	3.00	1.34	.572276
7	1.00	3.00	1.52	.699405
8	1.00	3.00	1.50	.612372
9	1.00	3.00	1.62	.696419
10	1.00	2.00	1.32	.430116
11	1.00	3.00	1.90	.763763
12	1.00	3.00	1.58	.786342
13	1.00	3.00	1.72	.693421
14	1.00	3.00	1.56	.666458
15	1.00	3.00	1.70	.750000
16	1.00	3.00	1.50	.629153
17	1.00	3.00	1.32	.610328
18	1.00	3.00	1.42	.553022
19	1.00	3.00	1.48	.653197

craniosacral findings (thus lending more credibility to the balance of the research project). Perusal of Table 5 reveals that the reliability coefficients are below acceptable levels (0.7) on parameters 3 and 10 in the cranial portion of the examination. This low reliability coupled with high percent of agreement is probably due to the scarcity of abnormal findings.

Table 6 gives the overall percentage of agreement for the total examination between the author and the other examiners, both individually and as an aggregate. In calculating the total percentage of agreement, a weighting system was applied so that the number of examinations done by each examiner is proportionately represented. Allowing ± 0.5 variance on the motion restriction rating scale for all 19 parameters, the overall agreement was 86 percent. The author considers this level of agreement acceptable to validate the reliability and reproducibility of the results of his craniosacral examinations.

APPENDIX B. EXAMINATION RESULTS

Subject No.	Physician	1	2	3	4	5	6	7	8	9	10	11	12	13	14	15	16	17	18	19
1	U	1	1	1	1	1	1	1	1	1	1	1	1	2	1.5	1	1	1	1.5	1
	G	1	1.5	1	1	1	1	1	1	1	1	1	1	1.5	2	1	1	1	2	1
2	U	1	1	1	2	1	1	1	1.5	1	2	1	1	2	1	1.5	1	1	1	2
	G	1	1	1	2	1	1	1	2	1	1.5	1	1	2	1	2	1	1	1	1
3	U	2	2	2	2	1	1.5	2	1	2	1	1	2	1	1	2	1	1	1.5	1.5
	G	1	1	1	1	1	1.5	2	2	1.5	1	1.5	2	1	1	2.5	1	1	1.5	1
4	U	1	1	2	1	1	1	2	1	2	1	1.5	1	2	1	1	1	1	1.5	1
	G	1	1	2	1	1	1	2	1	2	1.5	1	1	2.5	1	1.5	1	1	1.5	1
5	U	1.5	1	2	1	1	1	1	2.5	1	1	3	2	2	1.5	3	1	1	2	1
	G	1	1	3	1	1.5	1	1	2	2	1	3	2	1	1	3	1	1	2	2
6	U	2	2	2	1	1	1	2	1	1	2	1	1	3	1.5	1	1	1	1	1.5
	G	2	1	1	1.5	1	1	1.5	1	1	2	1	1	2	2	1	1.5	1	1	2
7	U	1	1	2	1	1	1	1	1	1	1	2	1.5	1.5	1	1	1	1	2	1
	G	1	1.5	2	1	1	1	1	1	2	1	2	1	2	1	1.25	1	1.25	1.5	1
8	U	1	1	2	1	1	1	1.5	1	1.5	1	1	1	2	1	1	1	1	1	2
	G	1	1	2	1	1	1	1.5	1	1	1	1	1	2	1	2	1.5	1	1	2
9	U	1	2	2	1	1	1	2	1	1	1	1	1	2	1	1	1	1.5	1	1
	G	1	2	2	1	1	1	2	1	1	1.5	1	1	1.5	1	1	1	1	1	1
10	U	1	1	2	1	1	1	1	2	1	1	1	1	2	1	1	1	1	1	1
	G	2	1	1.5	1.5	1	1	1	2	1	1	1	1	1.5	2	1	1	1	1	1
11	U	1	1	1	1	1	1	1	1	1.5	1	2	1.5	2	2	1	1	1	1.5	1
	G	1	1	1	1	1	1.5	1	1	1	1	2	1	1.5	1.5	1	1	1	1	1
12	U	2	1	2	1	1	1	1.5	2	2	1	1	1	1	1	1	1.5	1	1	1
	W	2	1	1	1	1	1	1	2	2	1	1.5	1	1	1	1	2	1	1	2
13	U	2	2	2.5	2	2	2	2	2	2	1	2	2	1	1	1	1	1	3	1
	W	1	2	2	2	2	2	1	2	2	1.5	2	2	1	2	1	2	1	3	2
14	U	2	1	2	1	1	2	1	1	1	1.5	2	1	2	1	2	1	2.5	2	2
	W	2	1	2	1	1	2	1	1	1	2	2	1	2	1	2	2	2	1	2
15	U	1	2.5	2	2	3	1	3	1	1	3	2	2.5	2	1	1.5	2	1	1	1
	W	1	2	2	1	3	1	3	1	1	2	2.5	2	2	1	2	1	1	1	1
16	U	1	3	3	1	1	2	1	3	3	1	3	3	3	1	3	3	1	2	2
	W	2	2	3	2	1	2.5	1	2.5	3	2	3	2.5	2.5	1	3	2	1	2	2
17	U	1	1	2	1	1	1	1	2	2	1	1	1	1	1	1	1.5	1	2	1
	W	1	2	2	1	1	1	1	2	2	1	1	1	1	1	1	2	1	2	1
18	U	2	2	2	2	1	2	1	1	2	1	2	2	1	2	1	1	2	1	2
	W	2	2	2	2	1	2	1	1	2	1	2	2	1	2	1	1	2	1	2
19	U	3	3	2	2	2	1	2	3	1	2	3	1	2	3	1	1	1	2	1
	W	3	3	3	2	2	1	2	3	1	2	3	1	2	2.5	1	2	1	2	1
20	U	2	1	2	3	2	1	1	1	2	1	2	1	3	1	2	1	2	1	1
	M	2	1	1	2.5	1	1	2	1	1	2	1	1	3	1	2	1	1	1	1
21	U	2	1	2	1	1	1	1	2	2	1	2	1	1	2	1	2	2	1	1
	M	2	1	2	1	1	1	1	2	1	1	2	1	1	2	1	2	1	1	1
22	U	2	1	2	1	1	1	2	1	3	1	2	3	1	1	1	1	1	1	1
	M	3	1	2	1	1	1	2	2	3	1	2	3	1	2	2	1	2	1	1
23	U	2	1	2	2	3	1	1	1	1	2	3	3	3	2	3	2	2	1	1
	M	2	1	1.5	1.5	3	1	1	1	1	1	3	3	3	2	3	1,5	1.5	1	1
24	U	1	2	2	2	2	2	1	3	1	1	1	2	3	1	3	1	2	1	2
	M	1	2	2	3	2	2	3	1	2	2	3	3	2	3	2	3	3	1	3
25	U	2	1	2	3	1	3	1	1	2.5	1	2.5	3	1	3	2	1	1	1	2
	M	2	1	1	3	2	3	3	1	3	1	3	3	1	3	3	3	3	2	3

Table 7 presents the data derived from the measurement of the CRI rate and the other body rhythms during each of the 50 examinations of the 25 children. Perusal of this data reveals that in only 5 times out of 50 measurements (10 percent) was the CRI rate within one cycle of another body rhythm of either examiner or subject. Therefore, 90 percent of the time the CRI rate was significantly different from the pulse and respiratory rates of the examiners and subjects. This finding provides evidence in favor of the CRI as an independent body rhythm. The author does not mean to imply that the CRI may not be the resultant modulation of other body rhythms, merely that ultimately it was significantly different 90 percent of the time.

CONCLUSIONS

First, it is possible to achieve an acceptable degree of interexaminer reliability and percentage of agreement between examiners utilizing craniosacral examination methods and techniques.

Second, this interexaminer reliability and percentage of agreement lends considerable evidence to the existence of a real and perceptible craniosacral motion system.

Third, craniosacral examination by an experienced and well-trained examiner may be considered reliable and reproducible. (The question of validity is reserved for subsequent investigations.)

Appreciation is expressed to the officials of the East Lansing schools and to Drs. John Haubenstricker and Vernon Seefeldt, of the Motor Coordination Clinic in the Department of Health, Physical Education and Recreation of Michigan State University, who have been so generous with their time and efforts in this research.

1. Winchell, C.A.: The hyperkinetic child. Greenwood Publishers, Westport, Conn., 1975
2. Beter, T.R., Cragin, W.E., and Drury, F.: The mentally retarded child and his motor behavior. Charles C. Thomas, Publisher, Springfield, Ill., 1972
3. Morris, P.R., and Whiting, H.T.A.: Motor impairment and compensatory education. G. Bell and Sons, London, 1971
4. Sutherland, W.G.: The cranial bowl. Free Press Co., Mankato, Minn., 1939
5. Wales, A.L.: The work of William Garner Sutherland. JAOA 71:788-93, May 72
6. Magoun, H.I., Sr.: Osteopathy in the cranial field. Journal Printing Co., Kirksville, Missouri, 1966
7. Magoun, H.I., Sr.: The temporal bone. Troublemaker in the head. JAOA 73:825-35, Jun 74
8. Woods, R.H.: Structural normalization in infants and children with particular reference to disturbances of the central nervous system. JAOA 72:903-8, May 73
9. Michael, D.K., and Retzlaff, E.W.: A preliminary study of cranial bone movement in the squirrel monkey. JAOA 74:866-9, May 75
10. Retzlaff, E.W., Michael, D.K., and Roppel, R.M.: Cranial bone mobility. JAOA 74:869-73, May 75
11. Dunbar, H.S., Guthrie, T.C., and Karspell, B.: A study of the cerebrospinal fluid pulse wave. Arch Neurol (Chicago), 14:624-30, Jun 66

Baker, E.G.: Alteration in width of maxillary arch and its relation to sutural movement of cranial bones, JAOA 70:559-64, Feb 71

Brierley, J.B., and Field, E.J.: Connexions of spinal subarachnoid space with lymphatic system. J Anat 82:153-66, Jul 48

Brierley, J.B.: Metabolism of the nervous system. D. Richter, Ed., Pergamon Press, New York, 1957

Brooks, C., Kao, F.F., and Lloyd, B.B.: Cerebrospinal fluid and the regulation of ventilation. F.A. Davis Co., Philadelphia, 1965

Brown, J.H.V., Jacobs, J.E., and Stark, L.: Biomedical engineering. F.A. Davis Co., Philadelphia, 1971

Dandy, E.: The brain. Harper & Row, New York, 1969

Davson, H.: Physiology of the cerebrospinal fluid. Churchill, London, 1967

Flexner, L.B.: Some problems of origin, circulation and absorption of cerebrospinal fluid. Quart Rev Biol 8:397-422, Dec 33

Frymann, V.M.: Relation of disturbances of craniosacral mechanisms to symptomatology of the newborn. Study of 1,250 infants. JAOA 65:1059-75, Jun 66

Gray, H.: Anatomy of the human body. Ed. 26. C.M. Goss, Ed. Lea & Febiger, Philadelphia, 1954

Hamit, H.F., Beall, A.C., Jr., and DeBakey, M.E.: Hemodynamic influences upon brain and cerebrospinal fluid pulsations and pressures. J Trauma 5:174-84, Mar 65

Leusen, I.: Regulation of cerebrospinal fluid composition with reference to breathing. Physiol Rev 52:1-56, Jan 72

Michael, D.K.: The cerebrospinal fluid. Values for compliance and resistance to absorption. JAOA 74:873-6, May 75

Miller, H.C.: Head pain. JAOA 72:135-43, Oct 72

Netter, F.H.: The nervous system. Ciba Pharmaceutical Products, Inc., New York, 1953

Pritchard, J.J., Scott, J.H., and Girgis, F.G.: The structure and development of cranial and facial sutures. J

Anat 90:70-86, Jan 56

Retzlaff, E.W., Michael, D.K., Roppel, R.M., and Mitchell, F.L.: The structures of cranial bone sutures. JAOA 75:607-8, Feb 76

Retzlaff, E.W., Roppel, R.M., and Michael, D.K.: Possible functional significance of cranial bone sutures. American Association of Anatomists, 88th Session, MSU-COM, March 24-27, 1975

Rubin, R.C., et al.: The production of cerebrospinal fluid in man and its modification by acetozolamide. J Neurosurg 25:430-6, Oct 66

Schaltenbrand, G.: Normal and pathological physiology of cerebrospinal fluid circulation. Lancet 1:805-8, 25 Apr 53

Thomas, L.M., et al.: Static deformation and volume changes in the human skull. Stapp Car Crash Proceedings, 12th Annual Conference, Detroit, October 22-23, 1968

Warwick, R., and Williams, P.L.: Gray's Anatomy. Brit. Ed. 35. W.B. Saunders Co., Philadelphia, 1973

Weed, L.H.: Positional adjustments of the pressure of cerebrospinal fluid. Physiol Rev 13:80-102, Jan 33

Weed, L.S.: The cerebrospinal fluid. Physiol Rev 2:171-22

Welch, K., Friedman, V.: The cerebrospinal fluid values. Brain 83:454-69, Sep 60

Wolstenholme, G.E.W., and O'Connor, C.M.: CIBA symposium on cerebrospinal fluid production, circulation, and absorption. Churchill, London, 1952

Accepted for publication in March 1977. Updating, as necessary, has been done by the authors.

This study has been funded in part by NIH Biomedical Research Support Grant No. GRSP 18-1976 and by an institutional grant from the AOA Bureau of Research.

Appendix K

Holism, Osteopathy and Biomechanics

JOHN E. UPLEDGER, D.O., F.A.A.O., Associate Professor, Michigan State University, College of Osteopathic Medicine, Guest Editor*

Recently I have presented material in several "Holistic Pain Control" seminars. There seems to be considerable amount of activity in this area by medical professionals around the world.

Almost without exception, I have been impressed that "Holism" translates to mean "multidisciplinary." It does *not* appear to me that "Holism" is interpreted to mean that the "Holistic physician" must search for and treat the primary cause of the problem.

This multidisciplinary approach means that impressive "Holistic Pain Control" Centers are being born which include such therapeutic modalities as:

Drug Therapy
Acupuncture
Transcutaneous Electrical Nerve Stimulation
Psychological evaluation and counseling
Pastoral counseling
Manual Medicine
Physiotherapy
Self Hypnosis (Positive imaging)
Surgical procedures
Physical Environmental Therapy
Nutritional Therapy
Psychosocial Environmental Therapy, and the like

Each of these modalities will produce some positive effect in selected cases. Taken in combination, the percentage of effectiveness is increased.

I am, however, disappointed that the very words "Holistic Pain Control" impart the philosophical approach under which many of these prestigious centers operate. It does not mean elimination of pain by finding and treating the cause. It simply means the reduction of pain to hopefully tolerable levels by the use of newer and more sophisticated technology as well as by combining various types of approaches. It does seem to mean masking the symptoms rather than identifying and treating the primary cause.

It is, however, obvious that an awareness of the importance of the neuromusculoskeletal system and biomechanics is developing as this symptom-oriented Holistic approach grows. Perhaps as these Holistically inclined physicians gain experience they will begin to realize that in a significant number of cases this magnificent *neuromusculoskeletal system contains the patient's complete medical history.* And that by intelligent study of this system, the dedicated physician is usually able to determine the cause of the pain, thus obviating the need for "Holistic Pain Control."

*Reprinted from Michigan Osteopathic Journal, November 1977, p. 11, by permission of the Michigan Association of Osteopathic Physicians and Surgeons, Inc.

Perhaps this approach, which attempts to identify and treat primary causes of symptoms and dysfunctions, can be named Holistic Diagnosis and Treatment.

On the other hand, perhaps it has already been named Osteopathic Diagnosis and Treatment and does not need further name change—simply application of the principles upon which the osteopathic profession was founded.

Ideally, osteopathic physicians have an advantage in that they are more intimately acquainted with the neuromusculoskeletal system by virtue of educational and philosophical experience than are other branches of the healing arts. Osteopathy does, in fact, possess all of the tools to practice Holistic medicine or healing. Osteopathic physicians begin their careers in the healing arts with this definite advantage.

The paranoia and insecurity which attacks many of our osteopathic physicians is indeed an unfortunate circumstance which has caused a de-emphasis upon (if not an embarrassment related to) the osteopathic use of the hands in diagnosis and treatment. It is time that we osteopathic physicians gained some pride in the use of our hands as the fine diagnostic and treatment tools they are. We understand very little of the untapped potential which the human organism possesses in terms of ability to perceive and understand patient problems.

I am telling you this because I want to make a plea for osteopathic physicians to begin to use the intelligence that their hands can provide when examining the neuromusculoskeletal system in the search for the cause of the patient problems.

References

ALLEN, B.K. and BUNT, E.A. 1977. *Dysfunctioning of the Fluid Mechanical Craniosacral System as Revealed by Stress/ Strain Diagnosis.* International Conference on Bioengineering, Cape Town, South Africa.

ARBUCKLE, B.E. 1977. *The Selected Writings of Beryl Arbuckle.* National Osteopathic Institute and Cerebral Palsy Foundation, Camp Hill, Pennsylvania.

BAKER, E.G. 1971. Alteration in Width of the Maxillary Arch and Its Relation to Sutural Movement of Cranial Bones. *JAOA.* 70:559-64.

BERING, E.A. 1955. Choroid Plexus and Arterial Pulsation of Cerebrospinal Fluid: Demonstration of Choroid Plexuses as a Cerebrospinal Fluid Pump. *Arch. of Neurol. Psychiatry* 73:165.

BETER, T.R., CRAGIN, W.E. and DRURY, M. 1972. *The Mentally Retarded Child and His Motor Behavior.* Springfield: Charles C. Thomas.

BRIERLEY, J.B. 1957. *Metabolism of the Nervous System.* Edited by D. Fichter. New York: Pergamon Press.

BRIERLEY, J.B. and FIELD, E.G. 1948. Connexion of Spinal and Sub-arachnoid Space with Lymphatic System. *J. of Anatomy.* 82:153-66.

BROWN, J.H.V., JACOBS, J.E. and STARK, L. 1971. *Biomedical Engineering.* Philadelphia: Davis Publishing Co.

CARPENTER, M. 1978. *Core Text of Neuroanatomy.* Baltimore: Williams and Wilkins Co.

CATHIE, A. 1974. The Fascia of the Body in Relation to Function and Manipulative Therapy. *Amer. Acad. of Osteopathy Yearbook.* pp. 81-4.

CIBA FOUNDATION. 1958. CIBA Foundation Symposium on Cerebrospinal Fluid Production, Circulation, and Absorption. Boston: Little, Brown Publishing Co.

CLEMENTE, C. 1975. *Anatomy: A Regional Atlas of the Human Body.* Philadelphia: Lea and Febiger.

CROOKS, C.M., KAO, F.F. and LLOYD, B.B. 1965. *Cerebrospinal Fluid and the Regulation of Ventilation.* Philadelphia: Davis Publishing Co.

DANDY, W. 1969. *The Brain.* New York: Harper and Row (Hoeber Medical Division).

DAVSON, H. 1967. *Physiology of the Cerebrospinal Fluid.* London: Churchill.

DUNBAR, H.S., GUTHRIE, T.C., and KARSPELL, B. 1966. A Study of the Cerebrospinal Fluid Pulse Wave. *Arch. of Neur.* 14:624.

FLEXNER, L.B. 1933. Some Problems of the Origin, Circulation and Absorption of Cerebrospinal Fluid. *Quart. Review of Biol.* 8:397-422.

FOLDES, F.F. and ARROWHEAD, J.C. 1948. Changes in Cerebrospinal Fluid Pressure Under the Influence of Continuous Subarachnoid Infusion of Normal Saline. *J. Clin. Invest.* 27:346.

FRYMANN, V.M. 1966. Relation of Disturbances of Craniosacral Mechanisms to Symptomatology of the New Born: Study of 1,250 Infants. *JAOA.* 65:1059-75.

_____. 1971. A Study of the Rhythmic Motions of the Living Cranium. *JAOA.* 70:928-45.

GRAY, H. 1954. *Anatomy of the Human Body.* 26th ed. Edited by Goss, C.M. Philadelphia: Lea and Febiger.

GRANT, J.C. 1951. *An Atlas of Anatomy.* Baltimore: Williams and Wilkins Co.

HAMIT, H.F., BEALL, A.C., and DeBAKEY, M.E. 1965. Hemodynamic Influences Upon the Brain and Cerebrospinal Fluid Pressures and Pulses. *J. of Trauma.* 5:174-84.

JACOB, S.W. and FRANCONE, C.A. 1974. *Structure and Function in Man.* Philadelphia: W.B. Saunders Co.

JONES, L.H. 1981. *Strain and Counterstrain.* Colorado Springs: Amer. Acad. of Osteopathy.

LEUSEN, I. 1972. Regulation of Cerebrospinal Fluid Composition with Reference to Breathing. *Physiology Review.* 52:1-56.

LIVINGSTON, R.B., WOODBURY, D.M. and PATTERSON,

J.L. 1965. Fluid Compartments of the Brain: Cerebral Circulation. Edited by Ruch, T. C. and Patten, H.D. *Physiology and Biophysics.* pp. 939-58. Philadelphia: W.B. Saunders Co.

MAGOUN, H.I. 1966. *Osteopathy in the Cranial Field.* Kirksville: Journal Printing Co.

_____. 1974. The Temporal Bone: Troublemaker in the Head. *JAOA.* 73:825-35.

_____. 1978. *Practical Osteopathic Procedures.* Kirksville: Journal Printing Co.

MARMAROU, A., SHULMAN, K. and LaMORGESE, J. 1975. Compartment Analysis of Compliance and Outflow Resistance of the Cerebrospinal Fluid System. *J. of Neurosurg.* 43:523-34.

McMINN, R.M.H. and HUTCHINGS, P.T. 1977. *Color Atlas of the Human Body.* Chicago: Year Book Medical Publishers, Inc.

MICHAEL, D.K. 1974. The Cerebrospinal Fluid: Values for Compliance and Resistance to Absorption. *JAOA.* 74:874-6.

MICHAEL, D.K. and RETZLAFF, E.W. 1975. A Preliminary Study of Cranial Bone Movement in the Squirrel Monkey. *JAOA.* 74:866-9.

MILLER, H. 1972. Head Pain. *JAOA.* 72:135-43.

MORRIS, C.R. and WHITING, H.T.A. 1971. *Motor Impairment and Compensatory Education.* London: G. Bell and Sons.

NETTER, F. 1953. *The Nervous System.* New York: CIBA Pharmaceutical Products, Inc.

OWMAN, C. and EDVINSSON, L., eds. 1977. *Neurogenic Control of the Brain Circulation.* The Proceedings of the International Symposium held in the Wenner-Gren Center, Stockholm. Oxford: Pergamon Press.

PRITCHARD, J.J., SCOTT, J.H. and GIRGIS, F.G. 1956. The Structure and Development of Cranial and Facial Sutures. *J. of Anatomy.* 90:70-86.

RETZLAFF, E.W., et al. 1976. Craniosacral Mechanisms. *JAOA.* 76:288-9.

RETZLAFF, E.W., et al. 1978. Temporalis Muscle Action in Parieto-Temporal Suture Compression. *JAOA.* 78: 127.

RETZLAFF, E.W., et al. 1979. Age-Related Changes in Human Cranial Sutures. *JAOA.* 79:115-6.

RETZLAFF, E.W., MICHAEL, D.K., ROPPEL, R. 1975. Cranial Bone Mobility. *JAOA.* 74:866-9.

RETZLAFF, E.W., MITCHELL, F.L. and UPLEDGER, J.E. 1977. Sutural Collagenous Bundles and Their Innervation in Saimuri Sciureus. *Anatomy Records.* 187:692.

RHODIN, J.A.G. 1974. *Histology: A Text and Atlas.* New York, London and Toronto: Oxford University Press.

RUBIN, R.C., et al. 1966. The Production of Cerebrospinal Fluid in Man and Its Modification by Acetozolamide. *J. of Neurosurg.* 25:430-5.

ST. PIERRE, R.S., et al. 1976. The Detection and Relative Movement of Cranial Bones. *JAOA.* 76:128.

SCHALTENBRAND, G. 1953. Normal and Pathological Physiology of Cerebrospinal Fluid Circulation. *Lancet.* 264:805-8.

SUTHERLAND, W.G. 1939. *The Cranial Bowl.* Mankato: Free Press Co.

THOMAS, L.M., et al. 1968. *Static Deformation and Volume Changes in the Human Skull.* 12th Annual Conference, Stapp Car Crash Proceedings, Detroit, Michigan.

WALES, A. 1972. The Work of William Garner Sutherland, D.O. *JAOA.* 71:788-93.

WARWICK, R. and WILLIAMS, P., eds. 1978. *Gray's Anatomy.* 35th British edition. Philadelphia: W.B. Saunders Co.

WEED, L.H. 1933. Positional Adjustments of the Pressure of Cerebrospinal Fluid. *Physiological Review.* 13:80-8.

WEED, L.S. 1922. The Cerebrospinal Fluid. *Physiological Review.* 2:171-80.

WELCH, K. and FRIEDMAN, V. 1960. The Cerebrospinal Fluid Values. *Brain.* 83:454-8.

WINCHELL, C.S. 1975. *The Hyperkinetic Child.* Westport: Greenwood Publishers.

WOODS, J.M. and R.H. 1961. A Physical Finding Related to Psychiatric Disorders. *JAOA.* 60:988-93.

WOODS, R. 1973. Structural Normalization in Infants and Children with Particular Reference to Disturbances of the Central Nervous System. *JAOA.* 72:903-8.

Index